Cognitiv

Second Ec

Entirely revised, rewritten and augmented with 17 completely new chapters, this new edition builds strongly on the aims of the previous edition to provide the latest scientific validation of cognitive behaviour therapy with practical treatment guidance for clinical child psychologists and psychiatrists working with disturbed children. Coverage ranges broadly from school refusal and adjustment to parental divorce through eating and sleeping disorders to substance abuse. It will be invaluable to clinicians wanting to provide ever more effective psychological treatment for children and families.

From a review of the first edition

'. . . clearly written by a number of international authorities in the field . . . This book will be useful to child psychiatrists and other child mental health professionals, as well as social workers, educationalists and school nurses. It is highly recommended for bench and departmental libraries.'

European Child and Adolescent Psychiatry

'. . . impressive . . . this book is likely to be read and consulted widely.'

Behaviour Research and Therapy

Philip J. Graham is Emeritus Professor of Child Psychiatry at the Institute of Child Health in London.

Cambridge Child and Adolescent Psychiatry

Child and adolescent psychiatry is an important and growing area of clinical psychiatry. The last decade has seen a rapid expansion of scientific knowledge in this field and has provided a new understanding of the underlying pathology of mental disorders in these age groups. This series is aimed at practitioners and researchers both in child and adolescent mental health services and developmental and clinical neuroscience. Focusing on psychopathology, it highlights those topics where the growth of knowledge has had the greatest impact on clinical practice and on the treatment and understanding of mental illness. Individual volumes benefit both from the international expertise of their contributors and a coherence generated through a uniform style and structure for the series. Each volume provides first an historical overview and a clear descriptive account of the psychopathology of a specific disorder or group of related disorders. These features then form the basis for a thorough critical review of the aetiology, natural history, management, prevention and impact on later adult adjustment. While each volume is therefore complete in its own right, volumes also relate to each other to create a flexible and collectable series that should appeal to students as well as experienced scientists and practitioners.

Editorial board

Already published in this series:

Cognitive Behaviour Therapy for Children and Families

Second Edition

Edited by

Philip J. Graham
Institute of Child Health, London, UK

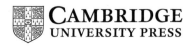

CAMBRIDGE
UNIVERSITY PRESS

PUBLISHED BY THE PRESS SYNDICATE OF THE UNIVERSITY OF CAMBRIDGE
The Pitt Building, Trumpington Street, Cambridge, United Kingdom

CAMBRIDGE UNIVERSITY PRESS
The Edinburgh Building, Cambridge CB2 2RU, UK
40 West 20th Street, New York, NY 10011–4211, USA
477 Williamstown Road, Port Melbourne, VIC 3207, Australia
Ruiz de Alarcón 13, 28014 Madrid, Spain
Dock House, The Waterfront, Cape Town 8001, South Africa

http://www.cambridge.org

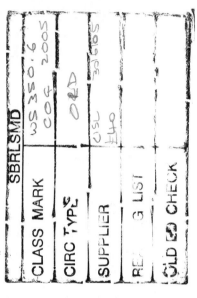

First edition published 1998
Second edition published 2005

Printed in the United Kingdom at the University Press, Cambridge

Typeface Dente MT 11/14 pt and Dax.   *System* LaTeX 2ε [TB]

A catalogue record for this book is available from the British Library

Library of Congress Cataloguing in Publication data

Cognitive behaviour therapy for children and families / edited by Philip J.Graham. – 2nd edn
       p.   cm. – (Cambridge child and adolescent psychiatry series)
Includes bibliographical references and index.
ISBN 0 521 52992 1 (paperback)
1. Cognitive therapy for children.   2. Cognitive therapy for teenagers.   3. Family psychotherapy.
I. Graham, P. J. (Philip Jeremy)   II. Series.
RJ505.C63C645   2004
618.92′89142–dc22   2003065834

ISBN 0 521 52992 1 paperback

Contents

viii   Contents

Contributors

Dr Jennifer L. Allen
Department of Psychology and Linguistics
Macquarie University
North Ryde
New South Wales 2109
Australia

Dr Renuka Arjundas
Newcastle Cognitive and Behavioural
Therapies Centre
Plummer Court
Carliol Place
Newcastle upon Tyne
NE1 6UR
UK

Dr Veira Bailey
Children's Department
Maudsley Hospital
Denmark Hill
London
SE5 8AF
UK

Professor Derek Bolton
Department of Psychology
Institute of Psychiatry
De Crespigny Park
Denmark Hill
London
SE5 8AF
UK

Dr David A. Brent
University of Pittsburgh School of Medicine
Western Psychiatric Institute and Clinic
3811 O'Hara Street
Pittsburgh
PA 15213
USA

Dr Trudie Chalder
Health Services Research and Academic
Department of Psychological Medicine
Guys, Kings and St. Thomas' School of
Medicine
103 Denmark Hill
London
SE5 8AZ
UK

Dr Cathy Creswell
Subdepartment of Clinical Health Psychology
University College London
London
WC1E 6BT
UK

Dr Jenny Doe
Luton Family Consultation Clinic
Trend House
Dallow Road
Luton
LU1 1LY
UK

Caroline L. Donovan
School of Psychology
University of Queensland
Brisbane
Queensland 4072
Australia

Jo Douglas
Ladymead
Loudwater Heights
Rickmansworth
Herts
WD3 4AX
UK

Dr Jonquil Drinkwater
The Park Hospital for Children
Old Road
Headington
Oxford
OX3 7LQ
UK

Dr Julie Elsworth
Dunstable Family Consultation Clinic
Dunstable Health Centre
Dunstable
LU6 3SU
UK

Dr Edna Foa
Center for the Treatment and Study
of Anxiety
3525 Market Street, 6th Floor
Philadelphia
Pennsylvania 19104
USA

Dr Martin Franklin
Center for the Treatment and Study
of Anxiety
3535 Market Street, 6th Floor
Philadelphia
PA 19104
USA

Dr Eilish Gilvarry
Centre for Alcohol and Drug Studies
Plummer Court
Newcastle Upon Tyne
NE1 6UR
UK

Dr Julie Goodman
Child Development Centre
Hotel Dieu Hospital
166 Brock Street
Kingston
Ontario K7L 5G2
Canada

Professor Philip J. Graham
The Institute of Child Health
30 Guilford Street
London
WC1N 1EH

Dr Jonathan Green
Academic Department of Child and
Adolescent Psychiatry
Booth Hall Children's Hospital
Charlestown Road
Blackley
Manchester
M9 7AA
UK

Professor Richard Harrington[†]
(died 22 May 2004)
Royal Manchester Children's Hospital
Hospital Road
Pendlebury
Manchester
M27 4HA
UK

Dr Martin Herbert
Quinta Park
Dousland
Devon
PL20 6NN
UK

Dr David Heyne
Faculty of Social and Behavioural Sciences
Leiden University
PO Box 9555
2300 RB Leiden
The Netherlands

Professor Neville King
Faculty of Education
Building 6
Monash University
Clayton
Victoria 3800
Australia

Dr John E. Lochman
Department of Psychology
University of Alabama
Box 870348
Tuscaloosa
AL 35487
USA

Dr John S. March
Child and Family Study Center
Duke University Medical Center
718 Rutherford Street
Durham
NC 27705
USA

Heather K. McElroy
Department of Psychology
Box 870348
University of Alabama
Tuscaloosa
AL 35487
USA

Professor Patrick McGrath
Department of Psychology
Dalhousie University
Pain and Palliative Care Service
IWK Grace Health Centre
Halifax
Nova Scotia B3H 3J1
Canada

Dr Robert J. McMahon
Department of Psychology
University of Washington
Box 351525
Seattle
WA 98195
USA

Dr Thomas O'Connor
MRC Social, Genetic and Developmental
Research Centre
Institute of Psychiatry
De Crespigny Park
Denmark Hill
London
SE5 8AF
UK

Dr Thomas H. Ollendick
Virginia Polytechnic Institute and State
University
Child Study Center
Department of Psychology
Blacksburg
VA 24061-0355
USA

Dr Dustin A. Pardini
Life History Studies, Suite 225
University of Pittsburgh Medical Center
Western Psychiatric Institute and Clinic
3811 O'Hara Street
Pittsburgh
PA 15213
USA

Dr William E. Pelham Jr.
Center for Children and Families
318 Diefendorf Hall
South Campus
3435 Main St. Building 20
State University of New York
NY 11794-2500
USA

Dr Sean Perrin
Institute of Psychiatry
De Crespigny Park
Denmark Hill
London
SE5 8AF
UK

Nancy C. Phillips
Department of Psychology
Box 870348
University of Alabama
Tuscaloosa
AL 35487
USA

Professor Ronald M. Rapee
Department of Psychology
Division of Linguistics and Psychology
Macquarie University
NSW 2109
Australia

Dr Dana M. Rhule
Department of Psychology
University of Washington
Box 351525
Seattle
WA 98195-1525
USA

Dr Ulrike Schmidt
Eating Disorders Research Unit
Institute of Psychiatry
De Crespigny Park
Denmark Hill
London
SE5 8AF
UK

Dr Patrick Smith
Institute of Psychiatry
de Crespigny Park
London
SE5 8AF
UK

Professor Susan H. Spence
School of Psychology
University of Queensland
Brisbane
Queensland 4072
Australia

Dr Paul Stallard
Department of Child and Adolescent
Psychiatry
Royal United Hospital
Coombe Park
Bath
BA1 3NG
UK

Dr Anne Stewart
Highfield Adolescent Unit
Warneford Hospital
Warneford Lane
Oxford
OX3 7JX
UK

Professor Bruce Tonge
Academic Research
Centre for Developmental Psychiatry
Clayton
Victoria 3168
Australia

Dr Jeremy Turk
Department of Psychiatry
St. George's Hospital Medical School
Cranmer Terrace
London
SW17 0RE
UK

Dr Kathryn S. Walker
Center for Children and Families
State University of New York at Buffalo
Building 20, 3435 Main Street
Diefendorf Hall, Room 318
Buffalo
New York 14214-2093
USA

Dr V. Robin Weersing
Yale Child Study Center
P.O. Box 207900
230 South Frontage Road
New Haven
CT 06520-7900
USA

Dr Miranda Wolpert
Dunstable Family Consultation Clinic
Dunstable Health Centre
Dunstable
LU6 3SU
UK

Professor William Yule
Department of Psychology
Institute of Psychiatry
De Crespigny Park
Denmark Hill
London
SE5 8AF
UK

1

Introduction

Philip J. Graham

Institute of Child Health, London, UK

In his historical account of the development of cognitive behaviour therapy
(CBT), Rachman (1997) describes three stages: the emergence of behaviour
therapy in the UK and the USA between 1950 and 1970, the growth of cognitive
therapy in the USA from the mid-1960s and the merging of behaviour and
cognitive therapy into CBT in both Europe and North America in the late 1980s.
The development of CBT in childhood and adolescence followed a similar, but
not identical course. First, behavioural therapies were developed rather earlier
in the children's field than with adults. For example, Mowrer and Mowrer (1938)
described a conditioning treatment for nocturnal enuresis before the Second
World War. Even earlier than this, Mary Cover Jones (1924) treated childhood
phobias with techniques such as desensitization. However, as in the adult field,
such techniques did not really become established until the 1950s and 1960s
when they were widely investigated and applied, especially with habit and phobic
disorders.

In contrast to the adult field, it is difficult to discern separate development of
purely cognitive therapy for children before the emergence of CBT. This may
be because it was assumed that children did not have the cognitive maturity to
benefit from a purely cognitive approach. However, in the mid- and late-1980s,
CBT for children and adolescents rapidly became established as a distinctive
form of therapy, especially after the publication of Philip Kendall's influential
textbooks on the subject (Kendall and Braswell, 1985; Kendall, 1991).

Although it may be difficult to discern a separate development of cognitive
therapy in the children's field, the 1970s and 1980s saw a considerable increase
in the study of cognitive development. Piagetian psychology, largely developed
between the 1930s and the 1950s, was subjected to considerable critical attention
(Bryant, 1976). The modest expectations of children's cognitive abilities that

Cognitive Behaviour Therapy for Children and Families, ed. Philip J. Graham.
Published by Cambridge University Press. © Cambridge University Press 2004.

emerged from Piaget's work were revised when it became clear that children could succeed in tasks in their natural environment much earlier than in the psychological laboratory. As Derek Bolton makes clear in Chapter 2 of this volume, the importance of distinguishing competence from performance was recognized, as was the significance of earlier experience and of context in the level of performance children were able to demonstrate. As O'Connor and Creswell suggest in Chapter 3, there is also much greater variation in the competence of children of the same age than Piaget acknowledged.

Despite the considerable modifications that have been made to Piagetian theory, as O'Connor and Creswell point out, recourse to this theory is still so widespread it could almost amount to an automatic thought among those considering the cognitive development of children. Yet, as they say, it is more appropriate to consider 'what cognition is involved in the production/maintenance of the problem in this particular case'. Such an approach would discourage the tendency to discount the possibility that CBT can be helpful with younger children merely because of their cognitive immaturity. If, as Stallard in Chapter 8 indicates, there is evidence that, by the age of 7 years, children are able to reflect competently on their own cognitive processes (Salmon and Bryant, 2002), there is no reason to think that they cannot participate in those frequently employed CBT techniques that require this particular cognitive capacity. Indeed, Stallard's chapter on the use of CBT with younger children suggests that, when comparing the effectiveness of CBT in children of different ages, there are no consistent findings that the young benefit less; sometimes, they seem to benefit more.

Since the first edition of this book was published in 1998, a number of other developments have occurred in the children's CBT field, some of which further differentiate it from that of adults. In particular, and this is not surprising in the light of the enormous growth of family therapy between the 1960s and 1980s, there is an increasing tendency to take account of the influence of other members of the family, especially parents, in the course disorders take. Wolpert, Doe and Elsworth, in Chapter 7, emphasize especially the ethical issues that arise in CBT when the views and interests of children and parents differ. But they also suggest that family therapy techniques, such as systemic interviewing, may have a useful part to play in the initial stages of therapy when exploring differences in perception between family members as to what they see as the problem and what they want done about it. These authors report on their own experience that other family techniques, such as reframing, may also be helpful in the application of CBT.

Working collaboratively with parents is seen as a central focus in the cognitive behavioural treatment of a number of disorders discussed in this book. But the involvement of parents goes further than involving them in the treatment of the child. Many of the chapter authors point to the need to work on the cognitions of parents if there is to be a successful outcome for the child. For example, Douglas, in Chapter 12 on feeding and sleeping disorders in young children, points to the need to correct parental irrational or distorted cognitions about food, cleanliness and patterns of sleep. Bailey takes a similar view when considering oppositional behaviour in Chapter 13, incorporating parent management training into the therapeutic repertoire required to help disobedient and aggressive younger children.

In a similar vein, Allen and Rapee, in Chapter 18 on anxiety disorders, point to the vicious cycle of transmission of fear from parent to child and from child to parent, often making it impossible to determine where the primary problem lies. (Incidentally, these authors also acknowledge the significance of genetic factors in the causation of anxiety disorders, which is another perspective that distinguishes the children's from the adult field.) Both they and Heyne, King and Ollendick, in Chapter 19 on school phobia, point to the importance of assessing parent and family functioning in the assessment of the presenting symptoms. Turk, in Chapter 15 on CBT in the management of children with developmental disabilities, proposes that family members should always be employed as co-therapists in treating the child, or indeed may be the focus of therapy themselves. Finally, Herbert in Chapter 11, discussing the management of distress and disorder in the children of separating and divorcing parents, puts parent training and counselling at the centre of his management approach, with such emphasis that one wonders whether he sees there is a place at all for therapy directed towards the children of separating parents.

Those using CBT with children are also obliged to take into account the context in which disorders occur if they are to have real hope of success. While the adult approach sometimes seems to be applied to adults as though they were living in a social vacuum, those dealing with children consistently manage the environment as much as they manage the child. The involvement of school staff in cases of school refusal and of the staff of inpatient units as those described by Green in Chapter 9 are the most obvious examples of situations in which the context has to be at the forefront of attention, but other chapter authors describe similar, if more attenuated, attention to family, school and the wider environment.

The differences between CBT approaches to children and adults should, however, not be exaggerated. Many of the authors in this book describe CBT approaches to children which are very similar to those used with adults. Reading the chapters by Harrington on depressive disorders (Chapter 16), March,

Franklin and Foa on obsessive disorders (Chapter 17), Chalder on chronic fatigue syndrome (Chapter 22), Arjundas and Gilvarry on substance and alcohol abuse (Chapter 26), Goodman and McGrath on pain management (Chapter 24) and Yule, Smith and Perrin on post-traumatic disorder (Chapter 20), one is struck not only by the similarity of symptomatology in children and adults but by the similarity of treatment approaches. All authors point to the necessity of using parents as co-therapist and to the relevance of context, but they all give primacy to the targeting of the child's or adolescent's symptomatology.

Another similarity between CBT in children and adults is the tension between treating the child as a unique individual and following a protocol that has been shown to be effective if applied in a standardized manner. Donovan and Spence, in Chapter 23, quote Hansen *et al.* (1998) who suggest that, when interventions are not tailored to the individual child, there is a reduced likelihood that: (1) the goals selected will be agreed upon by the child, parents and teacher; (2) the treatment will be fully explained and understood by all parties; (3) all parties will find the treatment agreeable; (4) the procedures will be gender and culture sensitive; and (5) achievement of the goals will lead to real improvement in the child's life. The resolution of this dilemma would seem to lie in researchers incorporating individualizing features of treatment into their standardized protocols.

Reading the chapters in this book, one is struck by the diversity of approaches that come under the broad rubric of CBT. Indeed, there seems to be significant overlap between CBT, behaviour therapy, interpersonal psychotherapy, problem-solving skills training, social skills training and family therapy. Nor are psychodynamic therapeutic skills irrelevant to the delivery of CBT. Schmidt, in Chapter 5 on motivational interviewing, describes techniques such as reflective listening for which a training in psychodynamic interviewing would be advantageous. Further, the evidence for the importance of non-specific factors, such as directiveness, warmth and a positive therapist–client relationship, so well described by Weersing and Brent in Chapter 4, is compelling.

The need to combine CBT with other forms of therapy is also evident from many of the contributions in this book. As far as the eating disorders are concerned, CBT alone may be sufficient in bulimia, in anorexia nervosa family therapy is a well-evaluated form of treatment that can be combined with CBT (Stewart, Chapter 21). In attention deficit hyperactivity disorder, medication is the first line of treatment for pervasively affected children, but CBT, often combined with stimulants, can be seen as the preferred approach where the condition is situation specific and associated with other disorders (Pelham and Walker, Chapter 14). The very promising results reported in the prevention and management of conduct disorders by McMahon and Rhule (Chapter 27) suggest that combinations of approaches, especially with intensive family case work or specialist foster care, can be effective in reducing recidivism.

Overlap between different forms of therapy there may be, but the last 6 years since the publication of the first edition of this book have seen further authoritative confirmation of the evidence for the effectiveness of CBT and allied approaches (often in comparison with other forms of therapy) in a wide range of conditions (Carr, 2000; Fonagy *et al.*, 2002). Hopefully, the next few years will see an expansion of training opportunities for therapists who wish to use this approach.

1.1   REFERENCES

Bryant, P. (1976). Piaget: causes and alternatives. In M. Rutter and L. Hersov (eds.), *Child Psychiatry: Modern Approaches*. Oxford: Blackwell Scientific Publications, pp. 239–54.

Carr, A. (ed.) (2000). *What Works with Children and Adolescents?* London: Routledge.

Fonagy, P., Target, M., Cottrell, D., Phillips, J. and Kurtz, Z. (2002). *What Works for Whom? A Critical Review of Treatments for Children and Adolescents*. London: Guilford Press.

Hansen, D. J., Nangle, D. W. and Meyer, K. A. (1998). Enhancing the effectiveness of social skills interventions with adolescents. *Education and Treatment of Children*, **21**, 489–513.

Jones M. C. (1924). The elimination of children's fears. *Journal of Experimental Psychology*, **7**, 383–90.

Kendall, P. C. (1991). *Child and Adolescent Therapy: Cognitive-Behavioral Procedures*. New York: Guilford Press.

Kendall, P. C. and Braswell, L. (1985). *Cognitive-Behavioural Therapy for Impulsive Children*. New York: Guilford Press.

Mowrer, O. and Mowrer, W. (1938). Enuresis: a method for its study and treatment. *American Journal of Orthopsychiatry*, **8**, 436–59.

Rachman S. (1997). The evolution of cognitive behaviour therapy. In D. Clark and C. Fairburn (eds.). *Science and Practice of Cognitive Behaviour Therapy*. Oxford: Oxford University Press, pp. 1–26.

Salmon, K. and Bryant, R. A. (2002). Posttraumatic stress disorder in children: the influence of developmental factors. *Clinical Psychology Review*, **22**, 163–88.

Part I

Developmental cognitive theory and clinical practice

2

Cognitive behaviour therapy for children and adolescents: some theoretical and developmental issues

Derek Bolton

Institute of Psychiatry, London, UK

2.1 Introduction

The term cognitive behaviour therapy (CBT) is used to cover a wide range of interventions in child and adolescent mental health, including (in no particular order) psychoeducation, anger management, anxiety management, behavioural operant methods, behavioural exposure methods, self-instruction methods, graded exercise, relaxation, social skills training, some kinds of parent training and cognitive restructuring in the style of adult CBT. There is a genuine question whether and in what sense this range and variety can be usefully seen as expressions of a unified model. In any case, it is common for authors on the theory and practice of CBT for children and adolescents to point out that the treatment model should take into account developmental issues, although it is less common for there to be detailed elaboration on what the developmental issues are that are crucial in relation to CBT for children and adolescents.

It turns out, this author believes, that there is a range of complicated theoretical issues, as well as a lack of data, underlying the question of developmental context of CBT. These issues include questions such as: given that behavioural methods can be used with children and can work well in some kinds of case, what is involved in adding 'cognitive' therapy? What is the real difference – in methods, or in the underlying models – between behaviour therapy for children and cognitive therapy? Is there a reasonable sense in which behaviour therapy modifies cognition and, therefore, is (a kind of) cognitive therapy? What does *talking* have to do with it? What kind of cognition does talking address that behaviour change does not? What kind of cognition does CBT with adults involve? Do children have that kind of cognitive capacity, and at what ages?

Cognitive Behaviour Therapy for Children and Families, ed. Philip J. Graham.
Published by Cambridge University Press. © Cambridge University Press 2004.

These issues are approached in this chapter by considering, first, what kind of cognition is involved in CBT with adults and CBT models of adult psychopathology and, secondly, the implications of cognitive developmental theory and research. It is apparent that the literatures involved in such an undertaking are very large indeed as well as complex, so what is presented here is selective and partial, and raises more questions than it suggests answers.

2.2   The theory of CBT as applied to adults

For detailed accounts of CBT theory, see, for example, Beck (1976), Beck *et al.*, (1985), Clark and Fairburn (1997), Clark and Beck (1999) and Salkovskis (1996b). A common characterization of the theory behind CBT, consistent with its background in cognitive psychology, is that behaviour is regulated by *appraisals of stimuli*, rather than by the stimuli themselves. 'Stimuli' mean events in the world, but also events within the body, and mental states of others and of the self. Appraisals may be verbal, but they may also be in sensori or sensori-motor code (e.g. threat perception is an appraisal that does not require verbal coding). 'Behaviour' involves motor behaviour, but also affective responses. A way of expressing the core working assumption of CBT is thus that appraisals – the meaning assigned to stimuli, or the way they are represented – are critical in the regulation of affect and behaviour.

CBT applies this working assumption to clinical problems, supposing that for problematic behaviour and emotion what is critical is regulation by appraisals. These maladaptive appraisals are of various kinds and levels, with technical names such as negative automatic thoughts, cognitive distortions, dysfunctional attitudes, core beliefs and compensation strategies including safety behaviours. Content varies according to the presenting problem and individual differences. Key maladaptive appraisals linked to problematic affect and behaviour may include, by way of illustration, the following: in antisocial behaviour, attribution of malign intent in the other and devaluation of the victim; in low mood and inactivity, the conviction 'I will fail/always have failed'; in anxiety and avoidance, various exaggerated perceptions of threat; and so on. A further crucial aspect of many CBT models is emphasis on the importance of appraisals that are secondary to the original behaviours, and the effects of these secondary appraisals. For example, a person may blame herself for being frightened to go out on her own and being dependent on others; or, again, a person may be self-critical because he seems to himself to be unable to make a lasting relationship. The secondary appraisals lead to further emotions and behaviour, such as shame and limiting of life-style, which commonly, and among other things, exacerbate the original problem.

The general CBT model may be applied to various kinds of presenting problems, including depression (Beck, 1976), various anxiety disorders such as social phobia, panic disorder and post-traumatic stress disorder (Clark, 1999), obsessive compulsive disorder (Salkovskis, 1999), hypochondriasis (Salkovskis, 1996a), bulimia (Vitousek, 1996), chronic fatigue (Sharp, 1997) and schizophrenia (Garety *et al.*, 2001).

Given a background model – at least the general model, or better, if available, a model for a specific kind of condition – how does CBT proceed? Assessment is conducted with the model in mind, to test out whether the model, or at least a part of it, is a reasonably good fit in the particular person's case and, if so, to elicit the details of its expression. This means trying to identify specific kinds and contents of negative automatic thoughts, the critical situations that trigger them, cognitive distortions, dysfunctional attitudes, core beliefs and safety behaviours, secondary appraisals and their further consequences and the functional relationship between them all (or as many as possible). The origins of false beliefs might also be considered – e.g. that they did make sense in the family of origin. The point of considering origins of beliefs, however, is secondary to the main point of assessment, which is to identify what has to change for the problematic affect and behaviour to change. Typically, in accord with the model, this will be an appraisal, a representation of reality, the self or of others, involving more or less of the kinds of thoughts and styles of cognition outlined in the general model – perhaps one core belief, perhaps a pattern of negative thinking or both.

As assessment proceeds, the model as applied to the particular person's case is gradually formulated, as much as possible in the client's own style and idiom, and shared between the therapist and the client. As the model is refined in a cooperative venture, the crucial appraisals driving the problems and hence what has to change are identified. Methods of change in CBT include variations on the following main themes: considering alternatives to problematic assumptions (appraisals), re-examining apparent evidence and counter-evidence in the light of these alternatives and carrying out experiments to test them – this latter theme including but not being restricted to behaviour therapy methods such as exposure, as interpreted in the cognitive model.

2.3   Relevance of early models of cognitive development: Vygotsky and Piaget

For detailed reviews of cognitive developmental theory, see, for example, Demetriou (1998), McShane (1991), Sameroff and Haith (1996) and Weinert and Perner (1996). Application of cognitive developmental theory to issues in CBT for children are rare, with notable exceptions including Ronen (1997), Holmbeck *et al.* (2000) and Piacentini and Bergman (2001). Two founding models of cognitive development, those of Vygotsky and Piaget, both remain highly influential, and both are highly relevant to the theory behind CBT, specifically in relation to the assumption of *fundamental linkage between cognition and action.*

In the developmental model developed by Vygotsky, cognition and action are seen as fundamentally *social,* and from this perspective there is an insight very close to the core theory behind CBT – namely, that *language has a key role in the regulation (or control) of action.* On this, Vygotsky said, for example (1981, pp. 69–70):

Children master the social forms of behavior and transfer these forms to themselves. With regard to our area of interest, we could say that the validity of this law is nowhere more obvious than in the use of the sign. A sign is always originally a means used for social purposes, a means of influencing others, and only later becomes a means of influencing oneself. According to Janet, the word initially was a command to others and then underwent a complex history of imitations, changes of functions, etc. Only gradually was it separated from action. According to Janet, it is always a command, and that is why it is the basic means of mastering behavior. Therefore, if we want to clarify genetically the origins of the voluntary function of the word and why the word overrides motor responses, we must inevitably arrive at the real function of commanding in both ontogenesis and phylogenesis.

In Piaget, the fundamental linkage between cognition and action is most clear in the sensori-motor stage, where they practically coincide, but it remains true in subsequent stages, including the mature formal operational attained during adolescence, characterized by abstraction, logic, theory and beliefs about beliefs, and which forms the basis of cultural practices of science, politics and so on. It is plausible to say that, in this development, the balance of influence shifts; at the beginning, cognition is very closely tied to action, and is made possible by action. By the time of maturity, however, cognition makes the practice possible.

While both developmental theories affirm the close connection between cognition and behaviour, they also both recognize that in development there is a loosening of cognition from action, so that in fact the former can in some sense run free of the latter, and this is particularly so as cognition develops from its sensori-motor origins by using conventional symbolism, i.e. language. Early in the development of language, cognition as verbally encoded can run free, at the level of grammatical or word play, in flights of fancy and in cultural practices of story-telling, spoken and written. The relationships of these kinds of representation to reality are complex and varied. The relevance of this point to CBT is that cognition in verbal code may be on a particular occasion divorced from sensori-motor and affective responses and, in this case, talking runs the risk of just talking and making no difference. This issue is relevant to CBT generally but it may be particularly relevant to therapy with children, insofar as they are in the process of forging the links between language, affect and behaviour.

Some of the first major work in cognitive therapy for children was based clearly on Vygotsky's developmental psychology – specifically on the idea that thought as inner speech becomes used for self-regulation of behaviour. This was the principle that underlay the development of 'self-instruction' therapy, aimed, for example, at enhancing problem-definition and problem-solving skills in impulsive children. Subsequent meta-analyses of treatment outcome studies found, however, that effect sizes for these treatments depended on the age of the children, with modest improvements prior to around the age of puberty and more clinically significant changes thereafter (Dush *et al.*, 1989; Durlak *et al.*, 1991). Interpretation of these meta-analytic studies was made in terms of Piagetian theory, with the inference that CBT may not be significantly effective for children until they have reached the formal operations stage at around adolescence.

In Piaget's theory, the 'formal operations' stage involves various, linked competencies, including facility with propositional logic and the predicate calculus, conceptual abstraction, meta-representation (thoughts about thoughts) and (explicit) systematic theory. For example, Inhelder and Piaget wrote (1958, pp. 339–40):

The adolescent is the individual who begins to build "systems" or "theories", in the largest sense of the term. The child does not build systems. His spontaneous thinking may be more or less systematic . . . but it is the observer who sees the system from outside, while the child is never aware of it since he never thinks about his own thought . . . The child has no powers of reflection, i.e. no second-order thoughts which deal critically with his own thinking. No theory can be built without such reflection. In contrast, the adolescent is able to analyse his own thinking and construct theories. The fact that these theories are oversimplified, awkward, and usually contain very little originality is beside the point.

These ideas are very relevant to assumptions of cognitive therapy, particularly relating to *meta-cognition*, the formulation of thoughts about thoughts, which pervades cognitive models, and to the notion of *systematic theory*, crucial to some cognitive therapy models of some disorders – e.g. Beck's model of depression, which implicates the person's theory about the self, world and future (Beck, 1976).

This points to a legacy of Piagetian developmental psychology, therefore, that there is a scepticism about the applicability of CBT to younger children, prior to adolescence. First-order cognition, it may be said, is found throughout living beings and certainly in young humans, but meta-cognition, according to Piagetian theory, kicks in later, at adolescence. This suggests that CBT will not do much for younger children, a theoretical conclusion used as noted above to interpret the findings of early meta-analytic studies of treatment outcomes. Conversely, this line of thought drawing out implications from Piagetian theory will also lend support to the idea that what is most effective for the younger children is behaviour therapy, *BT*, without (much) *C* (cognitive).

However, there are in fact plenty of reasons why we can no longer rest content with the negative conclusion suggested by Piagetian theory – most clearly the fact that the theory is old and that developmental psychology has moved on. However, the scientific progress has not been simply linear, just a matter of ever better and empirically more refined Piagetian-style theory. There have been changes internally to the general model – e.g. changes in estimation of what stages are reached at what ages – but these matters of detail have been subsumed within larger paradigm shifts. It was argued that Piagetian theory had confused competence with performance, which can be brought out by appropriately designed experiments, including at younger ages than predicted. This was coupled with increasing awareness that Piagetian theory had ignored major environmental influences that produced cognitive developmental changes in children, such as in the family or school. Further, paradigm shifts in psychology generally have affected developmental psychology – e.g. increasing dominance of the information-processing paradigm, and increasing emphasis on the domain-specificity of knowledge and the modularity of mind. The first breaks down cognition into many routines and subroutines, while the second emphasizes diverse systems dedicated to specific cognitive tasks. Both of these new paradigms focus away in several ways from general theories and statements about cognition and its developmental stages and focus instead on specifics and on processes of change.

The upshot of these various developments is that Piagetian cognitive developmental stage theory left the apparent implication that the application of CBT to pre-adolescent children would be radically limited – and then withdrew from the scene. This leaves a curious situation – familiar in CBT – in which a crucial assumption continues to work its effects, but is unavailable for testing. This threatens paralysis, at least in the theory, and suggests the need for a review, particularly in relation to *meta-cognition*.

2.4   Varieties of meta-cognition

Regulation of behaviour by *meta-cognition (or reflection about cognition)* typically in language is emphasized in CBT for adults, although in fact it covers many different sorts of thing. It seems that language is crucially involved in meta-cognition and in theory of mind development specifically, but the details and even the direction of causality remains unclear (see, for example, Astington and Jenkins, 1999). Here are a few things covered in CBT, starting with what was most emphasized by Piaget.

2.4.1   *Recognition of logical or evidential connection* between beliefs, for example that this follows from that, belongs with the other, that these various thoughts imply a general proposition, or form a theory

This is crucial to some cognitive models and techniques, particularly those that use the ideas of theory, core assumptions and so on, as, for example, in some cognitive therapy approaches to depression in adults. It may be plausible to say that this capacity for theorizing is relatively late in development, that 5-year-olds have little of it, but many adolescents develop it. There is evidence, for example, that development and application of the concept of inferential validity may be attained later in childhood and in adolescence (Moshman and Franks, 1986), but also evidence that pre-adolescents, even young elementary school children, are reasonably adept at crucial aspects of theory building and application, such as differentiation of hypothetical beliefs from evidence, in particular domains (Sodian *et al.*, 1991).

2.4.2   *Evaluation/appraisal* of thoughts (or statements) as being, for example, bad, clever, stupid, useless, shameful, embarrassing, mad, etc.

This kind of appraisal is of course crucial to most if not all cognitive therapy models and methods, and perhaps comprises most of the so-called 'negative automatic thoughts' (NATs) that are regarded as crucial in the interpretation of current experience and therefore in the regulation of current affect and behaviour. It may not matter much whether these evaluations are prefaced by a social qualifier – 'they will think I am . . .' – insofar as the distinction between what *they think* and what *I think* may have to be worked out. Indeed, like many clinicians working with children and families, the author has often wondered whether today's repeated, somewhat battering comments from parents to child become the child-as-adult's NATs, while, conversely, encouraging comments become the child-as-adult's positive ATs. This would be consistent with key elements of Vygotsky's developmental psychology noted earlier: that mental life is an internalization of social life, and specifically that thought is inner speech. In cognitive models of adult mental health problems, it is typically assumed that activation of NATs involves both trigger situations but also dysfunctional assumptions and possibly core beliefs. But the possibility raised by the above considerations is that developmentally there may be an immediate pathway from trigger situations to NATs, made by parental evaluation, without mediation by general propositions.

In any case, there is apparently no reason from the point of view of cognitive development to put a lower boundary on the age at which children can have – whether spontaneously or by internalizing – these kinds of appraisals about thoughts, or opinions or behaviour, or about the self that has or does these things. There may be developmental factors related to content, however, as well as individual differences. For example, more complex affective states and descriptions such as pride and shame seem to appear in the transition from early to middle childhood (Harter, 1996; Stevenson-Hinde and Shouldice, 1996).

2.4.3   Representation of controllability of mental states

Recognition that mental states may be under the person's control, although some kinds are easier to control than others, is another form of meta-cognition. There is evidence that this capacity is already shown by 7-year-olds, although with increasing development through subsequent childhood (Flavell and Green, 1999).

2.4.4   Representation of what cognitive states are regulating another's or one's own behaviour

This is a particularly interesting kind of meta-cognition, involving what has come to be called 'theory of mind'. It is used mainly for attributing reasons for action and for affect, expressed in statements of the form: 'I (or he) did what I (or he) did because I (or he) felt like thus-and-so/believed such-and-such' and 'I (or he) felt like thus-and-so because this or that happened to me (or him) and I (or he) believed such-and-such'. Very young children begin to give reasons of a sort once they have the capacity for sentence production, and subsequently in development the representation of one's own states, or another's, evolves to comprise a theory of the self – an interpretative narrative involving history, personality and plans – providing the basis for concepts of self-awareness, autonomy and responsibility. In other words, this very important meta-cognitive capacity admits of degrees and begins to develop much earlier than adolescence, in young childhood (Chandler and Lalonde, 1996). In this connection, there is also evidence that young children around 6 years of age pass advanced higher-order theory of mind false belief tasks ('where does Jane think John thinks the ball is?') (Sullivan et al., 1994).

Meta-cognition of all four kinds described above is crucial in CBT. The client typically has some account of the maladaptive behaviour and her relationship to it, and this meta-cognition of various kinds is itself likely to be involved in the problem. This is because meta-cognition, like cognition generally, generates affect and behaviour. Meta-cognition – whether right or wrong, reasonable or unreasonable, fair or unfair – in fact generates further activity, above and beyond the behaviour associated with the original cognition. For example, if I recognize that a succession of rejections are linked as such and form a generalization 'I am always rejected', then I will make the prediction: 'And the next time I will be too'. This is a new piece of information, over and above past individual instances. Or, if I judge my opinions or spontaneous thoughts to be bad or mad, then I am likely also to be ashamed or frightened, and act accordingly. If I judge – even though mistakenly – that anxiety cannot be controlled, then this will intensify my fear. Various kinds of errors are possible in relation to the fourth kind of meta-cognition considered above, i.e. representation of the cognitive states regulating one's own behaviour. For example, a child may believe he was angry at his friend because the friend was nasty to him, but he was in fact angry because the friend had something he wanted; or someone may believe that there is no information processing-regulating behaviour, such as physiological arousal, when there is, as in panic disorder, or that there is when there is not, as in early experiments on manipulating social factors in attribution (Schachter and Singer, 1962). But even though such meta-cognitive appraisals of this fourth kind may be wrong (in any of the above ways), they generate further behaviour consistent with them. In the illustrations just given, the associated further behaviour would be: self-righteousness and uninhibited anger, panic and an emotion appropriate to the situation. These are new behaviours caused by the thoughts about the thoughts, by thoughts about the information processing, or lack of it, regulating one's (first-order) behaviour. This has the consequence that if first- and second-order cognition coincide, if one is a correct representation of the other, there is integrity and certainty in action, while, if they diverge, there is more or less mischief, typical of the kind that CBT and other forms of psychotherapy try to help sort out (Bolton, 1995).

2.5 'What cognitive developmental level is needed for CBT?'

This final section brings considerations so far to bear on the above question (see Chapter 8), mainly with the effect of deconstructing it. The main point is that the prior and primary question is rather: 'what cognition is involved in the production/maintenance of the problem in the particular case?' The therapist needs to address only what is really involved, regardless of what the child's 'cognitive developmental level' may be. There is no need to worry about the general question whether, for example, children age 7, or this particular child of age 7, is or is not capable of, for example, meta-cognition involving theory use.

Rather, the therapist needs to find out whether such cognition is involved in the problem and address it if so; if not, there is no need.

This line of thought suggests that the emphasis should be firmly on assessment of the particular case, although of course the assessment is theory driven. We know mainly from the adult models what kind of cognitions to look for in particular kinds of presenting problem. For example, in the case of panic attacks, it should be determined whether the key trigger is an external situation or some internal, somatic sign, and what catastrophizing appraisals are being made. In a presentation of obsessive compulsion, the appraisals involved in obsessions should be identified, such as any meta-cognitive appraisals involving exaggerated perceived responsibility. In depression, what are the key triggering external situations (such as loss) or task demands? What negative thoughts does the person have in these situations, to do, for example, with being alone or not being able to cope? In inappropriate aggression, what are the key triggers, such as frustration or conflict, and how are they appraised, for example using external attribution?

Clinical experience suggests that children often do report cognition of these various kinds. Some of the most important recent research on the theory of CBT for children has been focused simply on the crucial empirical question: to what extent do children show the kind of cognitive style and content implicated in CBT models for adults? Results here have been promising: studies with non-clinical samples suggest that children and adolescents use cognitive appraisals associated with depression and anxiety similar to those found in adults (e.g. Garber *et al.*, 1993; Chorpita *et al.*, 1996; Hadwin *et al.*, 1997).

There are, of course, particular issues that arise in assessing young children. Simply asking about feelings and emotions in relation to problematic situations may be less useful for children than for adults, because children on average may find lengthy conversations more difficult and because they may be more focused on the present. This is not to say that clinical interview with children cannot elicit articulated accounts of problematic situations – clearly, this sometimes does work. The degree of success may depend on, among other things, the extent to which events and associated affect have been articulated and recalled in family conversation, as in non-clinical cases (Nelson, 1996). Otherwise, it is useful to apply the principle that cognition in a particular kind of context is best accessed in that context, and, so, enactment may help – e.g. exposure to anxiogenic stimuli may facilitate the expression of specific threat perceptions. Or, bearing in mind that the parents have experience of the child in the key situations while the clinician may not, the clinician can simply ask the parents whether the child has ever said anything in or about the situations in question.

Alternatively, an unforced multiple-choice paradigm may be used to facilitate recall and reporting. The therapist may wonder aloud – e.g. 'Well, when I get angry at my brother it's often because he did either this, that or the other' – or the therapist could invite the parents to wonder why they might be angry, the aim being that such a conversation, not with the child as the explicit focus, may cue the child to contribute their own opinion from their own case. This is something they often, although of course not always, will do. There are many other methods well known to child mental health workers, such as role play, story-telling and so on. The main aim of the CBT assessment is to find out what – if any – appraisals are actually driving the problematic affect and behaviour, judged by self-report, spontaneous or cued.

The main question for assessment, then, is what kinds and contents of appraisals are in practice at work in the generation and/or maintenance of the problems presented by the particular child. To the extent that this or that kind or content are operating, they can be addressed in the ways familiar in CBT for adults. To the extent that other kinds of cognitions or contents are not at work in the child, then – even if they are typically found in adults and are part of the model of the presenting condition in adults – it does not matter. In other words, the answer to the general question – what cognitive developmental level is needed for CBT? – is: whatever level is involved in generating the problem in the particular case.

The problem of cognitive development for CBT is then not primarily a matter of what developmental level is needed for applicability of the therapy, but is rather primarily a matter of what kinds and contents of appraisals are implicated in the generation and maintenance of clinical problems presenting in childhood in general, and what kinds and contents specifically in particular cases. Developmental research since the dominant period of Piagetian general stage theory suggests, as indicated above, that there are likely to be large individual variations in this respect, at any given chronological age, dependent on many factors including, for example, temperament and social and family context.

It is also the case that the younger children are, the less likely it is that they have the complex cognitive capacities and performance characteristic of adulthood. However, the considerations as above imply that this is in a key respect irrelevant to the issue of using CBT for children. If some aspect of cognitive therapy is not applicable to children because they have not yet developed the requisite cognitive processes – perhaps, say, meta-cognition or explicit systematic theory – then by the very same consideration there would be reason to believe that the mature cognitive processes implicated in models of adult mental health problems would not be operating in children. In other words, the same developmental theory that would counter-indicate cognitive therapy for children would at the same time imply that the cognition it addresses plays no prominent role in typical childhood disorders. It is consistent with this, for example, that meta-cognition in the form of explicit systematic theory apparently does not play a prominent role in common childhood anxiety and behaviour problems, and, by contrast, that clinical conditions frankly involving elaborate theorizing are rare in children, such as paranoid delusions or presentations of depression involving a theory of the self, world and future.

There may, however, be other requirements for the effective use of CBT that may be problematic particularly with children, but because of factors other than general cognitive developmental level. CBT assumes that cognition drives behaviour and affect and that it can be modified working primarily within the domain of verbally encoded information and command. One way in which these assumptions might be limited derives precisely from the implied reliance on the regulation of affect and behaviour by verbally encoded rules. As indicated earlier, language comes to have this function, but does not have it automatically or neces-sarily. Hence, the importance in assessment, emphasized above, of determining what verbally encoded rules the child does actually use. But suppose there are no verbally encoded rules? Suppose that the behaviour and affect of the child in the circumstances in question are innate – e.g. stranger anxiety in the very young child – or are regulated solely by principles of classical or operant conditioning – such as fear of dogs after being bitten – or instrumental aggression? These kinds of behaviours, in animals and children, run their course regardless of talking. Children typically may learn to override such behaviours by verbally mediated information and commands, but there is no reason a priori to suppose that this must happen in every case. It remains possible from a theoretical point of view, either because of a biological dysfunction or as an extreme of normal variation, that the behaviour of some children is regulated in high degree by immediate environmental contingencies, with little or no verbal mediation. Nothing in the theory predicts that these children can be taught verbal mediation that will over-ride motor responses. This of course is consistent with the findings cited earlier, that attempts to make good 'cognitive deficiencies' in impulsive behaviour by teaching verbal control have had limited success with younger children (Dush et al., 1989; Durlak et al., 1991), and with the current position that attention deficit hyperactivity is relatively unresponsive to psychological therapy includ-ing self-instructional methods (Hinshaw, 2000; Nolan and Carr, 2000). This kind of explanation of the ineffectiveness of CBT in children, however, is specific to particular kinds of problem and posits specific mechanisms (or absence of mech-anisms) outside of or at the limits of the normal range, and is not a matter of the 'general cognitive level of children'.

On the positive side, there may be particular positive indications for CBT in children and adolescents. By the time of adulthood, people have had the time, capacity and need to build up styles and systems of belief around problematic behaviour, including entrenched secondary appraisals that unfortunately exacerbate and maintain the problem. Because they are still developing, by contrast, the child and adolescent have views of themselves and the world that are less fixed and so far more open to new possibilities.

2.6 Conclusions

There is a good match in many respects between the working assumptions of CBT and some fundamental principles of cognitive development which is to do with the close connection between cognition and action and the role of language in mediating behaviour. Piagetian general stage theory seemed to imply, however, that meta-cognition, crucial in CBT, appears relatively late (in adolescence) and this has been used to interpret relatively poor outcome of early studies of CBT with young children. Yet, meta-cognition comes in various shapes and sizes, and many kinds if not all begin to have made their appearance already in young childhood. In general, Piagetian stage theory has been overtaken in various paradigm shifts, and, consistent with this, the general question 'what cognitive developmental level is needed for CBT?' is no longer viable. The main question is rather: 'what cognition is involved in the production/maintenance of the problem in the particular case?' There seems to be no reason why all or most cognitive therapy models and methods should not be applied to children, once they can use language, indefinitely far down the age range. They may or may not work in particular kinds of case, but failure to help much with impulsive behaviour for example, may be best viewed in relation to particular kinds of condition, rather than general models of cognitive development.

CBT for children is at an early stage of development and there is a pressing need for research in many areas, not only in the area of cognitive development. For example, more needs to be known in the normal, non-clinical case about the origins and determinants of the child's and adolescent's cognitive style and content. To what extent is the child's view of himself and the world learnt from significant attachment figures, and to what extent from verbal information and from modelling? How far is there a 'family cognition' as opposed to the various styles and views of several individuals? To what extent does the child acquire views from other informants and models, e.g. at school, from peers? Or does the child's cognitive style and content derive more 'from within', as a product of, for example, temperament and personal experience? In the clinical domain, there is much work to be done in individual case studies and in case series on the cognitive processes and content regulating affect and behaviour, on similarities and differences compared with models of problems in adults and on the construction of cognitive models of distinctive child mental health problems.

2.7 Acknowledgements

Early versions of this chapter were presented as part of a symposium on 'New developments in the understanding of cognition in children and adolescents', at the BABCP Annual Conference, Glasgow, June 2001, and at the Children's Department Seminar, South London and Maudsley NHS Trust, February 2002. The author is grateful to many colleagues for their helpful comments on previous versions, including Francesca Happé, Ulrike Schmidt and Ruth Williams. Errors that remain are the author's.

2.8 REFERENCES

Astington, J. W. and Jenkins, J. M. (1999). A longitudinal study of the relation between language and theory-of-mind development. *Developmental Psychology*, **35**, 1311–20.

Beck, A. T. (1976). *Cognitive Therapy and the Emotional Disorders*. New York: International Universities Press.

Beck, A. T., Emery, G. and Greenberg, R. L. (1985). *Anxiety Disorders and Phobias: A Cognitive Perspective*. New York: Basic Books.

Bolton, D. (1995). Self-knowledge, error and disorder. In M. Davies and A. Stone (eds.), *Mental Simulation: Evaluations and Applications*. Oxford: Blackwell, pp. 209–34.

Chandler, M. and Lalonde, C. (1996). Shifting to an interpretative theory of mind: 5- to 7-year-olds' changing conceptions of mental life. In A. J. Sameroff and M. M. Haith (eds.), *The Five to Seven Year Shift. The Age of Reason and Responsibility*. Chicago: University of Chicago Press, pp. 111–39.

Chorpita, B. F., Albano, A. M. and Barlow, D. H. (1996). Cognitive processing in children: relation to anxiety and family influences. *Journal of Clinical Child Psychology*, **25**, 170–6.

Clark, D. (1999). Anxiety disorders: why they persist and how to treat them. *Behaviour Research and Therapy*, **37**, S5–S28.

Clark D. M. and Fairburn C. B. (eds.) (1997). *Science and Practice of Cognitive Behaviour Therapy*. Oxford: Oxford University Press.

Clark, D. M. and Beck, A. T. (1999). *Scientific Foundations of Cognitive Therapy and Therapy of Depression*. New York: John Wiley and Sons.

Demetriou, A. (1998). Cognitive development. In A. Demetriou, W. Doise and C. F. M. van Lieshout (eds.), *Life-Span Developmental Psychology*. New York: John Wiley and Sons Ltd, pp. 179–270.

Durlak, J. A., Fuhrman, T. and Lampman, C. (1991). Effectiveness of cognitive behavior therapy for maladapting children: a meta-analysis. *Psychological Bulletin*, **110**, 204–14.

Dush, D. M., Hirt, M. L. and Schroeder, H. E. (1989). Self statement modification in the treatment of child behavior disorders: a meta-analysis. *Psychological Bulletin*, **106**, 97–106.

Flavell, J. H. and Green, F. L. (1999). Development of intuitions about the controllability of different mental states. *Cognitive Development*, **14**, 133–46.

Garber, J., Weiss, B. and Shanley, N. (1993). Cognitions, depressive symptoms, and development in adolescents. *Journal of Abnormal Psychology*, **102**, 47–57.

Garety, P., Kuipers, E., Fowler, D. Freeman, D. and Bebbington, P. (2001). A cognitive model of schizophrenia. *Psychological Medicine*, **31**, 189–95.

Hadwin, J., Frost, S., French, C. C. and Richards, A. (1997). Cognitive processing and trait anxiety in typically developing children: evidence for an interpretation bias. *Journal of Abnormal Psychology*, **106**, 486–90.

Harter, S. (1996). Developmental changes in self-understanding across the 5 to 7 shift. In A. J. Sameroff and M. M. Haith (eds.), *The Five to Seven Year Shift. The Age of Reason and Responsibility*. Chicago: The University of Chicago Press, pp. 207–36.

Hinshaw, S. P. (2000). Attention deficit/hyperactivity disorder: the search for viable treatments. In P. C. Kendall (ed.), *Child and Adolescent Therapy: Cognitive-Behavioral Procedures*, second edn. New York: Guilford Press, pp. 88–128.

Holmbeck, G. N., Colder, C., Shapera, W., Westhoven, V., Kenealy, L. and Updegrove, A. (2000). Working with adolescents: guidelines from developmental psychology. In P. C. Kendall (ed.), *Child and Adolescent Therapy: Cognitive-Behavioral Procedures*, second edn. New York: Guilford Press, pp. 335–85.

Inhelder, B. and Piaget, J. (1958). *The Growth of Logical Thinking from Childhood to Adolesence*. New York: Basic Books.

McShane, J. (1991). *Cognitive Development: An Information Processing Approach*. Oxford: Basil Blackwell.

Moshman, D. and Franks, B. A. (1986). Development of the concept of inferential validity. *Child Development*, **57**, 153–65.

Nelson, K. (1996). Memory development from 4 to 7 years. In A. J. Sameroff and M. M. Haith (eds.), *The Five to Seven Year Shift. The Age of Reason and Responsibility*. Chicago: University of Chicago Press, pp. 141–60.

Nolan, M. and Carr, A. (2000). Attention deficit hyperactivity disorder. In A. Carr (ed.), *What Works with Children and Adolescents: A Critical Review of Psychological Interventions with Children, Adolescents and Their Families*, Hove, UK and New York: Brunner-Routledge, pp. 65–101.

Piacentini, J. and Bergman, R. L. (2001). Developmental issues in cognitive therapy for childhood anxiety disorders. *Journal of Cognitive Psychotherapy*, **15**, 165–82.

Ronen, T. (1997). Cognitive developmental therapy with children. Chichester and New York: Wiley.

Salkovskis, P. M. (1996a). The cognitive approach to anxiety: threat beliefs, safety-seeking, and the special case of health anxiety and obsessions. In P. M. Salkovskis (ed.), *Frontiers of Cognitive Therapy*. New York: Guilford, pp. 48–74.

(ed.) (1996b). *Frontiers of Cognitive Therapy*. New York: Guilford.

(1999). Understanding and treating obsessive-compulsive disorder. *Behaviour Research and Therapy*, **37**, S29–S52.

Sameroff A. J. and Haith, M. M. (1996). Interpreting developmental transitions. In A. J. Sameroff and M. M. Haith (eds.), *The Five to Seven Year Shift. The Age of Reason and Responsibility*. Chicago: University of Chicago Press, pp. 3–15.

Schachter, S. and Singer, J. E. (1962). Cognitive, social, and physiological determinants of emotional state. *Psychological Review*, **69**, 379–99.

Sharp, M. (1997). Chronic fatigue. In D. M. Clark and C. B. Fairburn (eds.), *Science and Practice of Cognitive Behaviour Therapy*. Oxford: Oxford University Press, pp. 381–414.

Sodian, B., Zaitchik, D. and Carey, S. (1991). Young children's differentiation of hypothetical beliefs from evidence. *Child Development*, **62**, 753–66.

Stevenson-Hinde, J. and Shouldice, A. (1996). Fearfulness: developmental consistency. In A. J. Sameroff and M. M. Haith (eds.), *The Five to Seven Year Shift. The Age of Reason and Responsibility*. Chicago: University of Chicago Press, pp. 237–52.

Sullivan, K., Zaitchik, D. and Tager-Flusberg, H. (1994). Pre-schoolers can attribute second-order beliefs. *Developmental Psychology*, **30**, 395–402.

Vitousek, K. M. (1996). The current status of cognitive behavioural models of anorexia nervosa and bulimia nervosa. In P. M. Salkovskis (ed.), *Frontiers of Cognitive Therapy*. New York: Guilford, pp. 383–418.

Vygotsky, L. (1981). The genesis of higher mental functions. In J. V. Wertsch (ed.), *The Concept of Activity in Soviet Psychology*. New York: M. E. Sharpe Inc., pp. 144–88. Reprinted in K. Richardson and S. Sheldon (eds.) (1990), *Cognitive Development to Adolescence*. Hove: Lawrence Erlbaum Assoc., pp. 61–80.

Weinert, F. E. and Perner, J. (1996). Cognitive development. In D. Magnusson (ed.), *The Life-span Development of Individuals: Behavioural, Neurobiological, and Psychosocial Perspectives* (ed.). Cambridge: Cambridge University Press, pp. 207–22.

3

Cognitive behavioural therapy in developmental perspective

Thomas O'Connor and Cathy Creswell

Institute of Psychiatry, London, UK

Studies showing the effectiveness of cognitive behavioural therapy (CBT) for children have proliferated in recent years. Findings from these investigations provide clear evidence that CBT is an effective clinical tool for treating some of the more common psychological disorders in children and adolescence, principally anxiety and depression (Kendall, 1985; Harrington et al., 1998). Given that this first essential hurdle has been cleared, attention can now be directed towards two follow-on questions: what are the mechanisms underlying effective treatment and how do we understand the inevitable variation in treatment response? This chapter addresses these latter questions by appealing to developmental theory and research relevant to social cognitions and psychological disorders in children and adolescence.

The aims of the chapter are to outline why a developmental model of CBT is needed and how one might be constructed; to review illustrative findings from research on children's social cognitions and the extent to which CBT with children is informed by this research; to identify some of the obstacles blocking greater synthesis of developmental and clinical research relevant to CBT with children; and to draw implications for assessment and interventions.

3.1 What is a developmental approach?

Before considering what a development perspective can add to the practice of CBT with children, we first need to assess what it is. A developmental approach as applied to CBT with children can be characterized by several distinct features. A core consideration is the carrying forward of effects and the mechanisms involved, or, in other words, the nature of continuities and discontinuities in development. More broadly considered, psychopathology has been defined in

Cognitive Behaviour Therapy for Children and Families, ed. Philip J. Graham.
Published by Cambridge University Press. © Cambridge University Press 2004.

terms of the individual's development trajectory and whether it has veered off a normative developmental course (e.g. Bowlby, 1988). In other words, rather than (or perhaps in addition to) viewing psychopathology as a constellation of symptoms, it can be assessed according to the ability of the individual to meet the developmental challenges, such as the formation of positive peer relations in middle childhood. In terms of assessment, the focus should be not only on symptom expression but also on the individual's developmental course and projection of likely further disturbance. There are also implications of this approach for conceptualizing treatment. So, for example, prevention and intervention studies showing sustained or even continued improvements in children's adjustment after treatment (Barrett *et al.*, 1996; Silverman *et al.*, 1999) may be seen as the intervention altering the child's developmental trajectory and not simply reducing particular symptoms.

A second feature of a developmental approach as applied to CBT is to identify what it is about the children's developmental phase that might moderate treatment response or the way in which the intervention is delivered. The alternative (i.e. 'adevelopmental') position is that there is nothing specific about the child's cognitive, linguistic or social development that is pertinent to the delivery of the intervention or to understanding its effects. Few would accept this latter notion, although it is a hypothesis that is often not considered directly and rejected. So, for example, does the same kind of CBT intervention have different effects when delivered to children in different phases of development? If so, what accounts for these differences? Compared with mid-adolescents, do younger children need a form of CBT that makes less use of cognitive structuring? This would be the case if, for example, anxiety in younger children were not mediated by cognition/language (e.g. Prins, 2000).

More broadly, we might ask a parallel set of questions concerning the expression of psychopathology in children. For example, what does the finding that generalized anxiety has a later onset than separation anxiety tell us about the cognitive sophistication underlying the phenomenology of these disorders? Is it the case that *generalized* anxiety requires more sophisticated cognitive processes, i.e. those necessary for the child to generalize? Answering questions of this sort is complicated, but there are some illustrative findings. Thus, children's ability to generalize across contexts or show an understanding of constancy is evident in early childhood. However, whereas constancy of concrete and observable physical characteristics emerges in early childhood and constancy of gender and externally observable characteristics appears slightly later (Gouze and Nadelman, 1980), it is not until late childhood that children appreciate constancy of internal (psychological) characteristics (e.g. 8–9 years for self-identity in Guardo and Bonan, 1971). Accordingly, prior to middle childhood, children infrequently use trait terms to describe themselves and explain their own behaviour (Rotenberg, 1982). In a similar vein, compared with younger anxious children, older anxious children (adolescents) exhibit more trait anxiety and more worry (Strauss *et al.*, 1988). Finally, does the early onset of certain fears and phobias suggest a weaker cognitive basis than later emerging symptoms of anxiety (e.g. worry), and does this have any implications for the effectiveness of cognitive approaches?

Research into developmental changes in symptom expression has yet to elucidate what the clinical applications may be, but there are signs of progress. For instance, clinical wisdom and, increasingly, empirical research raise doubts about the position that depression should be defined similarly in children and adults (Garber, 2000). Progress towards a developmental understanding of treatment delivery has proceeded more slowly.

A third component of a developmental model seeks to place the child in his/her social context and to examine how the multiple social contexts in which the child is embedded (family, school, neighbourhood and subculture) influence his/her affect, cognition and behaviour. This is in contrast to the more 'insular' or individual focus in CBT. Applied to the clinic setting, a consideration of the child's social context may help explain why the child's cognitions and behaviour are resistant to change despite the application of sound clinical technique. Given the likely importance of social context, especially family processes, in working with children, this topic is developed further in a subsequent section.

A fourth component to a developmental model emphasizes the need to consider continuities between normal and abnormal behaviour rather than to assume a disjunction between the two. A corollary is that understanding normal variation may inform our understanding of abnormal behaviour and vice versa (Cicchetti and Cohen, 1995). It is well known that core 'symptoms' of the anxiety disorders, including fears and phobias, separation anxiety and obsessive-compulsive behaviour, all show strong age-based trends; furthermore, the age trends differ for each behaviour (Bolton, 1996; Evans *et al.*, 1997; Garber, 2000; Rapee, 2001). Thus, a fear of dogs would be considered within the boundaries of normal in early childhood, but the same fear (and accompanying behavioural avoidance) may have clinical significance in the older child or adolescent. A developmental hypothesis is that there may be similar mechanisms involved and that normative fear in childhood may be linked with non-normative fear in later childhood. To date, however, surprisingly few studies directly test this hypothesis.

3.1.1   How is development integrated in current practice and research on CBT?

The 'adevelopmental' model underlying CBT is illustrated in several ways. Thus, there is nothing about the theory (as generally defined) that predicts that younger children would be less responsive to CBT than older children or, more generally, how variation in treatment response might reflect the child's context or developmental phase. Additionally, the focus has traditionally been on the process of changing cognitions and behaviour in the 'here and now' and less on understanding their origins (although a possible exception to this may be more recent 'scheme-based' work for patients with complex problems).

Notwithstanding the lack of developmental emphasis in CBT, it cannot escape the treating clinician's attention that the child's development is relevant for the treatment. This clinical impression is reinforced by a number of recent conceptual articles and chapters discussing developmental issues in child CBT. However, writings on this topic typically appeal to vague notions about development that do not point to particular mechanisms or carry any particular clinical applications. As a result, what it is about development that is pertinent to applying CBT or understanding its (in)effectiveness is unclear; that is, whereas there is broad agreement that a developmentally informed model for CBT is needed, there is no consensus on what it is about development that is critical and how practice should be altered.

The ambiguous manner in which development is included in child CBT is illustrated in the case of age. As regards clinical practice, some consideration of the child's age is encouraged and there appears to be general agreement that older children may be more responsive to cognitive approaches whereas younger children may require more behaviourally oriented treatment techniques. However, there is as yet no clear formulation of why the child's age may moderate treatment response or shape the delivery of the treatment. This conceptual uncertainty is reflected in empirical findings. One meta-analysis of treatment response suggested age may be an important predictor, with larger effect sizes for adolescents and early adolescents than pre-adolescents (Durlak et al., 1991). In contrast, more recent studies reported that younger age (e.g. pre-adolescent versus adolescent) predicted a more positive response to treatment that involved a cognitive component (e.g. Southam-Gerow et al., 2001). In this case, older age may be associated with less positive results because the cognitive biases may have been more entrenched and more difficult to change (although the effects of age controlling for duration and severity of disturbance are often not reported; see also Cowen and Durlak, 2000); still other studies find no effect of age on treatment outcome. In short, the effect of age on treatment response is not robust and may differ across childhood disorders (Hudson et al., 2002).

The reason why age is not likely to move research on in any substantive way is that age is a proxy for a range of developmental processes, only some of which may be relevant to cognitively mediated therapy. We need to ask what it is indexed by age that explains variation in treatment response. In addition, a focus on age will obscure individual differences in social cognitive skills that may be only modestly associated with age, a topic discussed in more detail below. Consequently, we should not be too surprised to find that age is at best an inconsistent predictor of treatment response, and neither should we invest too much in findings that demonstrate that there is (or is not) a connection between age and treatment response. Importantly, the mixed findings concerning age as a predictor of treatment response do not mean that there may not be important developmental constraints on CBT, but simply that age is not a sensitive index of what these moderating factors are.

The remainder of this chapter will examine alternatives to age that may provide a developmental model to explain mechanisms of treatment and variation in treatment response.

3.2   Developmental–clinical research relevant to CBT with children: models and paradigms

One of the few consistencies among extant attempts to formulate a developmental model of CBT with children is an appeal to a grand normative developmental model of cognitive development as an explanation for age-based variation in treatment delivery and response, such as a Piagetian stage model. Indeed, the reliance on a Piagetian model in this area has all the qualities of an automatic thought: reflexive, pervasive, resistant to change or doubt and, most significant of all, without supporting evidence. There is, in fact, far less research into CBT or even the expression of symptomatology using a Piagetian stage model than the popularity of this notion would imply. There are various reasons why a general stage model has been found wanting, including a prioritization of normative developmental differences over attention to individual differences and a focus on 'core' cognitive processes rather than a consideration of intra-individual variation and the contextual nature of children's cognitions. This general issue is discussed in other chapters of this book (see Chapters 2 and 8) and are not further discussed here.

If general developmental models of cognitive development are limited in their application to the clinical context, what alternative approaches are there and are they likely to be of greater relevance? We consider alternative social cognitive models and paradigms that have been used extensively in developmental research and which may transfer to the clinic setting. By 'social cognition', we mean the cognitive processes concerning the child's social world. This blanket term covers a range of specific processes, including emotional understanding, empathy, social attribution and attachment representations, among others.

3.2.1   Social attribution and social information processing models

An extremely productive and clinically useful line of research assesses social information processing in young children. There are several examples of research of this kind, including the model of Dodge and colleagues (Crick and Dodge, 1994) and others (Garber and Flynn, 2001). The components of the social information processing model developed by Dodge are attending to, encoding and interpreting social cues (e.g. why did that child bump into me?); developing goals for one's own behaviour (e.g. what do I want to do now – given that I think the other child deliberately and provocatively bumped into me?); and generating potential solutions and evaluating their effects (e.g. what would happen if I hit back at him?) (Dodge, 1993). Support for the social information processing model has been reported by several research groups and with several clinical samples, although the model seems most often applied with aggressive and conduct disorder populations (Dodge and Frame, 1982).

There are, for the clinic setting, several advantages of this line of research. First, the methods used to derive distorted cognitions in children are easily imported into the clinic setting. Thus, the methods used in the research cited above could usefully be integrated with a standard clinic assessment. Secondly, there are now intervention and prevention programmes developed from the social information processing model. One of the better known examples of this is the Fast track prevention programme (Conduct Problems Prevention Research Group, 1992). Thirdly, not coincidentally, within this perspective, the development of treatment goals and strategies for accomplishing them is wholly consistent with the CBT model. Indeed, this approach may be thought of as a particular kind of CBT with children.

3.2.2   Attachment theory

Attachment theory (Ainsworth et al., 1978; Bowlby, 1982) was developed to explain how (and why) a child's experiences with caregivers shapes his/her social and personality development and intergenerational patterns of caregiving. A key component of the theory concerns the child's cognitive processing of experiences and the carrying forward of these cognitions, what Bowlby (1982) defined as an 'internal working model'. The internal working model is a representation or social–affective cognitive schema that the child develops in response to real-life experiences with the caregiver. Experiences are interpreted in, filtered by and organized into a cognitive schema that then shapes how the child comes to view self and others. The relevance for CBT is that, within the context of attachment theory, there is a model for understanding how distorted cognitive representational models about attachment relationships develop, how they are sustained and how they may increase vulnerability to psychopathology. Of further practical relevance is the fact that the methods used in attachment-based research can be adapted to the clinic setting, although in some cases this may require considerable training.

Assessments of attachment quality in infants and preschool-aged children are based on a laboratory-based measure of child and parent interactions in mildly and modestly stressful settings, the Strange Situation (Ainsworth *et al.*, 1978). Assessments of attachment quality in children older than preschool rely largely on a variety of projective story-stem and doll play approaches that tap into children's representations of self and caregiver (Bretherton and Mulholland, 1999; Green *et al.*, 2000). In these assessments, a child is shown toy figures and told the beginning of a story with an attachment theme (e.g. the child is hurt) and is asked to complete the story; the child is prompted for information about how the child and parent figures would feel and what would happen next. The content of the child's story is coded for instances of security (e.g. the child reports seeking out the parent, deriving comfort from him/her and returning to play), avoidance (e.g. the child makes no mention of the parent in his/her story and appears to comfort him/herself), and aggressive, controlling, chaotic or other themes. In some cases, the quality of his/her narrative is coded to reflect a coherent story with a clear beginning, middle and end (resolution) versus a jumbled or incoherent style in which the 'story line' is hard to follow. Several assessment protocol and coding methods have been devised (Bretherton *et al.*, 1990; Green *et al.*, 2000).

Separate lines of enquiry show how attachment representations shape children's interpretation and understanding of social and emotional experiences. In one study, 3-year-olds rated as having an insecure (i.e. non-optimal) child–parent attachment relationship showed a greater tendency to recall negative emotions in a recall test paradigm, whereas secure children showed greater recall of positive emotions to the same stimuli (Belsky *et al.*, 1996). The explanation provided was that insecure children are biased to attend to and focus on negative experiences, perhaps because that is more in keeping with their own experience or because it has been more adaptive to do so in the past. Another study of 2–6½-year-olds found that insecure attachment was associated with poorer understanding of negative emotions; compared with securely attached children, children with an insecure attachment had more difficulty explaining or making sense of negative emotions, as assessed by a laboratory task and from a naturalistic assessment of understanding emotions in others (Laible and Thompson, 1998). These two studies demonstrate how, from an early age, attachment representations influence how children process emotional experiences.

Whether or not these attachment cognitive 'biases' have direct input into the clinic context is, however, another matter. It would be premature and inaccurate to refer to insecurely attached children's cognitions as distortions; that is, insecurely attached children's cognitions of the parent as unavailable or unable to offer comfort and support consistently when needed may be *accurate*. The notion of 'distortion' may instead pertain to when these models or expectations are carried forward into, or transferred onto, other relationships, with peers, teachers or others. Thus, the transfer of cognitions and expectations of the parent as unavailable/insensitive to other relationships is likely to be one reason why insecurely attached children show increased problems in peer and social relationships and are at risk for behavioural/emotional problems. Nevertheless, despite the existence of cognitive biases, it would not be recommended and may, in fact, be clinically insensitive and even harmful to try to alter or challenge the insecure child's insecure cognitions, either in an adolescent or younger child (i.e. there is no point in trying to challenge the child's model of the parent as insensitive/psychologically unavailable if, in fact, that is the child's experience). Instead, the clinical prescription is to help the parent become more sensitively attuned and responsive to the child's attachment needs. In response to improved parental sensitivity, the child's cognitions of the parent as available and sensitive would be expected to alter. Significantly, within an attachment model, the clinical disturbance in the child may be conceptualized as incorporating a strong cognitive component, but the child's cognitions are not a direct target of clinical intervention. In this way, attachment theory provides a set of measures and concepts for understanding the cognitive processes associated with child adjustment and relationship problems, but proposes contrary treatment strategies (the exception being perhaps those CBT programmes that incorporate a family component to address parental behaviour towards the child). In fact, it may not be until adulthood that a focus on attachment cognitions *per se* is a focus for individual treatment within an attachment model.

3.2.3 Children's understanding of mind

Many cognitive models and paradigms have been devised in psychological research to study how young children understand the mind – their own and others' (Flavell, 1999). The focus of this research is the preschool years, or about

2–6 years of age. Several related concepts have been devised and operationalized within this conceptual framework and age window, including theory of mind, conceptual and interpersonal perspective-taking, empathy, emotion understanding and other concepts. At least in principle, research deriving from this tradition should have substantial relevance for developmental models of CBT. This is because much of this research and the theories underlying it can be thought of as trying to identify rudimentary processes in how children come to understand the connections between thoughts, feelings and behaviour. Additionally, as in the case of the attachment and social information processing models, the methods used in research on children's understanding of mind could be adapted to the clinic setting, although the limitation is that most of the established measures have been developed and validated on children of an age not normally considered for CBT (age under 6 years).

A question that hangs over this line of research is whether or not there is a link between the emergence of key social cognitive skills in young children (e.g. emergence of emotional understanding), which is the focus of research attention, and distortions of cognition and affect, which is the focus of clinical attention. It may be that the onset of social cognitions in early childhood and individual differences in distortions in cognitions (apparent after they have come on-line) are developmentally disconnected. Thus, for example, the meaning of conventional theory of mind assessments may be irrelevant outside of the age period of 3–5 years because children will *normally* attain this capacity (with the notable exception of those with autism and cognitive and language delay, who acquire it later in development). So, for example, children with conduct disorder appear to show no deficits in conventional theory of mind assessments (Happé and Frith, 1996). What is needed are assessments of emotional understanding, theory of mind, empathy and related constructs that extend well beyond early childhood to the age window in which children usually come to the attention of clinicians. Progress in this area is slow, although efforts to develop such measures for late childhood and adolescence have intensified in recent years (Happé, 1994; Bosacki and Astington, 1999). For now, research into emotional understanding, mentalizing and related concepts within the developmental psychology tradition has yet to be connected with the kinds of questions and samples that attract the attention of clinical researchers. So, for example, we do not yet know if individual differences in children's response to treatment are associated with individual differences in advanced emotional understanding and mentalizing. There are clearly prospects for greater synthesis, and this is a much-needed line of research.

This list of three models and paradigms for studying social cognition in children is not exhaustive. Instead, these models are highlighted because they have been extensively researched, have practical value and can be translated into a clinic assessment, and they may shed more light into the question of why and how CBT works than traditional models of general cognitive development.

3.3   Developmental–clinical research relevant to CBT with children: components and mechanisms

Whereas in the previous section we approached research into social cognition from the way developmentalists have conceived it, in this next section we will examine the research based on cognitive processes that has developed specifically out of a CBT framework. It is noteworthy that the ideas and methods in these two sections overlap only modestly.

3.3.1   Core components and mechanisms of CBT

CBT has been variably interpreted and applied in clinical practice. Dobson (1988) identified 22 different types of cognitive and cognitive behavioural therapy with differing rationales and various theoretical constructs. Therefore, it is necessary to define what we see as some of the core features of CBT before drawing links between the research literature and clinical practice. Several key features stand out. For example, Beck *et al.* (1979) emphasize how cognitive beliefs and information processing strategies produce characteristic (distorted) views of self, world and future. Of particular interest are three dimensions of cognition: schemata / dysfunctional beliefs (underlying predispositions constructed on the basis of previous experience), automatic thoughts (short internal dialogues that enable evaluation and interpretation of current experience and predictions about future events) and cognitive distortions or information processing biases (e.g. dichotomous thinking, over-generalization, selective abstraction, discounting positive events and catastrophizing). According to this model, primary thera-peutic effects should derive from the identification, testing and correction of distorted concepts and dysfunctional beliefs.

There is a growing research base examining these components of the CBT model in children. Results from some of these investigations are reviewed below.

Several studies have identified the presence of automatic thoughts in children with anxiety and depression (Brown *et al.*, 1986; Francis, 1988; Bogels and Zigter-man, 2000). There is some evidence, however, that the meaning of children's self-statements and attributions, one potential form of automatic thinking, may vary with development. In younger children, lack of ability as an explanation for poor performance may not reflect a stable characteristic of the self – as it would in adults – because ability is seen as something that can be increased with greater effort (Nicholls, 1978). Similarly, in younger children, luck does not represent an external attribute, but rather something that can be taken credit for (Weisz, 1981). Developmental changes in the meaning of children's self-statements may explain why Rholes *et al.* (1980) found that attributions are less strongly correlated with helplessness deficits in younger children (aged 3–5 years) than older children (aged 9–11 years).

More extensively investigated are cognitive distortions and processing biases in children with clinical disturbance or identified risk for disturbance, most often depression or anxiety (Vasey *et al.*, 1996; Garber, 2000). For example, attentional biases towards threat, based on the Dot Probe Task or Stroop Test, and increased vigilance to threat have been reported in clinically anxious children and adolescents, but it is not yet clear if there are developmental changes in visual attention to threat, at least in the age periods studied to date (Taghavi *et al.*, 1999).

An even greater number of studies examine information processing. Several lines of evidence indicate that anxious children interpret ambiguous information as threatening and make lower estimates of their own ability to cope with threat (Kendall, 1985). Within this paradigm, children are presented with a series of scenarios in which it is not quite clear what is happening; an interpretation is necessary in order to answer the questions that follow. For example, the child is told: 'You see a group of children from another class playing a great game. When you walk over to join in they are laughing.' The child is then asked to report what is happening and then prompted to report what s/he would do (from Barrett *et al.*, 1996). Typically, a forced choice is also presented in which the child is asked to select the interpretation that s/he would be most likely to make out of a threat, non-threat and neutral explanation of what is happening.

Studies using this and related methods consistently show that children with anxiety disorders or highly anxious non-clinical participants are more likely to interpret threat than their non-anxious peers. However, it is less clear if the tendency to interpret threat in these scenarios is specific to anxiety or a general feature of clinical disturbance (Barrett *et al.*, 1996; Bogels and Zigterman, 2000). Similar results have been reported using videotaped peer interaction vignettes (Bell-Dolan, 1995). As in the story vignettes, anxious children showed an increased tendency to misinterpret non-hostile as hostile intent and proposed more maladaptive responses to the scenarios, in particular more appeals to authority. With respect to physical threat, Prins (1986) found that high test-anxious children reported self-statements preoccupied with the threat of being hurt in an anxiety-provoking task.

Recent studies also note a tendency for anxious children to come to faster conclusions about threat (Muris *et al.*, 2000), to underestimate personal ability to cope (Bogels and Zigterman, 2000) and to experience more negative emotions and cognitions in response to the scenarios (Muris *et al.*, 2000). An alternative method of assessing interpretation biases uses the homophone paradigm, in which participants are presented words which have two meanings: one threatening and one non-threatening. Studies of this method suggest that anxious children make a threatening interpretation of ambiguous stimuli more often than non-anxious children (Taghavi *et al.*, 2000); this effect remained significant after taking depression into account, indicating some evidence for specificity.

Moreover, several studies connect meta-cognitive style and depression in children. Those styles thought to be associated with the maintenance and severity of depressive symptoms in adults include rumination, problem-solving and distraction (Nolen-Hoeksema, 1991; Nolen-Hoeksema *et al.*, 1992). Thus, whereas ruminating about depressive mood prolongs and worsens depression, engaging in problem-solving and distraction would be associated with less protracted and severe disturbance. The extent to which these cognitive styles were associated with persistence of depressive symptoms in children was investigated by Abela and colleagues (Abela *et al.*, 2002). They found that for both third graders (mean age 8 years 9 months) and seventh graders (mean age 12 years 10 months), self-reported rumination according to a questionnaire assessment predicted self-reported depressive symptoms over a 6-week period after controlling for the stability of depressive symptoms. No such effect was found either for self-reported problem-solving or for distraction. The findings are noteworthy in showing that at least some meta-cognitive styles observed in depressed adults are observable in middle childhood and, as in the case of adults and early adolescents, predict persistence and worsening of depression.

There are many other features of CBT that are an equally important part of the therapeutic process, including a 'here and now' emphasis, collaboration between the patient and therapist and an empirical focus (Beck *et al.*, 1979). How these components may be viewed within the context of a developmental model and what implications these ideas have for the delivery of CBT to young patients requires further attention.

In summary, what we know now is that many of the cognitive processes thought to underlie clinical disturbance and its treatment in adults are also found in children and adolescents. Indeed, compared with the substantial number of studies showing comparable cognitive deficits in children, adolescents and adults, it is surprising how few compelling demonstrations there are of developmental differences. Nevertheless, there are some notable shortcomings of the existing research base that need to be reconciled. First, much of the research is cross-sectional. Accordingly, we do not know if the cognitive processes identified in child populations are stable and mediate stability in symptomatology. Secondly, most studies are based on comparatively small samples. Thirdly, very few studies were designed with adequate power to test developmental hypotheses because of a limited age range sampled, small numbers of children of various ages or a failure to include a developmental marker of cognitive development (i.e. most studies rely on age as a marker of development and do not examine what features of cognitive development associated with age might account for age-based changes). Fourthly, most of the above studies were not based on a treatment design and so are only able to establish an association between cognitive processes and clinical symptoms. Furthermore, those treatment studies that were carried out have tended not to include the kinds of cognitive assessments reported in the observational studies cited above. Thus, even in the clinical research area, there is something of a division between research into the cognitive processes associated with disturbance and research into treatment effectiveness. In this regard, it is interesting to note that there is some evidence in children that cognitive processes of the type outlined above do not necessarily change in response to treatment. For example, Silverman *et al.* (1999) assessed children's negative cognitive errors before and after three different interventions for childhood phobias. They found a decrease in cognitive errors in all conditions, although only one treatment directly targeted cognitive components of anxiety. Similarly, Barrett *et al.* (1996) found that cognitive change was observed when CBT was incorporated as part of a family treatment model; children who received individual CBT did not show a parallel change. This leaves open the possibility that family treatment and not CBT as such was important for changing children's cognitions.

3.3.2 Treatment context

To the extent that a developmental perspective has been incorporated successfully into the practice of CBT with children, it may have less to do with the actual delivery of treatment and more to do with the context in which it is provided. This is the implication of findings from several clinical research groups that have experimented with the use of a family component to CBT with children (see Chapter 7). Incorporating a family component into treatment follows on from the demonstration that certain family processes accompany child anxiety. Dadds and colleagues (Dadds and Barrett, 1996; Shortt *et al.*, 2001) refer to one such process as the family's enhancement of the child's avoidant responses. Including the family as part of the treatment is suggested on the basis that family processes may be involved in the origins or maintenance of the child's anxiety and on the basis that the family is a central context for the child's development. The latter consideration would suggest that a family component would be a clinically helpful aid even if it were shown that the family did not display dysfunctional family processes associated with childhood anxiety; that is, the family would be considered to be an important component to treating the child simply because it provides such a central context for the children's development.

Several studies have shown that children who receive CBT plus a family component respond more positively than children who are treated with individual CBT. One of the more interesting results was that children (7–10 years) but not early adolescents (11–14 years) were likely to benefit from the inclusion of the family treatment component (Barrett *et al.*, 1996). The implication is that research seeking to identify how development may moderate treatment response may need to focus on the context in which the treatment is provided as much as on the treatment itself.

Focusing on the family context may also shed important insights into the mechanisms by which anxiety may be transmitted from parents to children. Research findings have suggested that several distinct processes operating in families may account for the familial nature of anxiety (Last *et al.*, 1987), including observation and imitation, modelling, vicarious learning or hearing about oneself from others and parenting practices (Parsons *et al.*, 1982; Goodman *et al.*, 1995; Garber and Flynn, 2001; Gerull *et al.*, 2002).

3.4 Suggestions for improving the integration of developmental theory, research and practice

This section takes as a starting point the poor fit between research into children's cognitions and the practice of CBT with children. This is an inevitable conclusion, evident in a more indirect form from publications in this area and in a more direct form from discussions with clinical colleagues and students. This section aims to consider how a better fit between research and practice might be accomplished.

3.4.1 Methods and meaning of research

One of the reasons for the tenuous links between research evidence and clinical practice of CBT with children is the complication of measuring social cognitive processes. For example, an important methodological lesson from research is that children's capacities to demonstrate social cognitive abilities are influenced by how they are assessed. A good illustration is in the area of measuring children's understanding of mixed emotions. Understanding mixed emotions, the notion that an event may provoke both positive *and* negative emotional reactions, is an important developmental landmark in children's understanding of emotion and the causes of emotions, and has wider implications for children's psychological development. The establishment of the point in development when children can be said to understand that events may provoke positive *and* negative emotions might seem to be a straightforward task. However, children's success at labelling mixed emotions in response to a particular event depends on how the task is presented. This is illustrated in a study of 50 6-year-olds by Brown and Dunn (1996). They found that, if the child was told that a character in a story felt both positively and negatively about a particular event, most (42 of the 50) children could give a plausible rationale for the positive and negative feeling; however, if children were not told how the character felt and were instead asked to tell the experimenter how the story protagonist may have felt, only 16 children spontaneously mentioned both a positive and negative feeling. An even smaller number of children (11 of 50) were able to give a spontaneous *personal* example of an event that made them feel both positively and negatively. So, as for the question 'when can a child understand mixed emotions?', we might well suppose the answer is around 6 or so years of age. However, that must be tied to the way in which we operationalize understanding of ambivalent emotions. If the question is instead posed as, 'when is the understanding of ambivalent feelings likely to have import into the clinical context?', it might be that the answer is not age 6 years but instead at the later assessments when children spontaneously report ambivalent feelings about events in their own lives (which may correspond more with how previous research suggested children understand mixed emotions).

A further potential limitation of extending current research into social cognitive processes to the clinic context is that many of the experimental assessments are affectively neutral (e.g. as in the case of Piagetian tasks) or, if there is affect involved, it is within a hypothetical context unrelated to the child (e.g. as in the case of emotional understanding tasks in which the child is asked to predict the emotion of a protagonist in a vignette). The applicability of commonly used methods and the findings from such methods to the clinical setting is likely to be compromised as a result of the 'impersonal' quality of the assessment. The fact that cognitive processes concerning neutral or hypothetical events may not translate to the individual psychology of the adult or child is to be expected. After all, it has been appreciated for some time that the cognitive vulnerabilities to depression (e.g. attributions of negative events to internal, stable qualities of the self) may not be continuously active but may emerge only in response to negative events or in the context of negative mood (e.g. Teasdale, 1988). Recent evidence suggests that children's cognitions, including those characteristic of possible clinical disturbance, may be best accessed in the context of negative mood. For example, in their study of 5-year-olds, Murray and colleagues (Murray *et al.*, 2001) found that negative cognitions (expressions of hopelessness or low self-worth) were spontaneously expressed only when negative mood was induced, in this case by a card game with a friend in which their winning or losing was experimentally manipulated. Negative cognitions were not observed while the child was winning but were observed when the child was losing. Furthermore, an association between exposure to maternal depression and negative cognitions was evident only in the setting in which the child was losing the card game. The findings of Murray *et al.* (2001) are significant in demonstrating that spontaneously expressed negative (depressogenic) cognitions are observed in children as young as 5 years, that these cognitions are more commonly observed among those at risk for depression and that these cognitions are emitted in the context of negative but not positive (non-negative) mood.

A third illustration concerns a distinction between competence and performance in assessments of social cognitive skills, and the role of context. Good illustrations are provided by the fact that children show wide intra-individual variation in their display of social cognitive sophistication, as seen in preschoolers' discussions with parents, peers and siblings (Brown *et al.*, 1996; see also Cole *et al.*, 1997), as do early adolescents in their use of emotional understanding and mentalizing ability when talking about positive versus conflicted relationships (O'Connor and Hirsch, 1999). The implication is that, for research on social cognitive processes to be more clinically useful, greater emphasis needs to be placed on the social, relationship or affective context in which they occur.

The general divide between developmental theory and clinical practice is as unnecessary as it is counterintuitive. This state of affairs is probably explained by a host of factors other than how research is conducted. For instance, there is a general lack of cross-fertilization of developmental and clinical findings in academic and applied journals, a tendency for clinicians not to read research reports and the counterpoint that 'basic' researchers have difficulty elucidating the clinical significance of their findings and disseminating their results outside the academic setting. In any event, efforts to redress this are much needed. This may take several forms, such as those implied above. Additionally, including a component on developmental theory in CBT training courses is a good start, as is including a focused discussion of developmental theory in applied and practitioner orientated texts (as exemplified in the current volume). What benefits these efforts will realize remain to be seen. Will knowledge of developmental theory make more effective cognitive behavioural therapists? Will knowledge of developmental research enable clinicians to identify those individuals who are most likely to respond to a course of CBT? Perhaps. At present, the strongest argument for adopting a developmental perspective is merely the promise of more effective clinical treatment.

3.5 Implications and recommendations for clinical practice

Deriving practical applications of developmental research for clinical practice with children is, as has been repeatedly noted, no straightforward task. Nevertheless, this final section considers some practical lessons from the preceding discussion and highlights how clinic-based research may play an especially important role in advancing theory.

3.5.1 Assessment, treatment and prevention

If there were cognitive preconditions to effective CBT, then it would be possible to develop a screening measure that would identify those children likely to respond to this form of treatment. Similarly, if the contextual factors that impeded CBT were known, then it would be a reasonably straightforward task to distinguish those children most likely to respond to the comparatively brief treatment delivered within a standard CBT framework. Unfortunately, despite many years of CBT practice with children, there is only limited progress on these two fronts. Consequently, recommendations for the clinic setting are necessarily speculative. Nonetheless, some speculations are provided.

We take as a starting point that there is a need to ascertain, as early as possible in the course of clinic contact, an assessment of the likelihood of treatment failure versus treatment success. The twin themes developed in this chapter are a consideration of the child's social cognitive sophistication and the child's context. As for the former, there are no clear indicators of treatment success. It is important to rule out some of the more obvious candidates, however. Thus, assessment of basic language and intellectual skills using traditional cognitive assessments may be important, particularly if there are doubts about the appropriateness of CBT because of, for example, the child's age. However, standardized tests assess only very broad intellectual abilities and may not be sensitive to the kinds of cognitive processes tapped by CBT.

Of the more specific kinds of social cognitive assessments available, those developed by Dodge and colleagues cited above seem applicable. Measures of the older child's emotional understanding, reflective capacity and ability to use mental states of self and other have not been systematically developed, but may be worth exploring. There is, for example, evidence from several sources that interview-based measures seem to work well from around 8 years of age, and it is possible that this would be the optimal context for ascertaining these kinds of social cognitive processes (e.g. Target et al., 1998; Humfress et al., 2002). Inevitably, however, in the absence of established measures or methods, clinicians will be faced with having to oversee their own experimentation on how best to elicit the child's ability to link thoughts, feelings and behaviour.

Recommendation for assessing the child's context is more obvious. Detailed assessment of the child's family and family relationships is routinely conducted, and its importance is supported by research findings. In addition to assessing symptomatology in the parents, which may both alter and complicate treatment, some assessment of the quality of parent–child relationship is indicated. Fortunately, there are specific guidelines on the dimensions of kinds of parent–child relationship quality that may be of particular interest. Findings suggesting how the family enhances the child's avoidance and so maintains and accentuates the child's symptoms are noteworthy (Barrett et al., 1996; Dadds and Barrett, 1996; Hudson and Rapee, 2001); there are, in addition, a number of other dimensions of the parent–child relationship that predominate research and are worth incorporating in a clinic assessment of the parent–child relationship, including warmth/support, conflict and monitoring/control and psychological autonomy (see O'Connor, 2002).

However speculative the specific recommendations for assessment might be, the recommendation from research for treatment are even less clear. At this point, perhaps the main point worth emphasizing is that *experiences in the clinical setting* have an illustrious history for generating hypotheses and spurring systematic clinical as well as basic research. Detailed case reports and case audit consideration of the origins of successes and failures in cases would be a helpful start in that direction.

3.6   Conclusions

In conclusion, we offer several summary statements. First, there is, to date, a poor fit between 'basic' developmental research into social cognitive processes and clinical/applied research on CBT with children. Furthermore, these lines of investigation rely on largely distinct models and paradigms. Secondly, perhaps as a consequence of the previous point, there is very limited empirical evidence for a developmental model underlying CBT with children. According to published reports, to the extent that the child's development has been successfully integrated within a treatment approach, it has been in terms of the context in which CBT is delivered (namely, as part of a family model or not) rather than in terms of how CBT itself may be modified. There are surprisingly few guidelines concerning what modifications need to be made for younger versus older children (though see Chapter 8) or what assessments should be carried out to determine the appropriateness of such modifications. Thirdly, a thesis underlying this chapter is that a developmental approach to assessment and intervention/prevention would help elucidate the mechanisms of change in CBT with children and identify the predictors of good versus poor response. It remains for future clinical research to test the hypothesis that a developmental model of CBT improves treatment success.

3.7   REFERENCES

Abela, J. R. Z., Brozina, K. and Haigh, E. P. (2002). An examination of the response styles theory of depression in third- and seventh-grade children: a short-term longitudinal study. *Journal of Abnormal Child Psychology*, **30**, 515–27.

Ainsworth, M. D. S., Blehar, M. C., Waters, E. and Wall, S. (1978). *Patterns of Attachment: A Psychological Study of the Strange Situation*. Hillsdale, NJ: Erlbaum.

Barrett, P. M., Dadds, M. M. and Rapee, R. M. (1996). Family treatment of childhood anxiety: a controlled trial. *Journal of Consulting and Clinical Psychology*, **64**, 333–42.

Beck, A. T., Rush, A. J., Shaw, B. F. and Emery, G. (1979). *Cognitive Therapy of Depression*. New York, NY: Wiley

Bell-Dolan, D. J. (1995). Social cue interpretation of anxious children. *Journal of Clinical Child Psychology*, **24**, 1–10.

Belsky, J., Spritz, B. and Crnic, K. (1996). Infant attachment security and affective-cognitive information processing at age 3. *Psychological Science*, **7**, 111–14.

Bogels, S. M. and Zigterman, D. (2000). Dysfunctional cognitions in children with social phobia, separation anxiety disorder and generalised anxiety disorder. *Journal of Abnormal Child Psychology*, **28**, 205–11.

Bolton, D. (1996). Developmental issues in obsessive-compulsive disorder. *Journal of Child Psychology and Psychiatry*, **37**, 131–7.

Bosacki, S. and Astington, J. W. (1999). Theory of mind in preadolescence: relations between social understanding and social competence. *Social Development*, **8**, 237–55.

Bowlby, J. (1982). *Attachment and Loss: Volume 1. Attachment*, 2nd edn. New York: Basic Books.
    (1988). Developmental psychiatry comes of age. *American Journal of Psychiatry*, **145**, 1–10.

Bretherton, I. and Mulholland, K. A. (1999). Internal working models in attachment relationships: a construct revisited. In J. Cassidy and P. Shaver (eds.), *Handbook of Attachment*. New York, NY: Guilford, pp. 89–111.

Bretherton, I., Ridgeway, D. and Cassidy, J. (1990). Assessing internal working models of the attachment relationship: an attachment story completion task for 3-year-olds. In M. T. Greenbergh, D. Cicchetti and E. M. Cummings (eds.), *Attachment in the Preschool Years*. Chicago: University of Chicago Press, pp. 273–308.

Brown, J. M., O'Keefe, J., Sanders, S. H. and Baker, B. (1986). Developmental changes in children's cognition to stressful and painful situations. *Journal of Pediatric Psychology*, **11**, 343–57.

Brown, J. R. and Dunn, J. (1996). Continuities in emotion understanding from three to six years. *Child Development*, **67**, 789–802.

Brown, J. R., Donelan-McCall, N. and Dunn, J. (1996). Why talk about mental states? The significance of children's conversations with friends, siblings, and mothers. *Child Development*, **67**, 836–49.

Cicchetti, D. and Cohen, D. J. (1995). Perspectives in developmental psychopathology. In D. Cicchetti and D. J. Cohen (eds.), *Developmental Psychopathology*. New York: Wiley, pp. 2–20.

Cole, D. A., Maxwell, S. E. and Martin, J. M. (1997). Reflected self-appraisals: strength and structure of the relation of teacher, peer and parent ratings to children's self-perceived competencies. *Journal of Educational Psychology*, **89**, 55–70.

Conduct Problems Prevention Research Group. (1992). A developmental and clinical model for the prevention of conduct disorder: the Fast Track program. *Development and Psychopathology*, **4**, 509–27.

Cowen, E. L. and Durlak, J. A. (2000). Social policy and prevention in mental health. *Development and Psychopathology*, **12**, 815–34.

Crick, N. and Dodge, K. A. (1994). A review and reformulation of social information processing mechanisms in children's social adjustment. *Psychological Bulletin*, **115**, 74–101.

Dadds, M. M. and Barrett, P. M. (1996). Family processes in child and adolescent anxiety and depression. *Behaviour Change*, **13**, 231–9.

Dobson, K. S. (1988). *Handbook of Cognitive-Behavior Therapies*. New York, NY: Guilford Press.

Dodge, K. A. (1993). Social-cognitive mechanisms in the development of conduct disorder and depression. *Annual Review of Psychology*, **44**, 559–84.

Dodge, K. A. and Frame, C. L. (1982). Social cognitive biases and deficits in aggressive boys. *Child Development*, **53**, 620–35.

Durlak, J. A., Fuhrman, T. and Lampman, C. (1991). Effectiveness of cognitive-behavioral therapy for maladapting children: a meta-analysis. *Psychological Bulletin*, **110**, 204–14.

Evans, D. W., Leckman, J. F., Carter, A. *et al.* (1997). Ritual, habit and perfectionism: the prevalence and development of compulsive-like behavior in normal young children. *Child Development*, **68**, 58–68.

Flavell, J. H. (1999). Cognitive development: children's knowledge about the mind. *Annual Review of Psychology*, **50**, 21–45.

Francis, G. (1988). Assessing cognitions in anxious children. *Behavior Modification*, **12**, 267–80.

Garber, J. (2000). Development and depression. In A. J. Sameroff, M. Lewis and S. M. Miller (eds.), *Handbook of Developmental Psychopathology*, 2nd edn. New York: Kluwer Academic/Plenum Press, pp. 467–90.

Garber, J. and Flynn, C. (2001). Predictors of depressive cognitions in young adolescents. *Cognitive Therapy and Research*, **25**, 353–76.

Gerull, F. C., Friederike, G. and Rapee, R. M. (2002). Mother knows best: the effects of maternal modelling on the acquisition of fear and avoidance behaviour in toddlers. *Behaviour, Research and Therapy*, **40**, 279–87.

Goodman, S. H., Adamson, L. B., Riniti, J. and Cole, S. (1995). Mothers' expressed attitudes: associations with maternal depression and children's self-esteem and psychopathology. *Journal of the American Academy of Child and Adolescent Psychiatry*, **33**, 1265–74.

Gouze, K .R. and Nadelman, L. (1980). Constancy of gender identity for self and others in children between the ages of three and seven. *Child Development*, **51**, 275–8.

Green, J., Goldwyn, R. and Stanley, C. (2000). A new method of evaluating attachment representations in young school-age children: the Manchester Child Attachment Story Task. *Attachment and Human Development*, **2**, 48–70.

Guardo, C. J. and Bonan, J. B. (1971). Development of a sense of self-identity in children. *Child Development*, **42**, 1909–21.

Happé, F. (1994). An advanced test of theory of mind: understanding of story characters' thoughts and feelings by able autistic, mentally handicapped, and normal children and adults. *Journal of Autism and Developmental Disorders*, **24**, 129–55.

Happé, F. and Frith, U. (1996). Theory of mind and social impairment in children with conduct disorder. *British Journal of Developmental Psychology*, **14**, 385–98.

Harrington, R., Whittaker, J., Shoebridge, P. and Campbell, F. (1998). Systematic review of efficacy of cognitive behaviour therapies in childhood and adolescent depressive disorder. *British Medical Journal*, **316**, 1559–63.

Hudson, J. and Rapee, R. M. (2001). Parent-child interactions and anxiety disorders: an observational study. *Behaviour, Research and Therapy*, **39**, 1411–27.

Hudson, J. L., Kendall, P. C., Coles, M. E., Robin, J. A. and Webb, A. (2002). The other side of the coin: using intervention research in child anxiety disorders to inform developmental psychopathology. *Development and Psychopathology*, **14**, 819–41.

Humfress, H., O'Connor, T. G., Slaughter, J., Target, M. and Fonagy, P. (2002). Generalised and relationship-specific models of social cognition: explaining the overlap and discrepancies. *Journal of Child Psychology and Psychiatry*, **43**, 873–83.

Kendall, P. C. (1985). Towards a cognitive-behavioral model of child psychopathology and a critique of related interventions. *Journal of Abnormal Child Psychology*, **13**, 357–72.

Laible, D. J. and Thompson, R. A. (1998). Attachment and emotional understanding in preschool children. *Developmental Psychology*, **34**, 1038–45.

Last, C. G., Hersen, M., Kazdin, A. E., Francis, G. and Grubb, H. J. (1987). Psychiatric illness in the mothers of anxious children. *American Journal of Psychiatry*, **144**, 1580–3.

Muris, P., Luermans, J., Merckelbach, H. and Mayer, B. (2000). 'Danger is lurking everywhere.' The relation between anxiety and threat perception abnormalities in normal children. *Journal of Behavior Therapy and Experimental Psychiatry*, **31**, 123–36.

Murray, L., Woolgar, M., Cooper, P. and Hipwell, A. (2001). Cognitive vulnerability to depression in 5-year-old children of depressed mothers. *Journal of Child Psychology and Psychiatry*, **42**, 891–9.

Nicholls, J. G. (1978). The development of the concepts of effort and ability, perception of academic attainment and the understanding that difficult tasks require more ability. *Child Development*, **49**, 800–4.

Nolan-Hoeksema, S. (1991). Responses to depression and their effects on the duration of depressive episodes. *Journal of Abnormal Psychology*, **100**, 569–82.

Nolen-Hoeksema, S., Girgus, J. S. and Seligman, M. E. P. (1992). Predictors and consequences of childhood depressive symptoms: a 5-year longitudinal study. *Journal of Abnormal Psychology*, **101**, 405–22.

O'Connor, T. G. (2002). Annotation: the "effects" of parenting reconsidered. Findings, challenges, and applications. *Journal of Child Psychology and Psychiatry*, **43**, 555–72.

O'Connor, T. G. and Hirsch, N. (1999). Intra-individual differences and relationship-specificity of social understanding and mentalising in early adolescence. *Social Development*, **8**, 256–74.

Parsons, J. E., Adler, T. F. and Kaczula, C. M. (1982). Socialization of achievement attitudes and beliefs: parental influences. *Child Development*, **53**, 310–21.

Prins, P. J. M. (1986). Children's self-speech and self-regulation during a fear-provoking behavioral test. *Behaviour, Research and Therapy*, **24**, 181–91.

  (2000). Affective and cognitive processes and the development and maintenence of anxiety and its disorders. In W. K. Silverman and P. D. A. Treffers (eds.), *Anxiety Disorders in Children and Adolescents: Research, Assessment and Intervention*. Cambridge, UK: Cambridge University Press, pp. 23–44.

Rapee, R. M. (2001). The development of generalized anxiety. In M. W. Vasey and M. M. Dadds (eds.), *The Developmental Psychopathology of Anxiety*. New York, NY: Oxford University Press, pp. 1045–95.

Rholes, W. S., Blackwell, J., Jordan, C. and Walters, C. (1980). A developmental study of learned helplessness. *Developmental Psychology*, **16**, 616–24.

Rotenberg, J. H. (1982). Development of character constancy of self and other. *Child Development*, **53**, 505–15.

Shortt, A. L., Barrett, P. M., Dadds, M. R. and Fox, T. L. (2001). The influence of family context and experimental context on cognition in anxious children. *Journal of Abnormal Child Psychology*, **29**, 585–96.

Silverman, W. K., Kurtines, W. M., Ginsburg, G. S., Weems, C. F., Rabian, B. and Serafini, L. T. (1999). Contingency management, self-control, and education-support in the treatment of childhood phobic disorders: a randomised clinical trial. *Journal of Consulting and Clinical Psychology*, **67**, 675–87.

Southam-Gerow, M., Kendall, P. C. and Weersing, V. R. (2001). Examining outcome variability: correlates of treatment response in a child and adolescent anxiety clinic. *Journal of Clinical Child Psychology*, **30**, 422–36.

Strauss, C. C., Lease, C. A., Last, C. G. and Francis, G. (1988). Overanxious disorder: an examination of developmental differences. *Journal of Abnormal Child Psychology*, **16**, 433–43.

Taghavi, M. R., Moradi, A. R., Neshat-Doost, H. T., Yule, W. and Dalgleish, T. (2000). Interpretation of ambiguous emotional information in clinically anxious children and adolescents. *Cognition and Emotion*, **14**, 809–22.

Taghavi, M. R., Neshat-Doost, H. T., Moradi, A. R., Yule, W. and Dalgleish, T. (1999). Biases in visual attention in children and adolescents with clinical anxiety and mixed anxiety-depression. *Journal of Abnormal Child Psychology*, **27**, 215–23.

Target, M., Fonagy, P., Shmueli-Goetz, Y., Datta, A. and Schneider, T. (1998). *The Child Attachment Interview (CAI) Protocol*, revised edn., VI, 1/5/99. University College London.

Teasdale, J. D. (1988). Cognitive vulnerability to persistent depression. *Cognition and Emotion*, **2**, 247–74.

Vasey, M. W., Elhag, N. and Daleiden, E. L. (1996). Anxiety and the processing of emotionally threatening stimuli: distinctive patterns of selective attention among high and low anxious children. *Child Development*, **67**, 1173–85.

Weisz, J. R. (1981). Illusory contingency at the state fair. *Developmental Psychology*, **17**, 481–9.

4

Psychological therapies: a family of interventions

V. Robin Weersing and David A. Brent

Yale Child Study Center, New Haven, Connecticut, USA

4.1 Psychological therapies: shared paths to success?

At last count, there were over 300 brand-name psychotherapies for youths (Kazdin, 2000). Although most of these interventions have never been tested in clinical trials, results of hundreds of studies indicate that youth therapy can be of significant benefit. In broad-based meta-analyses, effect sizes for child and adolescent psychotherapy are in the moderate to large range (Casey and Berman, 1985; Weisz *et al.*, 1987; Kazdin *et al.*, 1990; Weisz *et al.*, 1995), on par with the effects of adult therapy and many medical interventions (Weisz and Weersing, 1999). In addition to this global good news, in recent years the field has made strides in identifying empirically supported treatments (ESTs) with evidence of efficacy for specific youth problems and diagnostic profiles.

In 1998, the year of the last formal EST review, over two dozen promising treatments were identified for youth anxiety, depression and behavioural problems (see Lonigan and Elbert, 1998). The existence of this growing family of efficacious interventions raises a provocative question: how many therapies for youth are 'enough'? Or, phrased differently, how useful is new treatment development for the science and practice of psychotherapy?

For some diagnoses, such as bipolar disorder in childhood and adolescence, treatment development is still clearly the first order of business. However, for many youth problems, there is a growing consensus that expanding the family of psychotherapeutic interventions may be less useful than gaining deeper understanding of the treatments that we already have (e.g. Kazdin, 1995; Russell and Shirk, 1998; Weisz *et al.*, 1998; Kazdin, 2001). For instance, surprisingly little is known about *how* efficacious psychotherapies produce positive outcomes for youths and families. In 1990, Kazdin and colleagues reviewed the youth treatment

Cognitive Behaviour Therapy for Children and Families, ed. Philip J. Graham.
Published by Cambridge University Press. © Cambridge University Press 2004.

outcome literature and found than a mere 3% of studies included measures of therapeutic processes (Kazdin *et al.*, 1990). In a recent review of the youth EST literature, Weersing and Weisz (2002) upped the estimate to 10%, although they used a somewhat different definition of treatment mechanism. Understanding how therapy works would seem to be of great value, for researchers involved in testing models of psychopathology and intervention (e.g. Judd and Kenny, 1981; Weersing and Weisz, 2002) and for practitioners trying to implement treatments effectively in the strongest, 'purest' form possible (e.g. Scott and Sechrest, 1989). Investigations of therapy mechanism may also serve to shrink the list of 300+ treatments for children and adolescents in a useful way. It seems likely that there are fewer processes of therapeutic action than there are specific, identified treatment protocols, and we may be able to organize, synthesize and streamline our portfolio of interventions better by focusing on how the members of our therapeutic family are related at a mechanistic level.

In the remainder of this chapter, we will provide an overview of the existing literature linking therapeutic processes to the outcomes of child and adolescent treatment. We will exclude 'treatment mediation studies' – that is, investigations of therapeutic mechanisms of action specific to a single theoretical orientation or therapy programme (such as studies that investigate the role of cognitive change in producing the effects of CBT for youth depression). Readers are referred to Weersing and Weisz (2002) for a recent review of the child and adolescent treatment mediation literature. Therapy process research is based, in large part, on a generic model of therapeutic action, in which common elements of the treatment, such as the experience of a warm therapeutic relationship, are thought to account for a large proportion of outcome. Different therapy types (behavioural, psychodynamic) for different problems (anxiety, delinquency) are hypothesized to work through these same core mechanisms. Accordingly, in our review of youth process research, we include treatments from a wide range of theoretical orientations, treating a diverse set of youth and family problems.

4.2   Investigations of youth therapy process

The empirical investigation of youth therapy process has a 50-year history (Landisberg and Snyder, 1946), a legacy as long as therapy efficacy research with child and adolescent patients (Levitt, 1957). However, these two research enterprises appear to have developed on parallel tracks, rather than in concert. As mentioned previously, less than 3% of outcome studies include measures of general therapy processes, such as the therapeutic relationship (Kazdin *et al.*, 1990). Similarly, very few studies focusing on therapy process link these general therapy mechanisms to the out-of-session outcomes typically targeted in clinical trial research (Shirk and Russell, 1996).

Adult process–outcome research is much more extensive than the youth literature, with over 2300 adult process–outcome findings at last major count (Orlinsky et al., 1994). Results from this extensive body of adult research have been synthesized into several conceptual models, perhaps the most prominent of which is the generic model of psychotherapy (Orlinsky and Howard, 1987). As originally proposed, the generic model included five dimensions of therapy process hypothesized to affect outcome: (1) provisions of the therapeutic contract (e.g. therapy format, duration, frequency); (2) technical therapeutic operations; (3) development of a therapeutic relationship; (4) client self-relatedness (client motivation and openness to change); and (5) in-session impacts (therapeutic realizations). Orlinsky and Howard also identified various therapist, client and societal *inputs* (e.g. ethnicity) into the processes of psychotherapy and treatment *outputs* or outcomes. With some revision over time (Orlinsky et al., 1994), the generic model has served as a useful heuristic for organizing this body of work, incorporating new results into a meaningful context and generating new hypotheses for research.

Child therapy process research lacks such an organizing framework. One solution would be the exportation of the well-established generic model of psychotherapy from the adult literature to serve as a conceptual base for child therapy process research. In the authors' view, this has the potential to produce more confusion than clarity, as the generic model does not capture key pragmatic aspects of therapeutic work with children and adolescents. For example, unlike the adults of the generic model, children and adolescents seldom enter into their own therapeutic contracts, collaborate to fit the parameters of treatment to their self-perceived needs or arrive at treatment with self-identification of a problem and openness to change. Instead, children and adolescents are brought to treatment by their parents – if not against their will, often without the belief that anything is wrong with them and with little expectation that psychotherapy may be useful in their lives (Yeh and Weisz, 2001). Given this level of environmental control over youth's lives, the focus of 'child' treatments may be directed only tangentially at the youths themselves, as evidenced by the inclusion of both parent training (Patterson and Chamberlain, 1994) and family therapy (Alexander et al., 1976) in this review of child process research.

Given these concerns about the applicability of adult models of therapy process for children, we will organize our review of the youth process literature into thematic domains rather than around the Orlinksy and Howard model. We will also limit our review of purely descriptive youth therapy process studies and instead focus on investigations that attempt to tie therapy processes to changes in youths' distress, symptoms and functioning.

4.2.1   Early therapy process research

From the first study of child therapy process in the 1940s through the mid-1960s, child process research focused almost exclusively on characterizing the process of non-directive play therapy. Much of this early work appears to be microanalytic coding of all behaviour occurring during the play therapy hour, rather than selective measurement of therapist–child interactions thought to be theoretically significant components of change. In this early literature and later follow-up studies, some attempts were made to measure how these play therapy behaviours might vary over the course of treatment (Landisberg and Snyder, 1946), by developmental level of the child client (Lebo, 1952), between disturbed versus 'normal' children in simulated therapy (Moustakas and Schalock, 1955) and by type of play therapy – non-directive versus psychodynamic focused (Dana and Dana, 1969; Boll, 1971). In these first few decades of child therapy process research, no attempt was made to link descriptive measures of therapy process to post-treatment symptom change.

4.2.2   Therapist directiveness and client resistance

Since the mid-1960s, interest in comprehensively classifying all behaviours occurring during child therapy waned, replaced by an emphasis on investigating therapy processes thought to facilitate or impede positive outcome directly. A number of studies have investigated therapist levels of confrontation, guidance, teaching and structuring all under the general rubric of the 'directiveness' of therapist interpersonal style. It is interesting to note that all investigations of therapist directiveness uncovered in the authors' review have been conducted in the context of therapy with aggressive, impulsive or disruptive children and their families, and thus little is known about the relative merits of therapist directiveness with internalizing youngsters. An investigation of therapist *flexibility* in manualized CBT for child anxiety (Kendall and Chu, 2000) found no significant relationships between flexibility and outcome. However, germaneness of this study to discussion of directiveness is questionable, as flexibility seemed to be measured by personalization of the protocol to children's interests and talents (e.g. changing the media of a feelings dictionary) rather than by a permissive or client-led therapist interpersonal stance.

Within non-behavioural therapies for disruptive behaviour problems, there appears to be a positive effect of therapists taking a directive stance with their child clients. In the only published process–outcome study for this therapy type,

Truax and Wittmer (1973) found that higher levels of therapist confrontation of 'defence mechanisms' were significantly associated with better outcomes in psychodynamic group therapy with juvenile delinquents, including less time spent in jail over the study's 1-year follow-up period.

Across treatment type, directive therapist behaviours designed to keep children and families on-task and focused on the techniques of therapy appear to be beneficial. Having previously established the efficacy of their family systems treatment programme in reducing delinquent behaviour, Alexander *et al.* (1976) began a programme of research to uncover what therapist interpersonal variables might maximize positive outcomes within their treatment. Therapist structuring, a compound variable composed of therapist directiveness in treatment and personal self-confidence (both as rated by supervisors prior to therapists beginning therapy), accounted for 15% (after partialling out the effect of therapist interpersonal warmth) of variance in a composite outcome index – based on level of juvenile recidivism, continuation in treatment and quality of family communication. Similarly, Braswell *et al.* (1985) found that cognitive behavioural treatment (CBT) therapists' correction of impulsive children's performance on in-session exercises and therapists' directive attempts to involve children in the tasks of therapy through eliciting child feedback were significantly related to reductions in disruptive classroom behaviour at the end of treatment (as rated by teachers). Amount of time during the cognitive behavioural and behavioural protocol that therapists allowed to be spent on off-task behaviours, including child self-disclosure, bore a significant negative relationship to outcome.

While drawn from a very small number of studies, the evidence thus far appears to support the benefit of certain types of directive behaviours in child treatment. However, a programme of research on the process of parent training with families of seriously antisocial youth yields a nearly opposite set of results. Over the past 20 years, Patterson and colleagues have examined patterns of non-compliance with their behavioural parent-training intervention and delineated both the causes (family characteristics and directive therapist behaviours) and consequences (poor outcome and drop-out) of parent resistance to therapy. Patterson's structured, psychoeducational intervention teaches parents to alter their long-standing behaviour management strategies and methods of family communication. In an early article on resistance to this form of treatment, aptly subtitled 'a paradox for the behaviour modifier', Patterson and Forgatch (1985) demonstrated that directive therapist behaviours of teaching behaviour management techniques and confronting parents about problems in their discipline style led to an immediate increased likelihood of a parental resistant response (ranging in tone from direct authority challenges to voiced doubts about ability to comply with therapist instructions). This contingent relationship was demonstrated both in analyses of naturally occurring therapist–client interactions and through the use of a surreptitious ABAB design manipulating the directiveness of therapist behaviours in parent-training sessions. Additional studies have worked to establish: (1) the links between resistance to treatment on the one hand, and drop-out and poor outcome, on the other hand (Chamberlain et al., 1984); (2) the relationship between resistance and the 'working phase' of treatment, in which parents are challenged to begin implementing new discipline systems at home (Chamberlain et al., 1984; Stoolmiller et al., 1993); and (3) the reciprocal effect of parent resistance on future therapist behaviours, such as withdrawing effort from teaching social learning principles and disliking parents (Patterson and Chamberlain, 1994).

The apparent discrepancy between the consistent Patterson findings on the negative impact of therapist directiveness and the generally positive effects of therapist directiveness in other investigations lends itself to a variety of explanations. The Patterson studies may differ in three meaningful respects from the other investigations of therapist directiveness: (1) severity of child and family dysfunction, (2) intensity of therapist directive behaviours, and (3) level of structure of the therapy being provided. First, it is possible that participants in the Patterson investigations were particularly difficult to work with and 'prone' to treatment resistance. The only other parent- or family-focused investigation in this area is the work of Alexander and colleagues, and those authors indicated the delinquent adolescents in their sample engaged primarily in 'soft delinquency', whereas a number of participants in the Patterson studies (Patterson and Forgatch, 1985; Patterson and Chamberlain, 1994) were referred into therapy through the justice system. In addition to adolescent dysfunction, Patterson and colleagues also reported high rates of parental disturbance in their samples including widespread maternal depression and parental antisocial behaviour (including instances of physical abuse of the adolescents), both of which were significantly related to forms of resistant behaviour in-session and failure to complete parent homework assignments (Stoolmiller et al., 1993).

Secondly, aside from the possible non-comparability of the Patterson samples to the other investigations, the teaching and confronting behaviours in the Patterson studies may have been more intensely directive than the therapist structuring behaviours examined by other research teams (i.e. correction of errors, staying on-task, pointing out defence mechanisms, therapist self-confidence in opinions and suggestions). This explanation, that the Patterson therapists were either actually more directive or perceived as more directive by clients, is closely related to the third possible cause of the divergent sets of results.

The third cause relates to the fact that the effects of therapist directiveness may vary with the type of therapy being provided. The Patterson behavioural parent-training protocol is directive by its nature; therapists are cast as experts in child behaviour management, and a primary goal of the therapy is to educate parents and train them in the social learning model of child behaviour problems developed by the research team. Very directive therapists within highly structured therapies may exceed the 'optimal dose' of directiveness necessary to produce positive outcome. Findings from non-linear modelling analyses of the Patterson resistance data lend some support to this supposition; the shape rather than the absolute level of parent resistance to treatment has emerged as the important predictor of positive outcome – with a rise in resistance in the middle phase of treatment and a falling-off of resistance by the end predicting positive therapy outcome (Stoolmiller *et al.*, 1993). Given these data, it appears that, even within the structured Patterson parent-training protocol, therapists' directiveness may not be all bad and that some struggling on the parental side, matched by an optimal amount of pushing and perseverance on the therapist side, is both to be expected and desirable (Patterson and Chamberlain, 1994).

4.2.3 Therapist warmth and facilitative conditions

Another aspect of therapist interpersonal behaviour that has received attention in the child therapy process literature is therapist warmth, defined by supportive and empathic behaviours and by the projection of a warm, caring and respectful attitude. Although the constructs are clearly related, therapist interpersonal warmth is not synonymous with the therapeutic relationship between the therapist and child client (discussed later), in which the emphasis is on feelings of *mutual* warmth as well as active collaboration, engagement and agreement by both parties on the tasks and goals of treatment.

Many of the investigations of therapist warmth have been conducted by the same research teams that have examined the effects of therapist directiveness. Alexander and colleagues examined therapist warmth within their family systems treatment for delinquency and found that their index of therapist positive relationship skills (based on supervisors' ratings of therapist warmth, appropriate use of humour and ability to reflect and tie together family's affect and behaviour) accounted for more variance in child outcome than did therapist directiveness: 45% versus 15% (Alexander *et al.*, 1976). In the same study that first investigated the relationship between therapist directive behaviours and parental resistance, Patterson and Forgatch (1985) assessed the relationship between therapists' supportive and facilitative statements and parental compliance with the parent-training protocol and found that warm and facilitative therapist behaviours significantly decreased the likelihood of immediate parent resistance. Patterson and Forgatch did not probe this relationship by manipulating therapist warmth, and the links between these therapist behaviours and treatment outcome, presumably mediated through the level of client resistance to treatment, were not established.

Historically, the effects of therapist warmth have been most central to investigations of the process and outcome of non-behavioural child therapy. The client-centred tradition of therapy views the constant provision of high levels of therapist warmth combined with accurate empathic reflection of the client's experience (accurate empathy) and attentive tracking and reaction (genuineness or 'being there') as the necessary and sufficient mechanisms of change in treatment (Rogers, 1957). These three therapist behaviours are often termed the 'facilitative conditions' of treatment and their effects studied as a package. In this chapter, these investigations are summarized under the more general heading of therapist warmth, as we found several studies that investigated therapist warmth outside of the context of the other facilitative conditions, but we did not uncover child therapy studies examining genuineness or empathy that did not also examine warmth. Many of the early descriptive play therapy coding systems, briefly reviewed previously, included categories for therapist behaviours roughly analogous to warm affect, reflection or restatement and attentive observation among their comprehensive categorization of all therapist and child behaviours (e.g. Moustakas and Schalock, 1955).

The majority of research tying the effects of therapist facilitative conditions to non-behavioural child therapy outcome was conducted by Truax and colleagues during the late 1960s and early 1970s on group therapy with institutionalized juvenile delinquents. Overall, these investigations support the positive effects of high levels of the facilitative conditions on adolescents' self-concepts (e.g. Truax, 1971) and provide preliminary support for positive effects on functioning measures, such as time spent out of jail (e.g. Truax et al., 1970). The strongest and least ambiguous results from this line of work were obtained by Truax et al. (1966) in group therapy with female delinquents. Therapists were rated on their ability to provide facilitative conditions based on prior observations of their work with a similar sample of clients, and therapy groups were classified as being high or low in facilitative conditions before the beginning of treatment. On average, members of high groups improved across a broad spectrum of outcome measures – self-concept, acceptance of social rules, attitudes towards family and time spent out of institutions.

The relationship between therapist facilitative conditions and positive outcome observed with adolescents may also hold true with children. In a descriptive study of client-centred play therapy, Siegel (1972) observed that children provided with high versus low levels of facilitative conditions responded in-session over the course of treatment with more positive and insightful statements about themselves. In a process–outcome investigation of the effects of facilitative conditions, Truax *et al.* (1973) divided their therapists into high and low facilitative conditions categories (based on warmth and empathy; genuineness proved an unreliable measure). Neurotic children receiving therapy from high facilitation therapists were reported to be functioning significantly better at the termination of treatment, according to parent report, while low facilitation children significantly deteriorated, again according to the children's parents.

4.2.4 The therapeutic relationship

Our review of child therapy process research thus far has focused on therapist interpersonal styles that have been linked to treatment outcome. The study of the therapeutic relationship as a mechanism of change is an examination of the interaction between therapist and client styles and of behaviours, attitudes and feelings that are only partially within the power of therapists to manipulate. As such, the quality of the therapeutic relationship may be influenced by characteristics of children and adolescents, such as past history of trauma (Eltz *et al.*, 1995), and the development of positive therapeutic relationship may be conceived partly as a process of therapy, fostered by therapist behaviours and techniques, and partly as a function of pre-existing child and therapist characteristics outside the therapy process.

As defined by Bordin (1979), the therapeutic relationship generally is conceived as consisting of two main components: (1) the therapeutic bond, or mutual feelings of positive affectivity between the client and therapist; and (2) active collaboration, which is a shared vision of the goals of treatment and collaboration on the tasks of therapy necessary to accomplish those goals. Development of a strong therapeutic relationship has emerged as the single best process predictor in the adult psychotherapy literature (see Horvath and Symonds, 1991), correlating reliably at 0.20–0.30 with therapy outcome (e.g. Martin *et al.*, 2000). Shirk and Saiz (1992) have argued that the therapeutic relationship may be an even more significant contributor to outcome for children and adolescents due to the 'involuntary client' status of many children and adolescents at the beginning of therapy and the social deficits that are hypothesized to be central in the development and maintenance of many serious problems.

Certainly, children and parents often report the experience of a positive therapeutic relationship as a critical dimension of treatment, even in behaviourally focused interventions with very salient therapeutic techniques and homework exercises. For example, in a study by Motta and Lynch (1990), two-thirds of parents whose children received behaviour therapy for acting-out, inattention and school problems identified the therapeutic relationship as the most important component of their children's treatment protocol; not one of the parents rated the behavioural techniques employed as being of primary importance to outcome. Similarly, in a follow-up study of recall of participation in a CBT clinical trial for anxiety, 44% of children and adolescents identified the relationship they had developed with their therapists as the most important aspect of treatment (the most popular response; Kendall and Southam-Gerow, 1996). In contrast, dealing with their anxiety was rated most important by 39%. Therapy relationship problems have also emerged as a significant predictor of treatment drop-out from clinical trials of parent training for antisocial children (Kazdin and Wassell, 1998) and from eclectic therapy delivered in community child guidance clinics (Garcia and Weisz, 2002).

Yet, while the importance of a positive therapeutic relationship to clients seems clear, the actual effects of the relationship on symptoms and functioning are less well established. In the authors' review, ten published process–outcome investigations of the therapeutic relationship were found (see Table 4.1). In three of these studies, correlations of therapeutic relationship quality with outcome, while in a positive direction, were generally non-significant (Motta and Lynch, 1990; Motta and Tobin, 1992; Kendall, 1994). The remaining seven studies provide some evidence for a relationship-outcome link, but results are inconsistent across time, raters, definitions of the therapy relationship and outcome domains.

For example, Florsheim *et al.* (2000) predicted that positive relationships between delinquent teens and their therapists would predict symptomatic improvement and less recidivism across multiple types of placement programmes (e.g. group homes, therapeutic foster care settings). Contrary to expectations, positive ratings of the therapeutic relationship 3 weeks into treatment actually predicted worse outcomes (more internalizing and externalizing symptoms, more police contacts), while positive relationships 3 months into treatment predicted reductions in symptomatology and lower rates of recidivism. To unpack these results, a series of exploratory analyses testing the effects of alliance trajectory (getting worse, getting better) were conducted and concluded that change in therapeutic relationship was correlated with change in symptoms in a logical fashion: as alliances improved, so did symptoms and, as therapy relationships deteriorated, so did outcomes. However, Florsheim *et al.* collected therapy relationship and outcome measures on an assessment schedule that made it very difficult to determine if change in relationship predicted change in outcome, or if therapists and young people liked each other better as symptoms improved.

Table 4.1 Therapeutic relationship quality and treatment outcome

Study	Treatment type	Target problem	Significant effects?	Description
Motta and Lynch (1990)	Behaviour therapy	Disruptive behaviour	No	Parents rate relationship as important, but alliance does not correlate with cross-informant outcome ratings
Motta and Tobin (1992)	Behaviour therapy	Disruptive behaviour	No	Parents rate relationship as important, but alliance does not correlate with cross-informant outcome ratings
Kendall (1994)	CBT	Anxiety disorders	No	Relationship did not predict outcome, but therapists scored near ceiling of rating scale. At long-term follow-up, children and adolescents rate relationship as very memorable
Eltz et al. (1995)	Psychodynamic	Heterogeneous (inpatient sample)	Yes	Relationship predicted therapist- and patient-rated global outcome assessments. Maltreated patients formed worse alliances
Kazdin and Wassell (1999)	Parent training Parent training + child CBT	Disruptive behaviour	Yes	Parents' relationship with therapist and perceived relevance of treatment correlated with outcome. Composite variable including positive relationship 'protected' high-risk families from poor outcome
Kazdin and Wassell (2000)	Parent training Parent training + child CBT	Disruptive behaviour	Yes/No	Parents' relationship with therapist not directly correlated with outcome. Perceived relevance of treatment related to therapeutic change
Florsheim et al. (2000)	Multiple, usual care treatment models	Delinquency	Yes/No	Positive relationship early in therapy predicts poor outcome, but positive relationship rating 3 months into therapy predicts lower rates of recidivism
Noser and Bickman (2000)	Multiple, usual care treatment models	Heterogeneous (Fort Bragg sample)	Yes/No	Quality of relationship rated by children linked to positive changes reported by parents, providers and interviewers. Not predictive of outcomes rated by children themselves
Green et al. (2001)	Individualized inpatient care	Heterogeneous (inpatient sample)	Yes/No	Positive alliance with the child predicts good outcome, but positive relationship with parent predicts an increase in internalizing symptoms
Johnson et al. (2002)	Family therapy	Families at risk of losing custody of teenage children	Yes	Adolescent and parent ratings of relationship correlate with outcome. However, some problems with sample size, analyses and non-independence of ratings

Green *et al.* (2001) also found that positive ratings of the therapeutic relationships boded both well and ill in their sample of psychiatrically hospitalized youth. Warm relationships between children and therapists predicted positive post-hospitalization outcomes across informants (including school ratings of child behaviour), but positive relationships between parents and therapists were related to an increase in child internalizing symptoms. The results of Kazdin and Wassell (1999, 2000) demonstrate a different form of complexity. In their barriers to treatment model, they assess the effect of multiple practical and interpersonal barriers on therapy participation, attrition and outcome. Two of the components of the barriers to treatment construct correspond to the two-part therapy relationship definition advanced by Bordin (1979) – namely, the experience of a warm, supportive therapeutic alliance and agreement that treatment is relevant to the problem at hand (analogous to agreement on the tasks and goals of therapy). In two investigations, parents' belief that treatment was relevant was related significantly to reduction in youth antisocial behaviour, but in only one of these studies did the experience of a warm relationship predict good outcome.

4.3 Summary

The therapy process literature relevant to children and adolescents is sparse and scattered; however, a few consistent themes do emerge from this body of work. First, therapist interpersonal style is important to families. The quality of the therapeutic relationship, in particular, is very salient to both parents and children. Warm relationships are appreciated and remembered, sometimes many years later (Kendall and Southam-Gerow, 1996). The therapeutic relationship is viewed as being central to the experience of therapy across the broad family of therapeutic interventions and across many types of child problems (see Table 4.1). In addition, a poor therapy relationship may be a sufficient reason for families to cease participation in treatment – an even more potent reason than a perceived lack of symptomatic improvement (e.g. Garcia and Weisz, 2002).

Secondly, while general process factors are important to patients, it is less clear if these processes impact symptoms and functioning, and the evidence suggests that therapy process variables likely do not influence outcome in a simple, linear fashion. The studies of therapist directiveness provide a good illustration. Too little therapist directiveness may slow forward progress (e.g. Braswell *et al.*, 1985), but too much direction may promote negative reactions and treatment non-compliance (e.g. Patterson and Forgatch, 1985). Investigations of the therapeutic relationship show similarly complex (or perhaps inconsistent) patterns of results.

Thirdly, the design of most therapy process studies has not served to clarify these complex process–outcome relationships. With a few notable exceptions, such as the work of Patterson and colleagues, process and outcome are measured simultaneously, by the same rater and frequently at treatment termination. Given the correlation nature of most of these studies, this assessment strategy makes it impossible to determine the temporal order of changes in processes and symptoms, which is a key step in determining the causality of any observed process–outcome relationships.

4.4   REFERENCES

Alexander, J. F., Barton, C., Schiavo, R. S. and Parsons, B. V. (1976). Systems-behavioral intervention with families of delinquents: therapist characteristics, family behavior, and outcome. *Journal of Consulting and Clinical Psychology*, **44**, 656–64.

Boll, T. J. (1971). Systematic observation of behavior change with older children in group therapy. *Psychological Reports*, **28**, 26.

Bordin, E. S. (1979). The generalizability of the psychoanalytic concept of the working alliance. *Psychotherapy: Theory, Research, and Practice*, **16**, 252–60.

Braswell, L., Kendall, P. C., Braith, J., Carey, M. P. and Vye, C. S. (1985). 'Involvement' in cognitive-behavioral therapy with children: process and its relationship to outcome. *Cognitive Therapy and Research*, **9**, 611–30.

Casey, R. J. and Berman, J. S. (1985). The outcome of psychotherapy with children. *Psychological Bulletin*, **98**, 388–400.

Chamberlain, P., Patterson, G., Reid, J., Kavanagh, K. and Forgatch, M. (1984). Observation of client resistance. *Behavior Therapy*, **15**, 144–55.

Dana, R. H. and Dana, J. M. (1969). Systematic observation of children's behavior in group therapy. *Psychological Reports*, **24**, 134.

Eltz, M. J., Shirk, S. R. and Sarlin, N. (1995). Alliance formation and treatment outcome among maltreated adolescents. *Child Abuse and Neglect*, **19**, 419–31.

Florsheim, P., Shotorbani, S., Guest-Warnick, G., Barratt, T. and Hwang, W. (2000). Role of working alliance in the treatment of delinquent boys in community-based programs. *Journal of Clinical Child Psychology*, **29**, 94–107.

Garcia, J. A. and Weisz, J. R. (2002). When youth mental health care stops: therapeutic relationship problems and other reasons for ending outpatient treatment. *Journal of Consulting and Clinical Psychology*, **70**, 439–43.

Green, J., Kroll, L., Imrie, D. *et al.* (2001). Health gain and outcome predictors during inpatient and related day treatment in child and adolescent psychotherapy. *Journal of the American Academy of Child and Adolescent Psychiatry*, **40**, 325–32.

Horvath, A. O. and Symonds, B. D. (1991). Relation between working alliance and outcome in psychotherapy: a meta-analysis. *Journal of Counseling Psychology*, **38**, 139–49.

Johnson, L. N., Wright, D. W. and Ketring, S. A. (2002). The therapeutic alliance in home-based therapy: is it predictive of outcome? *Journal of Marital and Family Therapy*, **28**, 99–102.

Judd, C. M. and Kenny, D. A. (1981). Process analysis: estimating mediation in treatment evaluations. *Evaluation Review*, **5**, 602–19.

Kazdin, A. E. (1995). Bridging child, adolescent, and adult psychotherapy: directions for research. *Psychotherapy Research*, **5**, 258–77.

(2000). Developing a research agenda for child and adolescent psychotherapy. *Archives of General Psychiatry*, **57**, 829–36.

(2001). Progression of therapy research and clinical application of treatment require better understanding of the change process. *Clinical Psychology: Science and Practice*, **8**, 143–51.

Kazdin, A. E. and Wassell, G. (1998). Treatment completion and therapeutic change among children referred for outpatient therapy. *Professional Psychology: Research and Practice*, **29**, 332–40.

(1999). Barriers to treatment participation and therapeutic change among children referred for conduct disorder. *Journal of Clinical Child Psychology*, **28**, 160–72.

(2000). Predictors of barriers to treatment and therapeutic change in outpatient therapy for antisocial children and their families. *Mental Health Services Research*, **2**, 27–40.

Kazdin, A. E., Bass, D., Ayers, W. A. and Rodgers, A. (1990). Empirical and clinical focus of child and adolescent psychotherapy research. *Journal of Consulting and Clinical Psychology*, **58**, 729–40.

Kendall, P. C. (1994). Treating anxiety disorders in children: results of a randomized clinical trial. *Journal of Consulting and Clinical Psychology*, **62**, 100–10.

Kendall, P. C. and Chu, B. C. (2000). Retrospective self-reports of therapist flexibility in a manual-based treatment for youths with anxiety disorders. *Journal of Clinical Child Psychology*, **29**, 209–20.

Kendall, P. C. and Southam-Gerow, M. A. (1996). Long-term follow-up of a cognitive-behavioral therapy for anxiety-disordered youth. *Journal of Consulting and Clinical Psychology*, **64**, 724–30.

Landisberg, S. and Snyder, W. U. (1946). Nondirective play therapy. *Journal of Clinical Psychology*, **2**, 203–14.

Lebo, D. (1952). The relationship of response categories in play therapy to chronological age. *Journal of Child Psychiatry*, **2**, 330–6.

Levitt, E. E. (1957). The results of psychotherapy with children: an evaluation. *Journal of Consulting and Clinical Psychology*, **21**, 189–96.

Lonigan, C. J. and Elbert, J. C. (1998). Special issue on empirically supported psychosocial interventions for children (special issue). *Journal of Clinical Child Psychology*, **27**.

Martin, D. J., Garske, J. P. and Davis, M. K. (2000). Relation of the therapeutic alliance with outcome and other variables: a meta-analytic review. *Journal of Consulting and Clinical Psychology*, **68**, 438–50.

Motta, R. W. and Lynch, C. (1990). Therapeutic techniques vs. therapeutic relationships in child behavior therapy. *Psychological Reports*, **67**, 315–22.

Motta, R. W. and Tobin, M. I. (1992). The relative importance of specific and nonspecific factors in child behavior therapy. *Psychotherapy in Private Practice*, **11**, 51–61.

Moustakas, C. E. and Schalock, H. D. (1955). An analysis of therapist-child interaction in play therapy. *Child Development*, **26**, 143–57.

Noser, K. and Bickman, L. (2000). Quality indicators of children's mental health services: do they predict improved client outcomes? *Journal of Emotional and Behavioral Disorders*, **8**, 9–18.

Orlinsky, D. E. and Howard, K. I. (1987). A generic model of psychotherapy. *Journal of Integrative and Eclectic Psychotherapy*, **6**, 6–27.

Orlinsky, D. E., Grawe, K. and Parks, B. K. (1994). Process and outcome in psychotherapy – noch einmal. In S. L. Garfield and A. E. Bergin (eds.), *Handbook of Psychotherapy and Behavior Change*, 4th edn. New York: Wiley, pp. 270–376.

Patterson, G. R. and Chamberlain, P. (1994). A functional analysis of resistance during parent training therapy. *Clinical Psychology: Science and Practice*, **1**, 53–70.

Patterson, G. R. and Forgatch, M. S. (1985). Therapist behavior as a determinant for client non-compliance: a paradox for the behavior modifier. *Journal of Consulting and Clinical Psychology*, **53**, 846–51.

Rogers, C. R. (1957). The necessary and sufficient conditions of therapeutic personality change. *Journal of Consulting Psychology*, **21**, 95–103.

Russell, R. L. and Shirk, S. R. (1998). Child psychotherapy process research. In T. H. Ollendick and R. J. Prinz (eds.), *Advances in Clinical Child Psychology*, Volume 20. New York: Plenum, pp. 93–124.

Scott, A. G. and Sechrest, L. (1989). Strength of theory and theory of strength. *Evaluation and Program Planning*, **12**, 329–36.

Shirk, S. R. and Russell, R. L. (1996). *Change Processes in Child Psychotherapy: Revitalizing Treatment and Research*. New York: Guilford.

Shirk, S. R. and Saiz, C. S. (1992). Clinical, empirical, and developmental perspectives on the therapeutic relationship in child psychotherapy. *Development and Psychopathology*, **4**, 713–28.

Siegel, C. L. F. (1972). Changes in play therapy behaviors over time as a function of differing levels of therapist-offered conditions. *Journal of Clinical Psychology*, **28**, 235–6.

Stoolmiller, M., Duncan, T., Bank, L. and Patterson, G. R. (1993). Some problems and solutions in the study of change: significant patterns in client resistance. *Journal of Consulting and Clinical Psychology*, **61**, 920–8.

Truax, C. B. (1971). Perceived therapeutic conditions and client outcome. *Comparative Group Studies*, **2**, 301–10.

Truax, C. B. and Wittmer, J. (1973). The degree of therapist focus on defense mechanisms and the effect on therapeutic outcome with institutionalized juvenile delinquents. *Journal of Community Psychology*, **1**, 201–3.

Truax, C. B., Altmann, H., Wright, L. and Mitchell, K. M. (1973). Effects of therapeutic conditions in child therapy. *Journal of Community Psychology*, **1**, 313–18.

Truax, C. B., Wargo, D. G. and Silber L. D. (1966). Effects of group therapy with high accurate empathy and nonpossessive warmth upon female institutionalized delinquents. *Journal of Abnormal Psychology*, **71**, 267–74.

Truax, C. B., Wargo, D. G. and Volksdorf, N. R. (1970). Antecedents to outcome in group counseling with institutionalized juvenile delinquents: effects of therapeutic conditions, patient self-exploration, alternate sessions, and vicarious therapy pretraining. *Journal of Abnormal Psychology*, **76**, 235–42.

Weersing, V. R. and Weisz, J. R. (2002). Mechanisms of action in youth psychotherapy. *Journal of Child Psychology and Psychiatry*, **43**, 3–29.

Weisz, J. R. and Weersing, V. R. (1999). Psychotherapy with children and adolescents: efficacy, effectiveness, and developmental concerns. In D. Cicchetti and S. L. Toth (eds.), *Rochester Symposium on Developmental Psychopathology, Volume 9. Developmental Approaches to Prevention and Intervention*. Rochester, NY: University of Rochester Press, pp. 341–86.

Weisz, J. R., Huey, S. M. and Weersing, V. R. (1998). Psychotherapy outcome research with children and adolescents: the state of the art. In T. H. Ollendick and R. J. Prinz (eds.), *Advances in Clinical Child Psychology*, Volume 20. New York: Plenum, pp. 49–92.

Weisz, J. R., Weiss, B., Alicke, M. D. and Klotz, M. L. (1987). Effectiveness of psychotherapy with children and adolescents: a meta-analysis for clinicians. *Journal of Consulting and Clinical Psychology*, **55**, 542–9.

Weisz, J. R., Weiss, B., Han, S. S., Granger, D. A. and Morton, T. (1995). Effects of psychotherapy with children and adolescents revisited: a meta-analysis of treatment outcome studies. *Psychological Bulletin*, **117**, 450–68.

Yeh, M. and Weisz, J. R. (2001). Why are we here at the clinic? Parent-child (dis)agreement on referral problems at outpatient treatment entry. *Journal of Consulting and Clinical Psychology*, **69**, 1018–25.

Part II

Engagement and assessment

5

Engagement and motivational interviewing

Ulrike Schmidt

Institute of Psychiatry, London, UK

5.1 Introduction

In psychiatric and psychological practice, it is often assumed that when people present for an assessment the mere act of attendance suggests that the person has decided that he or she wants 'something', either a diagnosis or treatment. This also implies that the patient recognizes that something is wrong, that something distresses them and that they want to change or overcome their 'problem'. A further assumption is that it is the job of the health care practitioner to give information, advice or practical help, so as to induce positive change, improvement in health and reduce distress in their patient.

To a degree, these tacit assumptions have validity but often when working with young people, while their parents may fully subscribe to the above assumptions, there may be gross disparities between the goals of the parents and health practitioner on the one hand and those of the young person on the other. Some of these disparities result from developmental issues; others result from aspects of the disorder/problem itself that the young person presents with.

For example, one of the important developmental tasks of adolescence is for the young person to develop an individual identity and to become independent from their family of origin. To do and think things that go against adult authority and rules is a normal part of growing up. To attend a clinic and speak to a strange adult, who is seen as an extension of parental authority, about something that the adolescent either sees as 'not much of a problem' or would rather keep as a shameful and closely guarded private experience, is a difficult and uncomfortable thing to do and may be vetoed by the young person in principle.

There may also be important aspects of the disorder/problem behaviour that the young person positively values and is reluctant to give up. For example, Lucy, a 15-year old who was previously plump and teased by her peers about her weight, was brought to the clinic by her mother because she had been noted by her school to throw away her lunches, had lost some weight and admitted to her parents that she was making herself sick on a regular basis. Moreover, she sometimes cut her forearms when she had eaten more than she had allowed herself. She was not keen to have any treatment as she was very pleased with her new skinny appearance, which meant she was no longer teased and was allowed to be part of a popular group of girls at school and she had acquired her first boyfriend.

Health care professionals thus have to strike a difficult balance between what may be wanted by the patient and their parents and what they as clinicians judge may be needed. Cognitive behavioural therapy (CBT) is an action-orientated treatment which traditionally requires a willing and collaborating patient who is motivated to change. Engaging the young person to be able to make optimal use of everything that CBT has to offer is a crucial and difficult task.

Below, some theoretical concepts (e.g. models of behaviour change) and a clinical framework (based on motivational interviewing) are described, which are helpful when working with young people to engage them, which help them to develop personal change goals and which reduce ambivalence about and resistance to change.

5.2   Models of behaviour change

The transtheoretical model of change (Prochaska and DiClemente, 1982) recognizes that people do not make simple black or white decisions to change problematic behaviours. Rather, it holds that there is a gradual process, divided into phases. These are termed the 'stages' of change and connote the degree of readiness to work towards a goal. In this model, change is viewed as a progression from an initial *precontemplation* stage, where the person is not considering change, as they may not believe that they have a problem. In the *contemplation* stage, the individual is ambivalent about change and evaluates the pros and cons of change. In the *preparation* stage, planning and commitment to change are secured. In the *action* stage, the person makes specific behavioural changes to overcome their problem. From there, the person moves into the *maintenance* phase and then either exits their problem or relapses. It has been postulated that, for sustained change, people often have to go through the cycle of change several times.

Other aspects of the transtheoretical model are the 'processes' of change, i.e. the overt and covert activities an individual engages in to modify thinking, behaviour or affect in relation to a problem (Prochaska *et al.*, 1988). Further elements within the model are the decisional balance (balance of pros and cons for change), self-efficacy (DiClemente *et al.*, 1985) and temptations, all of which are thought to predict movement through the stages (Prochaska and Velicer, 1997). One important assumption of this model, which makes intuitive sense and for which there is some research evidence, is that any clinical intervention needs to be tailored to the individual's stage of change (DiClemente and Marden Velasquez, 2002). Thus, those in the earlier stages of change may benefit from being given additional information to help raise their awareness, whereas those in the determination stage may find it helpful to learn specific skills as to how to overcome their problem.

The transtheoretical model has been successfully applied to a variety of health behaviours, including smoking cessation, drug and alcohol use, weight control, fat intake, eating disorders, exercise acquisition and the take up of screening for mammography (for review, see Blake *et al.*, 1997; DiClemente and Marden Velasquez, 2002).

Critics of the transtheoretical model (Bandura, 1998; Davidson, 1998) have argued for a continuum measure of change rather than a categorical measure. Others have questioned the processes of change that have been defined.

Several other models include stages in behaviour change. For example, Weinstein (1988) distinguished five stages in the precaution adoption process. Gebhardt (1997) described four motivational stages in the health behaviour goal model. De Vries and Backbier (1994) describe change in attitudes, social influence and self-efficacy through motivational stages in their Attitude, Social Influence and Efficacy (ASE) model and Schwarzer (1992) has developed the Health Action Process Approach.

5.3   It is more than readiness that matters

Most of these models converge in suggesting that there are two components underlying readiness to change. These are: (1) recognition of the importance of a problem, which can also be termed willingness to change or conviction that change is needed; and (2) belief in one's ability, confidence or self-efficacy (Keller and Kemp-White, 1997; Rollnick, 1998; Rollnick *et al.*, 1999). The issue of importance relates to the question of why change is needed. This concept includes how the problem behaviour fits in with an individual's values and the expected outcomes of change. Confidence relates to a person's belief that they have the ability to master behaviour change. For example, a young person with chronic fatigue may desperately wish the fatigue to subside, but may not

Table 5.1   Questions with which to explore importance

'How important would you say is it for you to change . . .? On a scale of 0 to 10, where 0 not at all important and 10 is extremely important, where would you say you are?'

0   1   2   3   4   5   6   7   8   9   10

Not at all   Extremely

important   important

What would have to happen for it to become more important for you to change?

You have given yourself x on the scale. What would need to happen for your score to move from x to 10?

What stops you moving from x to 10?

What are the things that you take into account which make you give yourself as high a score as you do?

What are the good things about x behaviour? What are some of the less good things about x behaviour?

What concerns do you have about x behaviour?

If you were to change what would it be like?

believe they can do anything about it (high importance, low confidence). In contrast, a young person with obsessive compulsive disorder may not believe that it is worthwhile to give up egosyntonic rituals (low importance, high or low confidence).

5.4   How to measure importance and confidence

While sophisticated, disorder-specific, interview-based methods of the measurement of readiness to change exist, these measures of motivation are probably most useful as research tools, especially if they can be shown to predict outcome. In clinical situations, readiness to change is often rather fluid and can wax and wane within and between sessions. Thus, from a clinical point of view, it may not be reasonable to spend a great deal of effort measuring readiness accurately at one point in time. Rather, a clinician should be able to evaluate these concepts within the session whatever the agenda of the moment. This is particularly important at the start of treatment. Linear visual analogue scales (Tables 5.1 and 5.2), which measure the dimensions of importance and confidence on a continuum, are useful tools which can supplement therapeutic judgement (Keller and Kemp-White, 1997; Rollnick *et al.*, 1999; Miller and Rollnick, 2002). These concepts can be explored by the questions outlined in Tables 5.1 and 5.2.

Once the level of importance and confidence of one goal – e.g. to work with a therapist on a particular problem behaviour – has been established, then the

Table 5.2   Questions with which to explore confidence

How confident would you say you are, that if you decided to change . . ., you could do it? On a scale of 0–10, where 0 is not at all confident and 10 is extremely confident, where would you say you are?

0   1   2   3   4   5   6   7   8   9   10

Not at all   Extremely

confident   confident

What would make you more confident about making these changes?

Why have you given yourself as high a score as you have on confidence?

How could you go up higher so that your score goes from x to y?

How can I or anybody else help you succeed?

Is there anything that you found helpful in any previous attempts to change?

What have you learned from the way things went wrong last time you tried?

If you decided to change what might your options be? Do you know of any ways that have worked for other people?

What are the practical things you would need to do to achieve this goal? Are they achievable?

Is there anything you can think of that would make you feel more confident?

From Treasure and Schmidt, 2001.

intervention can be matched. The following techniques can be useful (from Treasure and Schmidt, 2001):

- *Low conviction* and *low confidence:* Find out where there are misconceptions or gaps in your patient's knowledge. Encourage your patient to think about aspects that they may previously not have considered. Provide information that is novel and relevant to the patient. The novelty aspect of information is very important to raise interest (K. Eammons, personal communication). For example, would they be interested in borrowing a new book or videotape? Emphasize their personal choice and freedom. Point out that you understand that their problem does not bother them at the moment. Reflect that you accept them whatever they decide about the possibility of change, but suggest to the patient that they might want to think about the issue. Make it clear that if they should become more interested in changing you would be there to help in any way you can and offer the support necessary.

- *Low conviction* and *high confidence:* Help the patient identify and discuss discrepancies between what he wants for himself in the future and where he is at in the present situation. Help him to recognize discrepancies and gaps in the information that he has. Discuss the patient's hierarchy of values and help him decide what is important in his life. Again, emphasize the patient's ultimate freedom of choice.

- *High conviction* and *low confidence:* Increase confidence by building on past experiences in which the patient has shown mastery in the face of difficulties and challenges. Work collaboratively with the patient on devising and implementing a change plan consisting of small manageable steps. Get the patient to define the size of each step, so that the plan is realistic and does not set him up for failure.
- *High conviction* and *high confidence:* Work with the patient to foresee and forestall difficult times. Offer information, practical advice and skills training as options, letting the patient decide what might work best in supporting his own efforts. Identify and remove obstacles to maintaining the desired course of action. Attend to progress by noting and affirming.

We have also found that it is useful to have an additional scale that measures how eager close others are to see change. This highlights the social context, in which change occurs. For example, conflict will arise if there is a great disparity between different family members in their readiness for change. Families with a young person with a problem may demand him/her to change instantly, which may lead to an 'antimotivational' environment, in which there is confrontation and high negative expressed emotion. Alternatively, differences in opinion between the parents about the urgency of the situation may paralyse any attempts to change. These examples illustrate the need for a broad exploration of the psychosocial environment.

5.5   Motivational interviewing

In parallel with the development of these various models to understand change, an empirically based, atheoretical form of therapeutic interaction, motivational interviewing (MI), has been developed (for review, see Miller, 1995, 1998, 2000; Miller and Rollnick, 2002). The techniques were based on observations about how therapist behaviour can influence outcome. For example, client resistance rates rose when a confrontational therapeutic style was used and fell with a client-centred approach. Miller developed a short intervention, 'the drinker's check-up', which operationalized some of the factors found to improve outcome. This 'check-up' with motivational feedback was compared with a confrontational approach. The outcome, in terms of drinking 1 year later, was worse in the group of patients who were given their feedback from the drinker's check-up in a confrontational manner (Miller *et al.*, 1993). In a further study, it was found that, if motivational feedback of the drinker's check-up was given as an initial intervention prior to entry into an inpatient clinic, patients were found to have a better outcome. The therapists for this group reported that their patients had participated more fully in treatment and appeared to be more motivated (Bien *et al.*, 1993; Brown and Miller, 1993).

5.6   What is MI? principles, definitions and techniques

MI has been defined as a client-centred directive method for enhancing intrinsic motivation to change by exploring and resolving ambivalence (Miller and Rollnick, 2002). It is a combination of style and technique.

The style and underlying philosophy borrow heavily from the ideas of Carl Rogers (1957) who emphasized warmth, empathy and unconditional acceptance as necessary conditions for a climate within which therapeutic change could take place. Thus, in MI: 'impetus for change is drawn from the client's own intrinsic motives and goals, and it is the client who gives voice to reasons for change. Direct persuasion, coercion, and other saliently external controls are avoided. The therapeutic relationship has a partnership character and the client's freedom of choice is emphasized' (Rollnick and Miller, 1995). Avoidance of confrontation or arguments is the aim of MI and resistance is seen as an interpersonal problem between therapist/client, and not as the client's problem. Resistance signals the need to 'change gear'.

Various metaphors have been used to describe the spirit of MI; one is that it is a dance rather than a wrestling match. Miller himself has drawn the analogy between MI and the gentle techniques used by Monty Roberts (1997), the original horse whisperer, to tame wild horses. The fable of the sun and the wind is also a useful analogy to describe the essence of MI: 'The sun and the wind were having a dispute as to who was the most powerful. They saw a man walking along and they challenged each other about which of them would be most successful at getting the man to remove his coat. The wind started first and blew up a huge gale, the coat flapped but the man only closed all his buttons and tightened up his belt. The sun tried next and shone brightly making the man sweat. He proceeded to take off his coat.' Therapists thus need to model themselves on the sun.

The four main principles of MI can be summarized as:

(1)   express empathy by using reflective listening to convey understanding of the client's position;

(2)   develop discrepancy between the client's most deeply held values and current behaviour;

(3)   roll with resistance by meeting it with reflection rather than confrontation; and

(4)   support self-efficacy by building confidence that change is possible.

The basic techniques of motivational interviewing are those of client-centred counselling:

(1)   *Reflective listening.* At the most basic level, reflection is used as an attempt to understand the patient's perspective. It is thus a kind of hypothesis testing. By reflecting, the therapist asks the patient: 'is this what you meant?' and this implies that the patient not the practitioner is an expert on their problem. Different types

of reflection (such as overshooting, undershooting, double-sided reflection) are used more strategically when clients are ambivalent or resistant to change (see section on resistance below). The use of reflection in MI sets it apart from CBT where Socratic questioning is used. Both methods, however, have similar goals – i.e. to aid guided self-discovery – especially if reflection is used strategically. It could be argued that reflection is less intrusive than Socratic questioning and may therefore be more appropriate in the early stage of a therapeutic encounter, especially with those who are reluctant to change.

(2) *Affirmation* Many young people who present with a problem may have had negative feedback from peers or family about their difficulty and may have developed negative views about themselves as a person. The use of affirmation may be helpful in restoring damaged self-esteem. Any attempt at affirmation needs to take into account the reluctance that adolescents sometimes have to being 'praised' and this may need to be done in a humorous or low-key manner, e.g. *'I have been very impressed with how openly you have talked about what are some very tricky issues.'*

(3) *Summarizing:* Intermittent summaries of what has been said give the therapist an opportunity to check out with the patient whether they have really understood what has been said. Moreover, summaries can be used strategically to emphasize. Alternatively, de-emphasize certain aspects of what has been said to guide the person gently towards greater problem recognition and motivation for change.

(4) *Asking open-ended questions:* The aim of this is to get the patient rather than the therapist to make a case for change by voicing concerns about their behaviour, intention to change and optimism for change. A number of questions / techniques that gently guide the person towards recognition of difficulties are listed next.

(5) *Focus on eliciting the patient's own concerns*
For example, *'your mum has brought you here and is clearly concerned. Are you worried at all about . . .?'* or: *'It seems that things have changed quite a bit since I last saw you. How is that affecting you?'* Probe for effects on physical and psychological well-being, ability to study/work, relationships with parents, peers, and boyfriends.
'What worries you about . . .? What concerns do you have about . . .?'
'What makes you think that you need to change?'
'What are the benefits of change?'
'If you decided to change, what would work for you? What makes you think that you can change?'

(6) *The good and the not so good of the problem*
Enquire about and acknowledge the positive and negative aspects of the disorder: e.g. *'what are the good things about your . . .? How has it helped you?'*

'Are there things you don't like about your . . . disorder? Has your problem with . . . stopped you from doing what you want to do?'

'What is the worst aspect of your . . .? What is the best . . .?'

(7) *Explore goals and values*

For example, *'if you compare where you are now in terms of how life is going and 5 years ago, what are the differences?'*

'Do you remember what life was like before your problem with . . . started?'

'What were your hopes, your goals, your strengths?'

'How has your 'problem' stopped you from moving forwards?'

(8) *Two possible futures*

For example, *'what would your future look like (say, in 5 years from now) if you made few changes in your life and your . . . continued?'*

'What would your future look like if you decided to make some changes in your life and things turned out really well?'

(9) *Emphasis on personal choice*

For example, *'what would you like to happen as a result of our meeting today?'*

(10) *Advice and feedback about health risks/problems*: Offer this where appropriate, without lecturing or threatening. The patient's permission for this may be required. For example, *'I have seen a number of young people with difficulties not dissimilar to your own – would you like me to tell you about the kinds of difficulties people with this type of problem tend to run into and what they have found helpful?'*

(11) *Offer a menu of change options*

For example, *'one option we have is to refer you to our practice counsellor to look at some of the issues we discussed in some more depth. Another option is to prescribe some medication, which might be helpful. Which option would you prefer?'*

5.7   Dealing with resistance

Within the MI paradigm, resistance is seen as resulting from an interaction between therapist and client, not as something that is located just within the client. This acknowledges that the therapist's behaviour can 'up- or down-regulate' the client's resistance. Resistance is most likely to occur when the client experiences a potential loss of freedom or choice (Moyers and Rollnick, 2002). This inevitably produces a desire to counteract the perceived loss of choice. MI can be helpful in responding to this type of resistance, while other more intrapersonal types of resistance may be less accessible with this method.

Two types of responses are used within MI to deal with resistance: either reflective or strategic. Examples of core techniques are given below:

(1)   *Expressing respect for the patient:* e.g. acknowledge their reluctance to come –
       'I appreciate that it was not an easy decision for you to come today.'

(2)   *Over- and undershooting:* These are two types of reflections that direct the person
       towards change. For example, if the patient states they do not really have a prob-
       lem, the therapist reflects this back, minimizing their desire to change further
       (undershooting). The aim is to get the client to disagree. Likewise, in the case of
       a client who paints a totally black picture of their difficulties, the therapist makes
       what the patient says even bigger, 'overshooting' again with the aim to get the
       patient to disagree.

(3)   *Reflecting back the emotion:* Rather than reflecting the contents of the patient's
       resistance, it can be helpful to reflect the underlying emotion, in order to help
       the patient feel more understood. For example, *'what would work for you if you*
       decided to change?' 'If I knew that I wouldn't be here now!'
       'You sound angry with the . . ., this anger could help you fight it' or: 'You feel confused
       and irritated by your . . . and you are uncertain what to do.'

(4)   *Double-sided reflection:* This is useful if the person is very ambivalent, and gives
       conflicting messages. For example, *'you don't think that your . . . is harming you*
       seriously now, and at the same time you are concerned that it might get out of hand for
       you later.'
       'You really like to keep your . . . under tight control and would hate giving up doing . . .,
       and you can also see that it is causing serious problems for your family and your studies.'

(5)   *Juxtaposing two important and inconsistent values:* This is useful as it increases
       client discrepancy. For example, *'I wonder if it's really possible for you to keep . . . and*
       continue with all your extra-curricular activities too.'

(6)   *Emphasizing personal choice/control*
       This needs to be done in a cautious and respectful manner. For example, *'maybe*
       you'll decide that it's worth it to you to keep on . . . the way you have been, even though
       it's costing you.'
       'It's up to you what you do about this.'
       'No one can decide this for you.'
       'No one can change your . . . for you. Only you can do it.'

(7)   *Reframing*
       Reframing reluctance to change by construing the patient's underlying motive
       for not wanting to change in a positive way acknowledges respect for the
       patient.

(8)   *Symptoms as a reward.* For example, *'you may need to reward yourself in the evenings*
       for studying very hard during the day.'

(9)   *Symptoms as a protective function.* For example, *'you don't want to impose additional*
       stress on your family by openly sharing concerns or difficulties in your life (give examples).

As a result, you carry all this yourself and absorb tension and stress by . . ., as a way of trying not to burden your family.'

(10)   *Symptoms as an adaptive function.* For example, *'your . . . can be viewed as a means of avoiding conflict or tension in your marriage. Your . . . tends to keep the status quo, to keep things as they are. It seems like you have been . . . to keep your family intact. Yet you seem to be uncomfortable with this arrangement.'*

(11)   *Using gentle paradox*
This needs to be done cautiously and with respect and warmth. For example, *'you haven't convinced me that you are seriously concerned.'*
'I'll tell you one concern I have. This treatment programme is one that requires a fair amount of motivation from people, and frankly, I'm not sure from what you've told me so far that you're motivated enough to carry through with it. Do you think we should go ahead?'
'I'm not sure how much you are interested in changing, or even taking a careful look at your . . . problems. It sounds like you might be happier just going on as before.'

(12)   *Shifting the focus*
Sometimes when faced with resistance, it can simply be helpful to switch to a different topic of conversation, so as to avoid a head-on collision. This will give time to build up an alliance and more difficult areas can be revisited later.

5.8   The evidence base of MI

MI facilitates behaviour change in many areas. The efficacy of interventions derived from MI has been summarized in two systematic reviews (Dunn *et al.*, 2001; Burke *et al.*, 2002). MI has been shown to be effective in the treatment of alcohol problems, abuse of drugs, smoking cessation, psychiatric treatment adherence, HIV risk behaviours and other domains, such as dietary change, exercise and other lifestyle changes.

In general, motivational interventions are more efficacious than no treatment and not significantly different from credible alternative treatments. In the area of alcohol and substance abuse, relatively brief motivational interventions yield moderate to large effects and good maintenance over time. Motivational interventions have been found to be efficacious both as stand alone treatments and as preludes to other treatments, such as CBT.

In Project Match (1997a), a very large study in people with alcohol problems comparing a four-session motivational intervention with 12 sessions of CBT or 12-step treatment, the brief motivational intervention was as effective as the longer intervention. In this study, one of the hypotheses was that patients in the precontemplation and contemplation stages would do better with motivational treatment whereas those in action would do better with a skill-based intervention. In the short term, no matching between approach and stage of change was found. However, the 15-month outcome of the less motivated group who were allocated to motivational enhancement therapy was better than that in the two other forms of treatment (Project MATCH, 1997b). In a study of bulimia nervosa comparing four sessions of motivational enhancement therapy with four sessions of CBT as a prelude to further group CBT, no evidence to suggest that stage matching contributed to the outcome was found (Treasure *et al.*, 1999; M. A. Katzman *et al.*, unpublished data). Although the idea of matching different types of treatment to different clients has an intuitive appeal, it is probably overly simplistic to assume that measurement of one specific variable at one point of time within a complex intervention might have a large effect on outcome.

Motivational interventions have been successfully used in adolescents, both as preventative interventions in young people who had initiated risky behaviours and as a prelude to other treatments such as CBT or residential treatment. Results, as yet, are mostly preliminary, but promising (Baer and Peterson, 2002), echoing the findings from the adult literature.

5.9   Therapist behaviours of MI

Rollnick and Miller (1995) were able to define specific and trainable therapist behaviours that they felt led to a better therapeutic alliance and better outcome. A good motivational therapist needs to be able to:

(1)   understand the other person's frame of reference;
(2)   express acceptance and affirmation;
(3)   filter the patient's thoughts so that motivational statements are amplified and non-motivational statements are dampened down;
(4)   elicit client's self-motivational statements: expressions of problem recognition, concern, desire, intention to change and ability to change;
(5)   match processes to stage of change, ensuring they do not jump ahead of the client; and
(6)   affirm the client's freedom of choice and self-direction.
    Points (1), (3), (4) and (5) cover issues relating to the transtheoretical model of change. They explore the reasons that sustain the behaviour and aim to help the client shift the decisional balance of pros and cons into the direction of change. Points (2) and (6) cover the interpersonal aspects of the therapeutic relationship. The therapist needs to provide a warm, optimistic setting and take a 'one-down' position by emphasizing the client's autonomy and right to choose, but be ready to offer expert advice and skills once the patient is ready to 'go'.

Broadly speaking, MI seems to work by reducing client 'negativity' (Miller, 1999), and in Project Match (1997b) it seemed to be particularly useful for helping angry clients. Low levels of resistance predict change (Miller *et al.*, 1993) and have a more powerful effect than increasing the number of positive statements about change. Resistance often follows confrontation. The typical proportion of time therapists spend in confrontation before training in MI is 5–15%. Unless confrontational therapist behaviour is reduced with training, there is little change in client outcome.

5.10   Adapting motivational strategies for working with young people in assessment and engagement for CBT

There are a number of advantages of using motivational techniques in young people attending for treatment. A clinical style that is respectful, acknowledges choice and ambivalence and does not increase resistance is a logical choice. MI not only minimizes conflict but also uses ambivalence to develop motivation for change. Baer and Peterson (2002) commented that there is often a common curiosity and openness to philosophical questions among young people which might make MI particularly helpful. Furthermore, MI tends to support personal change goals rather than parental- or therapist-based goals, which naturally supports exploration of world views and continued efforts towards autonomy.

There are a number of challenges when translating standard techniques of MI for use in young people. Only in a minority of cases is it the young people themselves who seek help. Young people are often coerced into treatment and are often angry. These feelings will conflict with engagement in any interview. This problem can be minimized by the therapist openly acknowledging in a respectful manner how difficult it must have been for the young person to attend. Ingersoll and colleagues (2000) suggest that an important early task for the counsellor is to distinguish himself or herself from other adults with more traditional messages. This may be achieved by providing information that is different from that to which the young person has previously been exposed.

The therapeutic style of MI requires the therapist to take their cue from the patient, to ask open questions and to reflect on the answers with an equal balance of power between client and therapist. Young adolescents may find this approach somewhat alien and threatening. They tend to be wary, suspicious and sensitized to being misunderstood. In this context, the therapist may need to give more structure to the session and not only rely on open questions at the beginning. The therapist will be judged as to whether he or she understands the problem during the process of information exchange and so the content and approach should include expert guidance. As Baer and Peterson (2002) say: 'Essentially, rapport and alliance will develop when the *experience* of the interview is different rather than by hearing the therapist's intentions that it will be so.'

Personalized feedback about the problem and attached risks and the consequences if left untreated can be presented in chart form to give comparisons with the norm or by summarizing the discussions of the assessment in a letter to the patient. The author and colleagues compared a motivational assessment interview followed by a personalized feedback letter with a standard assessment followed by a general practitioner's letter in adults presenting to a community mental health team. Those who received the motivational assessment and personalized feedback felt more satisfied with the assessment, more understood and more involved in their care and these changes tended to persist until several months after the assessment (Humfress *et al.*, 2002). Feedback can be helpful for showing patients the degree of severity of their difficulty and to initiate discussions about what the recommended treatment is at a particular stage. This facilitates a collaborative approach and reduces the potential for direct confrontation between patient and therapist.

One of the tenets of MI is that the client should take personal responsibility to choose whether he or she will decide to change. Clearly, for many problems faced by young people, this is neither a realistic, desirable or ethical option and there may be a legal framework prohibiting this sort of approach.

One way to use this within a motivational framework is for the therapist to bring in the concept of 'a higher power or authority' constraining the action of both therapist and patients. This means that the therapist does not have to use direct confrontation or coercion but approaches the controversial area indirectly through society's rules. An example of using this type of intervention is as follows: '*The rules of good medical practice for the management of anorexia nervosa suggest that the patient should be weighed at every session. You and I have to abide by those rules. You do not have to see your weight if you choose. How should we do it?*'

We have already mentioned above that there is often great disparity between family members in terms of the importance they place on the problem. Parents may differ in how concerned they are about the young person's difficulties and what should be done about them. These different views can lead to high levels of confrontation at home, which counteracts the motivational approach of the clinic. An intervention which involves teaching the family the basic principles of MI exists. In addition to developing communication skills, family members are also taught how to reinforce non-symptomatic behaviour and to remove attention from problematic behaviour. These techniques are based on the Community Reinforcement Approach (CRAFT; Meyers *et al.*, 1998) which, in the alcohol and substance misuse field, has been shown to be highly effective in engaging unmotivated clients in treatment (Meyers *et al.*, 1999; Miller *et al.*, 1999; Meyers *et al.*, 2002).

Beyond the initial assessment, the author and colleagues have found that young patients find it helpful to discuss motivational aspects of their difficulties through the use of written exercises – e.g. getting them to write two letters to the future, one imagining themselves without their difficulty, the other imagining they still have the difficulty, or writing a letter to their problem as a friend or as an enemy (Schmidt *et al.*, 2002).

Miller (1999) in discussing some of the limitations of motivational interviewing pointed out that, even at the point where someone recognizes the importance of change and has the confidence to change, it may still not be possible for them to take action to change if they think they are not worth 'saving'. This taps into the area of powerful, maladaptive core beliefs, which are self-sabotaging. In such cases, therapeutic efforts may need to concentrate on identifying and modifying these core beliefs before the motivation to change pathological behaviours can be revisited. Thus, therapy will be a process of iterative cycles of assessment and movement.

5.11   REFERENCES

Baer, J. S. and Peterson, P. L. (2002). Motivational interviewing with adolescents and young adults. In W. R. Miller and S. Rollnick (eds.), *Motivational Interviewing. Preparing People for Change*, 2nd edn. New York: Guilford Press, pp. 320–32.

Bandura, A. (1998). Health promotion from the perspective of social cognitive theory. *Psychology and Health*, **13**, 4.

Bien, T. H., Miller, W. R. and Boroughs, J. M. (1993). Motivational interviewing with alcohol outpatients. *Behavioural and Cognitive Psychotherapy*, **21**, 347–56.

Blake, W., Turnbull, S. and Treasure, J. L. (1997). Stages and processes of change in eating disorders. Implications for therapy. *Clinical Psychology and Psychotherapy*, **4**, 186–91.

Brown, J. M. and Miller, W. R. (1993). Impact of motivational interviewing on participation in residential alcoholism treatment. *Psychology of Addictive Behaviors*, **7**, 211–18.

Burke, L., B., Arkowitz, H. and Dunn, C. (2002). The efficacy of motivational interviewing and its adaptations. In W. R. Miller and S. Rollnick (eds.), *Motivational Interviewing. Preparing People for Change*, second edn. New York: Guilford Press, pp. 217–50.

Davidson, R. (1998). The transtheoretical model. In W. R. Miller and N. Heather (eds.), *Treating Addictive Behaviours*, 2nd edn. New York: Plenum.

De Vries, H. and Backbier, E. (1994). Self-efficacy as an important determinant of quitting among pregnant women who smoke: the Ø- pattern. *Preventive Medicine*, **23**, 167–74.

DiClemente, C. C. and Marden Velasquez, M. (2002). Motivational interviewing and the stages of change. In W. R. Miller and S. Rollnick (eds.), *Motivational Interviewing. Preparing People for Change*, 2nd edn. New York: Guilford Press, pp. 201–16.

DiClemente, C. C., Prochaska, J. O. and Gibertini, M. (1985). Self efficacy and the stages of self change in smoking. *Cognitive Therapy and Research*, **9**, 181–200.

Dunn, C., Deroo, L. and Rivara, F. P. (2001). The use of brief interventions adapted from motivational interviewing across behavioral domains: a systematic review. *Addiction*, **96**, 1725–42.

Gebhardt, A. G. (1997). *Health Behaviour Goal Model: Towards a Theoretical Framework for Health Behaviour Change*, Ph.D. thesis. The Netherlands: University of Leiden.

Humfress, H., Igel, V., Lamont, A., Tanner, M., Morgan, J. and Schmidt U. (2002). The effect of a brief motivational intervention on community psychiatric patients' attitudes to their care, motivation to change, compliance and outcome: a case control study. *Journal of Mental Health*, **11**, 155–66.

Ingersoll, K. S., Wagner, C. C. and Gharib, S. (2000). *Motivational Groups for Community Substance Abuse Programs*. Richmond, VA: Mid-Atlantic Addiction Technology Transfer Center / Center for Substance Abuse Treatment.

Keller, V. F. and Kemp-White, M. (1997). Choices and changes: a new model for influencing patient health behavior. *Journal of Clinical Outcome Management*, **4**, 33–6.

Meyers, R. J., Miller, W. R., Hill, D. E. and Tonigan, J. S. (1999). Community reinforcement and family training (CRAFT): engaging unmotivated drug users in treatment. *Journal of Substance Abuse*, **10**, 291–308.

Meyers, R. J., Miller, W. R., Smith, J. E. and Tonigan, J. S. (2002). A randomized trial of two methods for engaging treatment-refusing drug users through concerned significant others. *Journal of Consulting and Clinical Psychology*, **70**, 1182–5.

Meyers, R. J., Smith, E. J. and Miller, W. R. (1998). Working through the concerned significant other. In W. R. Miller and N. Heather (eds.), *Treating Addictive Behaviours*, 2nd edn. New York: Plenum.

Miller, W. R. (1995). Increasing motivation for change. In R. K. Hester and W. R. Miller (eds.), *Handbook of Alcoholism Treatment Approaches*, 2nd edn. Needham Heights, MA: Allyn and Bacon.

(1998). Enhancing motivation for change. In W. R. Miller and N. Heather (eds.), *Treating Addictive Behaviours*, 2nd edn. New York: Plenum.

(1999). Updates, education and training. *Motivational Interviewing Newsletter*, **6**, 1–6.

(2000). Rediscovering fire: small interventions, large effects. *Psychology of Addictive Behaviors*, **14**, 6–18.

Miller, W. R. and Rollnick, S. (2002). *Motivational Interviewing: Preparing People for Change*, 2nd edn. New York: Guilford Press.

Miller, W. R., Benefield. R. G. and Tonigan, J. S. (1993). Enhancing motivation for change in problem drinking: a controlled comparison of two therapist styles. *Journal of Consulting and Clinical Psychology*, **61**, 455–61.

Miller, W. R., Meyers, R. J. and Tonigan, J. S. (1999). Engaging the unmotivated in treatment for alcohol problems: a comparison of three strategies for intervention through family members. *Journal of Consulting and Clinical Psychology*, **67**, 688–97.

Moyers, T. B. and Rollnick S. (2002). A motivational interviewing perspective and resistance in psychotherapy. *Journal of Clinical Psychology*, **58**, 185–93.

Prochaska, J. O. and DiClemente, C. C. (1982). Transtheoretical therapy: toward a more integrative model of change. *Psychotherapy: Theory Research and Practice*, **19**, 276–88.

Prochaska, J. O. and Velicer, W. F. (1997). The transtheoretical model of behaviour change. *American Journal of Health Promotion*, **12**, 38–48.

Prochaska, J. O., Velicer, W. F., DiClemente, C. C. and Fava, J. (1988). Measuring processes of change: applications to the cessation of smoking. *Journal of Consulting and Clinical Psychology*, **56**, 520–8.

Project Match Research Group (1997a). Matching alcoholism client heterogeneity: post treatment outcomes. *Journal of the Study of Alcohol*, **58**, 7–29.

Project MATCH Research Group (1997b). Project MATCH secondary a priori hypotheses. *Addiction*, **92**, 1671–98.

Roberts, M. (1997). *The Man Who Listens to Horses*. New York: Ballantine Publishing Group.

Rogers, C. (1957). The necessary and sufficient conditions for therapeutic personality change. *Journal of Consulting Psychology*, **21**, 95–103.

Rollnick, S. (1998). Readiness and confidence: critical conditions of change in treatment. In: W. R. Miller and N. Heather (eds.), *Treating Addictive Behaviours*, 2nd edn. New York: Plenum.

Rollnick, S. and Miller, W. R. (1995). What is motivational interviewing? *Behavioural and Cognitive Psychotherapy*, **23**, 325–34.

Rollnick, S., Mason, P. and Butler, C. (1999). *Health Behaviour Change. A Guide for Practitioners*. Edinburgh: Churchill Livingstone.

Schmidt, U., Bone, G., Hems, S., Lessem, J. and Treasure, J. (2002). Structured therapeutic writing tasks as an adjunct to treatment in eating disorders. *European Eating Disorders Review*, **10**, 1–17.

Schwarzer, R. (1992). Self efficacy in the adoption and maintenance of health behaviours: theoretical approaches and a new model. In Schwarzer, R. (ed.), *Self Efficacy: Thought Control of Action*. New York: Hemisphere.

Treasure, J. and Schmidt, U. (2001). Ready, willing and able to change: motivational aspects of the assessment and treatment of eating disorders. *European Eating Disorders Review*, **9**, 1–15.

Treasure, J. L., Katzman, M., Schmidt, U., DeSilva, P., Todd, G. and Troop, N. (1999). Engagement and outcome in the treatment of bulimia nervosa: first phase of a sequential design comparing motivation enhancement therapy and cognitive behavioural therapy. *Behaviour Research and Therapy*, **37**, 405–18.

Weinstein, N. D. (1988). The precaution adoption process. *Health Psychology*, **7**, 355–86.

6

Cognitive case formulation

Jonquil Drinkwater

The Park Hospital for Children, Oxford, UK

The field of cognitive behaviour therapy (CBT) for children and adolescents is rapidly evolving and is at an interesting stage of development. The majority of random controlled trials (RCTs) on CBT for a range of disorders have been behaviourally orientated rather than focusing on cognition. The more cognitive approaches to CBT have yet to be evaluated and are at the case study stage. In line with the developmental stage of the field, cognitive case formulation is not an area that has attracted much interest in child and adolescent CBT, and there is little literature on it. However, cognitive case formulation is currently the subject of an interesting debate in the adult CBT literature and this will be summarized here.

This chapter will describe the nature of cognitive case formulations, and the issues to be considered when carrying out cognitive case formulations with children and adolescents. It will discuss using newer approaches to cognition in CBT for children and adolescents and the role of the family in cognitive case formulations. The need for research in a range of areas will be outlined, including its role in the development of cognitive models for children and adolescents. Finally, a case example will be given which illustrates the use of a cognitive case formulation. The treatment based on this cognitive case formulation will then be contrasted with a more behaviourally orientated CBT case study.

Overall, it will be argued that, for the field of CBT for children and adolescents to progress, it is essential that we develop cognitive models and evaluate the more cognitively orientated formulations and treatments derived from them.

Cognitive Behaviour Therapy for Children and Families, ed. Philip J. Graham.
Published by Cambridge University Press. © Cambridge University Press 2004.

6.1   What is a cognitive case formulation in CBT?

Conceptualizing psychological problems can be defined as the process by which the therapist and patient are able to form a joint understanding of the unique position of the individual's current difficulties (Freeman 1992; Persons, 1989; Butler, 1998; Tarrier and Calam 2002). A cognitive case formulation in CBT provides an overall picture, explains symptoms and generates hypotheses about maintaining factors, core beliefs or underlying mechanisms, origins and the future. It helps develop a treatment plan, in particular the choice of a specific intervention, and also helps to determine a criterion of change. It is helpful in dealing with hitches in treatment such as non-compliance, blocks and relationship issues. In order to be most effective, a cognitive case formulation needs to be parsimonious, easy to understand and explain, and helpful in choosing what to do and predicting difficulties, as well as, most importantly, 'fitting' the understanding of both the therapist and the patient.

Persons (1989) has introduced the helpful notion of problems being on two levels in case conceptualization: first, 'overt difficulties' which are everyday problems encountered by the individual such as anxiety or relationship problems; and, secondly, the 'underlying psychological mechanisms' which relate to the beliefs the individual holds that drive and maintain the overt difficulties. Overt difficulties can be conceptualized with the patient in the form of a vicious circle including the cognitive, physiological, emotional and behavioural elements of the problem. The underlying psychological mechanisms concern the beliefs held by the individual as a result of their early experiences.

It is important to differentiate between cognitive theory and cognitive case formulations in CBT. Cognitive theory provides general explanations and hypotheses, while a cognitive case formulation is idiosyncratic. A cognitive case formulation is specifically tailored to the individual, provides the bridge between theory and clinical practice and guides the treatment plan (Butler, 1998; Persons and Davidson, 2001). The cognitive case formulation remains a hypothesis and is open to adjustment and validation throughout therapy. Most importantly, it is always shared between the therapist and patient. The complexity and content of the cognitive case formulation shared with the child or adolescent will of course vary depending on their developmental level.

Williams *et al.* (1997) have proposed an aid to cognitive case formulation called 'mind maps' which might help some children and adolescents to remember their formulation. Mind mapping is an approach that allows a therapist to structure, organize and integrate information in the cognitive case formulation in a clear and easily updateable way. Mind maps are colourful, branching pictures or diagrams that can help memory, thinking and organization of ideas and information. They use images or key words to anchor information and, by using different modes of memory storage, they increase the modalities and ways in which information can be remembered.

Kinderman and Lobban (2000) have summarized another approach to sharing formulations with patients which may be useful with adolescents. Formulations can be developed and presented as they evolve, with interventions evolving in parallel. Early in the therapeutic process, simple formulations are presented which are systematically elaborated as therapy progresses. This involves developing, collaboratively with patients, successive layers of formulation. Each of these layers builds on and incorporates the previous one yet involves an incremental increase in complexity, depth and information content.

6.2   Issues to be considered when carrying out cognitive case formulations with children and adolescents

A number of important issues need to be considered when undertaking cognitive case formulations with children and adolescents. First, cognitions are in the process of developing throughout childhood and adolescence, influenced by a number of contextual factors including families, peers and schools. Secondly, the cognitive case formulation needs to be appropriate to the developmental level of the child. This is also true of the components and style of intervention (see Chapter 8), Finally, the role of the family in contributing to the development and maintenance of distorted cognitions, as well as contributing to protective factors and promoting change, is an important factor to consider. Developmental research has begun to identify the links between parental and child cognitions (Garber and Robinson, 1997). However, some fundamental research on cognitive models for children and adolescents would greatly enhance our ability to develop effective case formulations that incorporate these factors.

6.3   Cognitive case formulation-based or manual-based treatment for children and adolescents

The current debate in the adult CBT literature has been summarized by Tarrier and Calam (2002). They remark that there has been a tendency in adult CBT for cognitive case formulation to be adopted by the clinician who deals with the heterogeneity of clinical work compared with the clinical researcher who, through clinical trials, evaluates the efficacy of specific treatments. Evaluating involves restricting patients in the trial to a homogenous group and assessing a standardized treatment, usually manual based, a process which has been accused of becoming increasingly distanced from clinical practice. Tarrier and Calam (2002) summarize the current debate in adult CBT in two key questions: first, should standardized treatment or cognitive case formulation protocols be used in clinical research; and, secondly, should standardized treatment or cognitive case formulation protocols be used in clinical practice? Persons (1991) has advanced a strong argument for a type of research protocol that includes case formulation and ideographic assessment within a treatment protocol and efficacy trial.

In child and adolescent CBT, this debate is not taking place and it is suggested that one of the major reasons for this is that the cognitive case formulation approach has not been widely adopted by either clinicians or researchers. There is, however, a debate about the use of manuals in general, which has been summarized by Ollendick and King (2000). They suggest that adhering to a treatment manual might seem at odds with adapting the formulation approach for individuals but it need not be. They propose two questions: first, how does the manual provide a general framework for treating this individual and, secondly, what aspects of this particular client will facilitate my use of the treatment manual?

Much of the outcome research on CBT with children and adolescents has been based on manuals (for example, March and Mulle, 1998). There are many issues about using CBT manuals for children and adolescents. First of all, as with the whole field of child and adolescent CBT, there is no consistent definition of CBT. CBT is an umbrella term that covers different behavioural and cognitive techniques undertaken in different permutations. Linked to this, there has been no component analysis to determine which are the effective components of CBT. The manuals have been largely behavioural with little emphasis on cognitive processes, and few research studies have focused on producing and measuring the element of cognitive change. Some manuals also assume a uniform developmental level, although the age group they are aimed at is quite wide. Even when there is a family component, it is not modified to take into account the particular role any individual family is playing in the development and maintenance of the problem. However, it is suggested that, overall, one of the most significant problems may be the lack of cognitive case formulations.

Kendall and colleagues (Kendall, 1994; Kendall *et al.*, 1997, 2001) have produced a series of manuals which have been very influential in the field of child and adolescent CBT. In particular, their manual for anxiety has been the basis for much subsequent research (Barrett *et al.*, 1996; King *et al.*, 1998; Last *et al.*, 1998; Mendlowitz *et al.*, 1999; Silverman *et al.*, 1999; Barrett *et al.*, 2001). The manual is for a 16 session programme for individuals: sessions 1–8 are the training segment and sessions 9–16 are the practice segment. The strategies used are mainly behavioural, with the only cognitive components being identification and modification of self-talk. This cognitive technique dates back to the early work of Meichenbaum (1977). The manual was written for individual therapy; however, there is no element of individual cognitive case formulation. This therapy has had relatively good outcome but it is argued that unless the field moves on, as a number of the chapters in this book suggest, from a heavy reliance on old-fashioned approaches to cognition we will not be able to enhance treatment outcome any further. It is argued here that the way to enhance the outcome of CBT for children and adolescents is for all treatment to be based on individual cognitive case formulations, whether or not the treatment is manual based, and for a wider range of cognitive interventions to be used.

6.4 Newer approaches to cognition

Cognitive models are needed which incorporate important developmental and family factors and empirical studies which test predictions from these cognitive models. We can adapt adult cognitive models that identify the key cognitive abnormalities and the cognitive and behavioural maintaining factors. We can also develop new cognitive models that include both developmental and main-tenance factors. Research into cognitions could look at the content, distortions, specificity and development of cognitions in children and adolescents. It could also investigate how cognitions and cognitive change can be sensitively measured. Research also needs to explore how the current use of behavioural techniques impacts and modifies cognition. Another key area is the development of schemas in individuals and families and their intergenerational transmission.

There is great variability in both the nature and extent of the cognitive compo-nent in CBT for children and adolescents. Obsessive compulsive disorder (OCD) is an area where there are interesting examples of both the more behavioural and the more cognitive approaches to CBT. The more behavioural approach is described in Chapter 17. The more cognitive approach has been based on the cognitive theory of OCD developed by Rachman (1997) and Salkovskis (1999). The cognitive theory of OCD suggests that people who suffer from obsessional problems misinterpret intrusive thoughts as a sign that they may be responsible for harm to themselves or to others. This interpretation moti-vates neutralizing behaviours, which can strengthen and maintain the threat/responsibility appraisals. Treatment involves procedures which reduce such misinterpretations.

Case studies have been undertaken with adolescents using the cognitive approach to OCD. Shafran and Somers (1996) used this approach in the treatment of two adolescents with good outcome. Williams *et al.* (2002) treated a series of six adolescents using cognitive case formulations and the cognitive approach. They found that during the course of treatment appraisals of responsibility changed at the same time as changes in symptom levels. These initial studies are very interesting and suggest the need to investigate further a more cognitive approach to the treatment of adolescents with OCD.

6.5   The role of the family in CBT

The role of the family is important in both cognitive case formulations and interventions based on them. There are many ways in which family factors can be included when developing a cognitive case formulation. It is possible to undertake separate cognitive case formulations for each parent and sibling as well as the child, or to combine these factors into a single formulation. The therapist may choose to focus solely on specific aspects of family involvement – e.g. to identify key distorted parental beliefs which are also present in the child – or may choose to identify only aspects of parent and sibling behaviour which are maintaining the child's disorder.

It is proposed here that it is important to consider the role of the family in the development and maintenance of distorted cognitions at all levels of a cognitive case formulation. Families have an important role in the development of schemas. They may also have a role in triggering and maintaining problems both through their cognitions (e.g. selective attention, attribution, expectancies and assumptions) and their behaviours such as reassurance and overprotection. Johnstone and Patenaude (1994) have proposed that the causal attributions which parents make regarding children's behaviour influence their responses to the child. To take the example of depression, White and Barrowclough (1998) found that depressed mothers made more spontaneous causal attributions about their children's problem behaviour and perceived these causes as being more personal and unique to the child, more stable and more under the child's voluntary control. The tendency to attribute child behaviour problems to factors that were idiosyncratic or personal to the child was predictive of both a diagnosis of depression and to higher depression scores on a standardized measure. The authors suggest that these attributions may mediate coping responses and hence may influence parenting behaviour. Interestingly, Garber and Robinson (1997) have shown that, after controlling for the level of depression, there remain differences between attributional style and perceived self-worth in the children of depressed mothers. Taking these two findings together, it is proposed that the cognitions and behaviour of the parent towards the child might have led to the formation of negative schema in the child. These negative schema might be maintained by the continuing negative cognitions and behaviour of the parent. In turn, the negative schema of the parent might be maintained by the negative cognitions and behaviour of the child.

Involving families in cognitive case formulations is at an early stage of development. As discussed previously, much of CBT outcome research in children and adolescents does not in any case involve interventions based on cognitive case formulations. However, it is interesting to review research on those CBT interventions which have included family members to see if there is evidence that involving families enhances the effectiveness of CBT. Barrett *et al.* (1996, 2001) compared individual CBT with CBT plus family anxiety management (FAM). Both groups showed significant improvement compared with a waiting list control, and self-report and clinician ratings indicated added benefits from CBT plus FAM. However, their 6-year follow-up showed that CBT plus FAM was no more effective than CBT alone. Cobham *et al.* (1998) found the inclusion of a family component increased efficacy only for those children who had at least one anxious parent. Mendlowitz *et al.* (1999) found parental involvement to be superior with regard to the child's active coping strategies, but not in child anxiety levels. Spence *et al.* (2000) found CBT effectiveness was not significantly greater when a family component was added.

Albano and Kendall (2002) make these mixed findings even more interesting by their comment that parents are also involved in individually delivered CBT interventions based on Kendall's manual. They comment that the clinician assesses each individual situation and 'doses' the parental involvement. Thirteen randomized controlled trials have been based on Kendall's manual and provide strong support for its effectiveness. However, as there has been no component analysis of Kendall's CBT package, and the amount of involvement of the parents has varied between individuals, the contribution of parental involvement to its effectiveness cannot be determined.

Turning more specifically to cognition, Nuata *et al.* (2003) compared CBT alone with CBT plus cognitive parent training (CPT) and found no additional effect of CPT. The authors comment that, as they had no measure to assess changes in parental cognitions, they were not able to assess whether parental cognitions changed, although this did not affect the anxiety of the child, or whether these cognitions did not change at all. The current status of research findings into the cognitive aspects of family involvement in CBT suggest that we have limited ideas about what cognitive change is necessary to improve outcome. It is not clear what cognitive change, if any, is being produced by current interventions, and we have no idea how to maintain cognitive change that is produced.

It is proposed that the lack of cognitive case formulations is another factor which may partly explain the mixed findings in treatment interventions involving families. A cognitive case formulation including the family factors would guide the treatment intervention. The therapist has many choices about how to involve the family in the treatment intervention. The therapist might choose not to involve the family but work only with the individual, as, for example, with an adolescent. This individual intervention could still involve looking at family factors. It is suggested that as current CBT interventions involving the family are not usually based on a cognitive case formulation this limits the effectiveness of these interventions and contributes to the mixed findings. Furthermore, if the child and family have little or no understanding of their formulation, this might contribute to the effectiveness of the intervention decreasing over time, or even lead to relapse. Hence, the issue of the involvement of families in both cognitive case formulation and interventions for children and adolescents is at an interesting stage of development.

6.6   A case example of a cognitive case formulation for anxiety

While recognizing the need to develop new cognitive models for children and adolescents, it is important not to dismiss adult cognitive models and the range of techniques used to modify cognition based on these models. Piacentini and Bergman (2001) reviewed the cognitive process thought to underlie the development and maintenance of anxiety disorders across the age span and the cognitive and behavioural treatment interventions that arise from this framework. Their review proposes that, although the study of cognitive process related to anxiety has focused on adults, the available data appear to support the notion that these cognitive processes play a similar role in childhood anxiety. This conclusion is supported by the work of Shafran and Somers (1996) and Williams et al. (2002).

A major problem is that the multi-component treatment packages (e.g. Kendall, 1994; Kendall et al., 1997) span a wide age range, including both children and adolescents, but use simple cognitive concepts such as modification of self-talk. It is proposed that adolescents, in particular, can benefit from cognitive case formulations based on adult cognitive models and the wide range of cognitive interventions which are based on these models. A case example will be described which aims to illustrate a cognitive case formulation and treatment interventions based on it which are largely cognitive rather than largely behavioural.

John is a 14-year-old boy with presenting problems of panic attacks, fear of illness and death, depression and family problems. He is the youngest of three children by a wide margin and feels isolated and unloved. A year before the onset of John's problems, his mother had an affair and blamed John and his siblings for the subsequent break-up of the marriage. John's father always worried about people being ill and dying. He is very concerned with his and other people's health, particularly since one of his brothers had suffered an early stroke. John's early history included an episode of anxiety problems when he was 10, which was treated with graded exposure.

John's current problems began following his second uncle having a heart attack. Shortly afterwards, John describes going to the toilet and looking at the carpet and thinking it sloped upwards. He thought that there was something wrong with his head and panicked. He began to have panic attacks twice a day and started avoiding going out, checking himself for odd symptoms, asking for repeated reassurance, trying to control his breathing, trying to distract himself by tapping his legs and sitting down when he felt anxious. He became depressed as he felt helpless to overcome his panics and thought they were ruining his life.

The first element of the conceptualization was for the panic attacks and was based on the cognitive theory of panic (Clark, 1986). This theory suggests that individuals panic as they have a tendency to interpret a wide range of bodily sensations in a catastrophic fashion. The sensations which are misinterpreted are mainly those involved in normal anxiety responses such as palpitations or breathlessness. The catastrophic misinterpretation involves perceiving these sensations as indications of an immediately impending physical or mental disaster such as a heart attack, or loss of control of thoughts and madness. In John's case, the trigger for his first panic attack was looking down quickly and thinking the carpet sloped upwards. He had the thought 'What if this is caused by a brain tumour?' and his belief rating for this thought was 100%. He became anxious and experienced dizziness, sweating and shaking as part of an anxiety response. He made the catastrophic misinterpretation that these symptoms meant he was dying.

The second element of the conceptualization was for his health anxiety. The cognitive theory of health anxiety states that bodily signs, symptoms, variations and medical information tend to be perceived as more dangerous than they really are, and that a particular illness is believed to be more probable than it really is (Salkovskis and Warwick, 1986). At the same time, people are likely to perceive themselves as unable to prevent the illness, unable to affect its course and having no effective means of coping with the perceived threat. If the sensations or signs are not those that increase as a result of anxiety, or the person does not regard the feared catastrophe as immediate, then the reaction will be health anxiety. However, if the symptoms that are misinterpreted are those that occur as part of anxiety-induced autonomic arousal, and the interpretation is that the symptoms are the signs of an immediate catastrophe, the symptoms will increase and a panic attack is the more likely response.

In John's case, he had both panic attacks and health anxiety. Triggers for his health anxiety included missing when reaching for something or moving his head suddenly. He would have thoughts such as 'I have a brain tumour, brain haemorrhage or multiple sclerosis.' The psychological factors maintaining his beliefs included, first of all, cognitive factors such as focusing on body sensations, a preoccupation with health worries and a bias towards confirmatory evidence of illness. Another factor was increased physiological arousal resulting from the perception of threat. Finally, there were a number of behavioural factors maintaining his health anxiety such as reassurance seeking, avoiding going out, tapping his legs, checking his eyesight and specific safety behaviours such as sitting down and moving slowly.

The role of the family was considered in the development and maintenance of John's problems at all levels of the cognitive case formulation. His early experience of relationships within the family were involved in the development of his core beliefs. To give specific examples, illness in the family and his father's health anxiety were important in the development of his beliefs and assumptions about health, and father and son shared several of these. His cognitions about being unloved and no-one looking after him were understandable in the context of his parents' marital problems and his mother's negative and rejecting statements and behaviour over many years. The critical incident was another example of ill health in the family, and the maintaining factors included his family repeatedly giving John reassurance when he asked for it.

Throughout assessment and treatment, the conceptualization was refined and modified. An overall conceptualization was developed which included family factors and brought together early experience, core beliefs, dysfunctional assumptions, the critical incident and the current problem in four systems: cognitive, behavioural, affective and physiological. All aspects of the conceptualization were arrived at jointly with John (Figure 6.1).

A treatment plan was developed based on this conceptualization. The next section will describe only the techniques used to modify cognition derived from the adult cognitive model. The panic attacks were tackled first and the treatment was based on the techniques used by Clark (1996). These involve, first of all, identifying catastrophic interpretations of bodily sensations and then generating

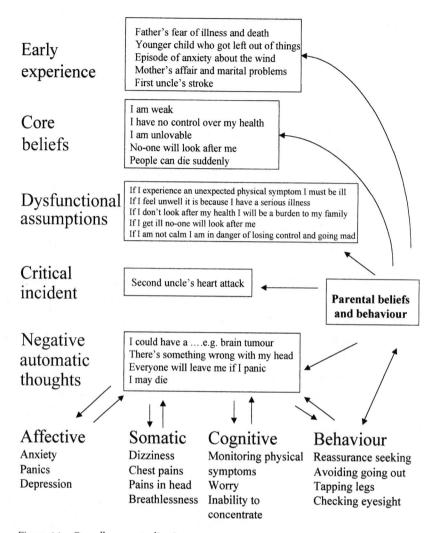

Figure 6.1   Overall conceptualization.

alternative, non-catastrophic interpretations. Then, the validity of catastrophic and non-catastrophic interpretations is tested by discussion and behavioural experiments. Behavioural experiments were set up to show John that the feared catastrophe did not happen. All of John's symptoms were elicited and worked through systematically – e.g. feelings of distancing and unreality. As always in the cognitive approach to CBT, the aim of the behavioural experiments was to change cognition.

A range of cognitive techniques was used for John's problems including cognitive restructuring. John also had thought–fact fusion as he believed that if he thought something it must be true. For example, he believed if he had the thought that his sister would have a heart attack it would happen, or if he thought he had lung cancer it must be true. Examples were worked on in the session to show that thinking something does not mean it is true. Humorous examples were included such as: if you think the moon is made of blue cheese, does that mean it is true?

Imagery modification was undertaken as John had a recurrent image of falling down on the pavement and nobody helping him. We worked on unpacking the meaning in the image, and then helped John to transform the image to change the meaning. After transformation, his image included friends picking him up and saying to him that it was just an image. Naturally occurring disconfirmatory evidence was also used. One example was John thought that if he did not set his alarm clock he would never wake up in the morning. One morning his alarm clock did not ring and this was used as evidence to disconfirm his thought. Other aspects of therapy included working together on stopping as many maintaining factors as possible such as avoidances (e.g. avoiding going out of the house) and safety behaviours (e.g. sitting down so he couldn't fall down).

Intervention on the family factors was carried out only with John and his adult older sister as both parents refused to attend for sessions. John's older sister was involved in the development of the cognitive case conceptualization and the subsequent intervention based on it. She helped John address some of the family factors' including the role of their father's health anxiety and the effect of their parents' marital problems on the development and maintenance of John's problems. She was also actively involved in decreasing reassurance seeking. The treatment had good outcome as measured on standardized questionnaires and improvement was maintained at 1-year follow-up.

It is interesting to compare this case study with one published by Ollendick (1995) which used a more behavioural approach to CBT. Ollendick's case study also involved a 14-year-old patient with panic, combined in this case with agoraphobia. The treatment involved, first of all, examining the nature of panic and the differences between it and anxiety. Subsequent sessions involved teaching relaxation techniques and developing positive self-statements and self-instructional strategies derived from Meichenbaum (1977). An exposure hierarchy of agoraphobic situations was developed and *in vivo* exposure sessions occurred with the therapist or the parent outside clinic sessions (Table 6.1).

Both single case studies had good outcome. However, the nature of the cognitive elements and the range of cognitive techniques used in the case study described here based on cognitive models are strikingly different. Research is needed to explore how the current use of behavioural techniques impacts on

Table 6.1 The techniques used to modify cognition in each of the case studies

Ollendick (1995)	Case study

• Identification of anxious self-statements
• Replace them with coping self-statements
	(1) Explaining the cognitive model
	(2) Joint cognitive case formulation
	(3) Behavioural experiments to test cognitions
	(4) Cognitive techniques:
	   • cognitive restructuring
	   • thought–fact fusion
	   • modification of imagery
	   • using naturally occurring
	    disconfirmatory evidence
	(5) Stopping avoidances and safety
	   behaviours which prevent cognitive
	   change
	(6) Education about anxiety, including
	   anxious cognitions, and specific illnesses

and modifies cognition, e.g. the use of exposure within a cognitive framework. These two case examples highlight the current marked differences in the field.

6.7 The way forward

CBT is committed to empirical validation both in terms of its basic theoretical premises and treatment outcome. The issues around cognitive case formulation are no different and should be resolved by reference to empirical findings. Fundamental research is needed to develop cognitive models that, unlike current adult cognitive models, include the development as well as the maintenance of psychological problems. Adult as well as child and adolescent CBT would benefit greatly from these models and the treatments derived from them.

Further research is also needed in a range of different areas. Some of these include: a comparison of cognitive case formulation-based versus manual-based treatment; CBT with a more behavioural approach versus a more cognitive approach; the role of the family in cognitive case formulations and the interventions derived from them; large RCTs which compare CBT against active comparison treatments; and longitudinal studies. It is suggested here that shifting towards a more cognitive approach to CBT, including using individual cognitive case formulations, may be an effective way forwards for child and adolescent CBT.

6.8   REFERENCES

Albano, A. M. and Kendall, P. C. (2002). Cognitive behavioural therapy for children and adolescents with anxiety disorders: clinical research advances. *International Review of Psychiatry*, **14**, 129–34.

Barrett, M., Dadds, M. R. and Rapee, R. (1996). Family treatment of childhood anxiety: a controlled trial. *Journal of Consulting and Clinical Psychology*, **64**, 333–42.

Barrett, M., Duffy, A. L., Dadds, M. R. and Rapee, R. (2001). Cognitive-behavioural treatment of anxiety disorders in children; long term (6 year) follow-up. *Journal of Consulting and Clinical Psychology*, **69**, 135–41.

Butler, G. (1998). Clinical formulation. In A. S. Bellack and M. Henson (eds.), *Comprehensive Clinical Psychology*, Volume 6. Elsevier.

Clark, D. M. (1986). A cognitive approach to panic disorder. *Behaviour Research and Therapy*, **24**, 461–70.

(1996). Panic disorder: from theory to therapy. In P. M. Salkovskis (ed.), *Frontiers of Cognitive Therapy*. New York: Guilford Press, pp. 318–44.

Cobham, V. E., Dadds, M. R. and Spence, S. H. (1998). The role of parental anxiety in the treatment of childhood anxiety. *Journal of Consulting and Clinical Psychology*, **66**, 893–905.

Freeman, A. (1992). The development of treatment conceptualisations in cognitive therapy. In A. Freeman and F. M. Dattillio (eds.), *Comprehensive Case Book of Cognitive Therapy*. New York: Plenum.

Garber, J. and Robinson, N. S. (1997). Cognitive vulnerability in children at risk for depression. *Cognition and Emotion*, **11**, 619–35.

Johnstone, C. and Patenaude, R. (1994). Parent attributions for inattentive-overactive and oppositional-defiant child behaviours. *Cognitive Therapy and Research*, **18**, 261–75.

Kendall P. C. (1994). Treating anxiety disorders in children: results of a randomised clinical trial. *Journal of Consulting and Clinical Psychology*, **62**, 100–10.

Kendall, P. C., Brady, E. U. and Verduin, T. L. (2001). Comorbidity in childhood anxiety disorder and treatment outcome. *Journal of the American Academy of Child and Adolescent Psychiatry*, **40**, 787–94.

Kendall, P. C., Flannery-Schroeder, E., Panichelli-Mindel, S. M. *et al.* (1997). Therapy for youth with anxiety disorders: a second randomised clinical trial. *Journal of Consulting and Clinical Psychology*, **65**, 366–80.

Kinderman, P. and Lobban (2000). Evolving formulations: sharing complex information with clients. *Behavioural and Cognitive Psychotherapy*, **28**, 307–10.

King, N. J., Tonge, B. J., Heyne, D. *et al.* (1998). Cognitive-behavioural treatment of panic disorder with agoraphobia in adolescents: a controlled evaluation. *Journal of the American Academy of Child and Adolescent Psychiatry*, **37**, 395–403.

Last, C. J. Hansen, C. and Franco, N. (1998). Cognitive-behavioural treatment of school phobia. *Journal of the American Academy of Child and Adolescent Psychiatry*, **37**, 404–11.

March, J. S. and Mulle, K. (1998). *OCD in Children and Adolescents. A Cognitive-Behavioural Treatment Manual*. New York: Guilford Press.

Meichenbaum, D. (1977). *Cognitive-Behaviour Modification: An Integrative Approach*. New York: Plenum.

Mendlowitz, S. L., Manassis, K. Bradley, S. *et al.* (1999). Cognitive-behavioural group treatments in childhood anxiety disorders: the role of parental involvement. *Journal of the American Academy of Child and Adolescent Psychiatry*, **38**, 1223–9.

Nuata, M. H., Scholing, A., Emmelkamp, P. M. G. and Minderaa, R. B. (2003). Cognitive-behavioural therapy for children with anxiety disorders in a clinical setting: no additional effect of a cognitive parent training. *Journal of the American Academy of Child and Adolescent Psychiatry*, **42**, 1270–8.

Ollendick, T. H. (1995). Cognitive behavioural treatment of panic disorder with agoraphobia in adolescents: a multiple baseline design analysis. *Behavioural Therapy*, **26**, 517–31.

Ollendick, T. H. and King, N. J. (2000). Empirically supported treatments for children and adolescents. In P. C. Kendall (ed.), *Child and Adolescent Therapy: Cognitive-Behavioural Procedures*. New York: Guilford Press.

Persons, J. B. (1989). *Cognitive Therapy in Practice. A Case Formulation Approach*. New York: Norton.

Persons, J. B. (1991). Psychotherapy outcome studies do not accurately represent current models of psychotherapy. *American Psychologist*, **46**, 99–106.

Persons, J. B. and Davidson, J. (2001). Cognitive-behavioural case formulation. In K. Dobson (ed.), *Handbook of Cognitive-Behavioural Therapies*, 2nd edn. New York: Guilford Press.

Piacentini, J. and Bergman, R. L. (2001). Developmental issues in cognitive therapy for childhood anxiety disorders. *Journal of Cognitive Psychotherapy: An International Quarterly*, **15**, 165–82.

Rachman, S. J. (1997). A cognitive theory of obsessions. *Behaviour Research and Therapy*, **35**, 793–802.

Salkovskis, P. M. (1999). Understanding and treating obsessive-compulsive disorder. *Behaviour Research and Therapy*, **37**, 29–52.

Salkovskis, P. M. and Warwick, H. M. C. (1986). Morbid preoccupations, health anxiety and reassurance: a cognitive behavioural approach to hypochondriasis. *Behaviour Research and Therapy*, **24**, 597–602.

Shafran, R. and Somers, J. (1996). Treating adolescent obsessive-compulsive disorder: applications of the cognitive theory. *Behaviour Research and Therapy*, **36**, 93–97.

Silverman, W. K., Kurtines, W. M. and Ginsburg G. S. *et al.* (1999). Treating anxiety disorders in children with group cognitive-behavioural therapy: a randomised clinical trial. *Journal of Consulting and Clinical Psychology*, **67**, 995–1003.

Spence, S. H., Donovan, C. and Brechman-Toussaint, M. (2000). The treatment of childhood social phobia: the effectiveness of a social skills training based cognitive-behavioural intervention, with and without parental involvement. *Journal of Child Psychology and Psychiatry*, **41**, 713–26.

Tarrier, N. and Calam, R. (2002). New developments in cognitive-behavioural case formulation. Epidemiological, systemic and social context: an integrative approach. *Behavioural and Cognitive Psychotherapy*, **30**, 311–28.

White, C. and Barrowclough, C. (1998). Depressed and non-depressed mothers with problematic preschoolers: attributions for child behaviours. *British Journal of Clinical Psychology*, **37**, 358–98.

Williams, C., Williams, S. and Appleton, K. (1997). Mind maps: an aid to effective formulation. *Behavioural and Cognitive Psychotherapy*, **25**, 261–7.

Williams, T. I., Salkovskis, P. M., Forrester, E. A. and Allsop, M. A. (2002). Changes in symptoms of OCD and appraisal of responsibility during cognitive behavioural treatment: a pilot study. *Behavioural and Cognitive Psychotherapy*, **30**, 69–78.

Part III

Client groups

7

Working with parents: some ethical and practical issues

Miranda Wolpert and Julie Elsworth

Dunstable Health Centre, Dunstable, UK

Jenny Doe

Luton Family Consultation Clinic, Luton, UK

7.1 Introduction

While there have been increasing attempts to respond to Kendall's call to 'unravel the role of parental involvement in the outcome of child therapy' (Kendall, 1994), there is still little solid research evidence to guide clinicians as to how best involve parents in cognitive behavioural therapy (CBT) for children and young people. It has been suggested that parents can be conceived as being involved in CBT with their children in three broad possible roles: facilitator, co-therapist or client (Stallard, 2002b). What research literature there is suggests that involving parents in one or more of these roles may be beneficial in the short-to-medium term for a range of presenting problems, and particularly for younger children, although the long-term gains are less clear (Barrett *et al.*, 1996; Fonagy *et al.*, 2002).

The majority of the literature on CBT for children and young people continues to reflect its 'adult' roots in terms of its primary focus on individual work with children themselves. While recent works have stressed the need to adopt a systemic perspective (e.g. Friedburg and McClure, 2002; Stallard, 2002a) there has been little detailed discussion of how this might be achieved. Moreover, there has been little examination of what factors need to be taken into account when determining the nature and extent of parental involvement, how parental roles might be negotiated and agreed with the parents themselves or how wider or more complex family issues might be addressed.

In this chapter, we will explore some of the tensions that arise when trying to apply CBT to work with children in the context of working with their families

Cognitive Behaviour Therapy for Children and Families, ed. Philip J. Graham.
Published by Cambridge University Press. © Cambridge University Press 2004.

Table 7.1 Theoretical, practical and ideological underpinnings of cognitive behavioural therapy

Theoretical underpinnings	Key techniques (adapted from Beck, 1995)	Ideological underpinnings
• Focus on how thoughts, feelings and behaviour all affect each other	• Base interventions on an ever-evolving formulation in cognitive (and behavioural) terms	• Commitment to openness and partnership
• Individual focus • No interest in unconscious motivation	• Requires sound therapeutic alliance • Emphasizes collaboration and active participation • Goal orientated and problem focused	• Principle of minimum invasiveness • Belief in resilience • Problems are continuum with normal difficulties encountered
• Change is not necessarily dependent on knowing ultimate cause, although this may be explored	• Initial emphasis is on the present • Educative and focus on relapse prevention • Time limited • Structured sessions	• Optimistic about possibilities of change
• It is necessary to understand the relationship between thoughts, feelings and behaviour in relation to the problem	• Teach client to identify, evaluate and respond to unhelpful thoughts and beliefs • Use range of techniques to change thinking mood and behaviour e.g. Socratic questioning, relaxation techniques, exposure and response prevention, emotional recognition	• Client-determined goals

and discuss how these tensions might be addressed. The authors have not set out to review specific structured programmes for parents, which are dealt with in relation to specific presenting problems in other chapters. Rather, the aim is to concentrate on the ethical and practical issues raised by trying to adopt a systemic perspective when using CBT in relation to children and young people.

Our thinking on these issues has developed largely out of the authors' clinical work, in which it is rare for children to attend without some family involvement. In clinical practice, the authors often find it valuable to draw on other therapeutic traditions, such as family therapy and narrative therapy, to enable effective use of CBT with children and their families. The authors have come to view many aspects of these therapeutic techniques as compatible with CBT theory and practice, and feel that they may present one possible starting point for developing a distinctive cognitive behavioural approach, embedded in systemic practice, to working with families and the wider system.

Although 'parents' are referred to throughout this chapter, carers, guardians or other adults who may be in *loco parentis* are also included.

7.2   Tensions arising out of trying to apply CBT to work with family systems

In Table 7.1, some of the key components of CBT theory, practice and ideology are teased out. Theory, practice and ideology are consistent with each other when working with an individual self-determined client. However, when working with systems rather than individuals, the links between theory, practice and ideology of CBT can raise specific challenges for clinicians. For example, how should the principle of 'client-determined goals' (column 3; Table 7.1) be interpreted when working with parents and children? Who should be regarded as the client? If a child is referred because he is refusing to attend school and, during assessment, he makes it clear that he does not wish to return to school despite his parents' wish that he do so, whose views should take priority? If a mother brings her child to therapy and reports that her divorced husband does not feel his daughter needs to change her behaviour, how should the therapist address this?

In terms of the principles of 'minimum invasiveness' and 'individual focus' (columns 1 and 3; Table 7.1), how can these be balanced against the need to look at wider family issues in some cases? If a child is referred because of high levels of anxiety and the parents spend much of the assessment session arguing and berating each other, do these marital issues need to be addressed before the child can be seen individually? If a family requests individual CBT for the child, saying the child's behaviour is causing all the many problems in family members, how should the therapist tackle this? If a therapist has child protection concerns, does this mean individual CBT is not appropriate?

In terms of the principles and practice of promoting 'collaboration' and 'partnership' (columns 2 and 3; Table 7.1) how is this best to be achieved with different family members? Should professional correspondence be copied to all family members or just to some? Should absent partners be contacted routinely or not? If one or both of the parents' first language is not English, how should the clinician accommodate this? If individual CBT for the child is deemed to be the treatment of choice, what is the best way to involve parents? Should parents be present in sessions or not? On what basis should the clinician decide on this?

These clinical challenges can be grouped as relating to one of three areas of potential tension, which can be termed 'domains of ethical concern':

(1)   challenges arising out of the need to balance different viewpoints;

(2)   challenges arising out of the need to address family issues while maintaining an individual focus; and

(3)   challenges arising out of the desire to promote genuine collaboration with different members of the system.

The issues grouped under each domain are summarized in Table 7.2.

These challenges face most clinical contacts with children, not just those with CBT focus, and some of the comments below would relate to any clinical contact with children and their families. As yet, CBT has not developed a distinctive way of responding to these challenges (Kendall and Morris, 1991). This chapter will draw out those aspects that may present the way forward for a distinctive CBT approach to these issues and will highlight those areas that need further research. We will explore each of these domains in turn.

7.2.1   Balancing competing views

In offering CBT to an individual child or young person, the therapist is situated in a complex nexus of professional, legal and ethical responsibilities that requires him or her to collaborate with parents (*The Children's Act, 1989*), respect the views and rights of children (Royal College of Psychiatry, 1997; *The Human Rights Act, 2000*) and collaborate where possible with other professional systems. Any young person's contact with a mental health service is likely to involve a complex system of relationships between parents, children and professionals (Glaser, 1996). Those involved in a child's contact with a mental health professional might include one or more parents, carers, other adult family members, guardians, others with corporate or statutory responsibility for the child's welfare, consult organizations/professionals as well as referred children themselves.

Table 7.2 Domains of ethical concern in using CBT with children and parents

Domain of ethical concern	Example where trying to apply CBT principles may raise difficulties	Key questions that need to be addressed
Balancing viewpoints	How can the commitment to openness and partnership be maintained in the face of competing viewpoints?	Who gives consent to treatment? Who determines the goals and outcomes of treatment? What should be done when the views of different family members are in conflict?
Addressing family issues	The principle of minimum invasiveness may mean that underlying family problems may not be addressed which may be detrimental to the best interests of the child	How can family issues best be assessed and dealt with? Is it appropriate to maintain an individual focus when working with children and their families?
Promoting genuine collaboration	There may be a lack of clarity about the role of parents in relation to therapy – parents may be spoken of as 'co-therapists' but really treated as patients Is it possible to be truly collaborative with all family members bearing in mind the power differentials existing between adults (therapists and parents) and children?	How can it best be determined and acknowledged what role should parents play in an intervention? How can involvement in decision making by all relevant family members best be optimized?

There may be little concordance between these different groups as to how they see the problem (Angold *et al.*, 1987; Klein, 1991), what they want in relation to particular episodes of clinical care or how they judge the success of the outcome (Hennessy, 1999). In relation to each of these aspects of the work, all of these groups may have competing views, wishes and interests (Pearce, 1994). Thus, in most routine work with children, the clinician is involved in balancing different views and goals. Clinicians need to tread a delicate line in trying to achieve balance between: (1) respecting the rights and wishes of young people; (2) respecting the rights of parents; (3) fulfilling a professional obligation to protect young people; and (4) ensuring full access to appropriate health care (Fuggle *et al.*, 2001).

At its most extreme, differences of opinion between children and their parents may lead to conflict around consent for treatment that may raise complex legal and ethical issues. Although such stark differences of opinion do not arise in the vast majority of cases, clinicians need always to be mindful of who is consenting to treatment and how this is being assessed. Therefore, the formal issues around consent will be addressed, before more common issues arising from the need to balance competing views in everyday clinical work with children and their families using CBT are explored.

7.2.1.1   Family members' roles in giving consent to treatment

CBT should only be undertaken when there is informed consent given by the child and/or by relevant others. Clinicians need to start any clinical work with children and families with a clear understanding as to who is providing consent for treatment.

Where the children are competent to make an informed choice themselves, their views (rather than those of their parents or other stakeholders) should be primary, as long as the therapist does not regard them as against the child's own best interests (British Medical Association, 1995; Royal College of Psychiatrists, 1997). Refusal by a competent child who consistently expresses a wish not to participate in an intervention, which is considered to be in his/her best interests, may require adjudication by a court. In practice, overriding a competent child's wishes in this circumstance is likely only to be justifiable in circumstances where there is a significant threat to life or long-term significant harm and where the benefits of an intervention are relatively clear.

In general, published guidance suggests that young people aged 16–18 years are presumed to be competent to give consent unless there are explicit reasons for invoking legal procedures, such as the use of the Mental Health Act. For children and young people under 16 years, either a child, a parent, a local authority (for children in care) or a court can provide consent. For this group, there is not a presumption of competence to give consent and the clinician is required to assess whether the patient is competent to provide consent if the issue arises. A competent young person should have 'sufficient understanding and intelligence to enable him/her to fully understand what is being proposed' (*Gillick* v. *West Norfolk and Wisbech Area Health Authority*, 1986). This requires an understanding of the risks and benefits of the intervention beyond the immediate discomforts and inconveniences that treatment may entail.

Where children are not considered to be competent to provide consent, either a parent, local authority or a court can determine treatment in line with the clinician's view of the child's best interests. Parental responsibility rests with the mother of the child. The father also has parental responsibility if he was married to the child's mother at the time of birth or if he has registered to have 'parental responsibility'. Parental responsibility is not abnegated if a child is in care to the local authority or adopted.

While everyone with parental responsibility should ideally be involved in decision making, disagreements between parents do not necessarily prevent decisions being made. The Children's Act states that 'where more than one person has parental responsibility for a child, each of them may act alone'. Where those sharing responsibility disagree on an issue, the onus is on the person objecting to the course of action to seek a court order to prevent it (Bainham, 1998). If parents are separated, it is good practice to keep the absent parent informed where possible, but there is no legal requirement to do so and this will have to be balanced against other factors and always judged in relation to the best interests of the child. Careful handling is often needed to avoid treatment decisions being caught up in conflicts between parents (FOCUS, 1999).

7.2.1.2   Involving family members in decision making

Regardless of who has given consent to treatment, we believe that any intervention should be carried out in a way that supports both the child and parents in active participation in decision making. This requires that children be provided with clear information tailored to their developmental level and their views about key aspects of the intervention plan be elicited. Similarly, parents should be provided with accessible information that takes into account their language requirements and any other specific relevant factors. Information provided should include the nature of planned work, likely benefits and risks and any possible alternatives to what is planned. In addition, clear agreements should be reached about the nature of confidentiality the child will be afforded in any individual work. The creation of individual contracts, written with each individual child and their family, has been found useful in some child service settings as one means of addressing these issues (Maguire *et al.*, 2001; Wolpert *et al.*, 2001). Others have found this to be helpful in individual cases, although excessively bureaucratic if applied universally.

In many cases, it may also be necessary and desirable to involve other interested systems, such as schools or social services, in decision making – although this should only be done with relevant family members' consent.

7.2.1.3   Working with different views of the problem

Determining whose goals and issues should be prioritized is often an ongoing and complex negotiation in CBT with children and their families. The authors believe it is important at the outset of therapy to elicit and acknowledge any differences in the view of the problem before working towards finding a way of agreeing common understanding and goals. In exploring differences of view, Stallard (2002b) has suggested that the therapist needs to maintain a 'detached, objective and impartial position'. Others have argued that a position of objective impartiality may be unobtainable, but that therapists need to be as aware as possible of their own biases and views and try to manage different perspectives by allowing them space to be heard, and by offering their own views and thoughts as appropriate (Wilkinson, 1998).

Drawing on systemic interview techniques and understandings may be of help in initial meetings with families as a way of opening up and exploring differences in perception between family members as to what they see as the problem and what they want done about it (Watzlawick *et al.*, 1974; Hoffman, 1981; McGoldrick, 1998). The work of Pearce and Cronen (1980), in particular, can be seen as applying a cognitive approach to family communication by exploring and elucidating how underlying beliefs (both individual and shared) may influence the behaviour and relationships of individual members.

'Reflexive questioning', a form of questioning used in family therapy (Tomm 1987a,b), can be employed to help family members challenge their own beliefs and cognitions. Reflexive questions are defined as: 'questions asked with the intent to . . . (activate) . . . the reflexivity among meaning within pre-existing belief systems that enable family members to generate or generalize constructive patterns of cognition or behaviour on their own' (Tomm, 1987a). While the language is different from that of CBT, the underlying principles could be seen as similar in that, by challenging false beliefs and cognitions, the individual members in the family are encouraged to come up with more constructive alternative understanding.

The technique of 'reframing' that arises out of the systemic literature may also be powerfully employed with families in helping them come to a shared view of the difficulties. 'Reframing' involves the therapist in encouraging family members to apply new meanings, which facilitate the development of a more positive slant on particular behaviours or events. For example, a child labelled as aggressive by his parents may be referred to, in another context, as passionate. If the therapist refers to the 'aggressive outbursts' as 'passionate outbursts', alternative meanings may be given to the same behaviour (Wilkinson, 1998).

Where possible, the aim is for the therapist and all family members to come to a view of the difficulties that does not involve blaming the referred child or other family members, but that positions all family members as collaborating to overcome the difficulties. Michael White's use of externalizing conversations, which use interview techniques to emphasize a shared way forward and do not dwell on issues of causation, seems to the authors to be concordant with general

CBT theory and practice (see Table 7.1) and provides a useful way forward in this regard (White and Epston, 1990). March (see Chapter 17) draws on the work of Michael White in helping parents understand their child's obsessive compulsive disorder as something outside the child's or parent's control that they can all work on together (March and Mulle, 1998).

7.2.2   Addressing family issues

We recommend that, wherever possible, clinicians should undertake a thorough assessment of the child, their family and the school context before any decision is made about whether individual CBT may be appropriate.

The aim of this family assessment is to assess the nature of the problem, clarify different people's views and help arrive at a shared formulation of the problem and action plan. It is not within the scope of this chapter to suggest how best to undertake a full family assessment – readers are referred to Wilkinson (1998) and Carr (1999) for useful overviews of this topic. However, it is perhaps worth reiterating that such an assessment does not just serve to provide information for the clinician, it can also be used in attempts to develop a shared formulation of the difficulties that all family members can agree on.

In terms of the distinctive CBT aspects of this assessment in relation to working with parents, two related but separate questions need to be addressed: to what extent can the presenting difficulties be understood as linked to family issues, and to what extent is direct intervention with the parent(s) indicated?

In terms of assessing how far the presenting difficulties can be understood as linked to family issues, it is widely accepted that for many difficulties parental views and behaviours influence the development of difficulties in the child (Carr, 1999). For example, anxious children are more likely to have parents with a range of anxiety problems, and family processes have been shown to contribute to avoidant responses in anxious children (Barrett et al., 1996). Similarly, in relation to disruptive and conduct-disordered children, there is much evidence to show the powerful effects of parental behaviours and cognitions in the development and course of such difficulties (Kazdin, 1995).

In some cases, family assessment may indicate that family issues are so significant as to preclude CBT as an approach in the first instance. If there are significant child protection concerns, these may need addressing prior to any therapeutic intervention being offered. Similarly, family assessment may reveal major parental mental health issues or marital stresses that need addressing as a primary focus. However, it is our view that, even if family factors are implicated as contributing to the presenting difficulties, this does not necessarily mean that the parents should be the primary focus of the intervention. Individual CBT with the child may still be appropriate, although the clinician may need to determine how best to address parental and/or family issues alongside work with an individual child.

There is little available research in this area to guide the clinician as to how to determine when it is best to work directly with parents alone, when with the child alone and when with a combination of child and parents. Negotiating family involvement is a complex and sensitive task. Demanding intensive family involvement when this runs counter to the wishes and views of key family members can lead to resentment and non-compliance with treatment. Conversely, when the clinical situation requires it, the failure to address family issues may seriously limit the potential benefits of CBT with an individual child.

There is a range of possible configurations of parental involvement in therapy including: the child being seen alone with minimal parental involvement, the child being seen along with their parents, the whole family being seen or the parents being offered separate/parallel interventions. The role of parents in any of these scenarios can vary from facilitator, to co-therapist to client/patient in their own right. Clearly, there are many possible variations and parents can be involved in their child's CBT in different ways during the course of a single intervention. In the light of what limited evidence there is available, the authors have started to construct a very crude tentative hierarchy of parental involvement, described below, to help guide decision making in clinical practice.

7.2.2.1   Parent as facilitator – child offered individual CBT with parent not present or infrequently seen

Most commonly, the role of parents in CBT has been conceived as that of a facilitator to aid the transfer of skills from clinical sessions to the home environment. In this model, it is assumed that the parents will have limited involvement in the intervention programme itself. They may not be present in sessions, but may meet with the therapist infrequently for updates, speak on the phone or have one or two educational sessions of their own (Kendall, 1994). Even within this approach, it has been found that there may be some advantages to keeping parents as informed as possible about their children's progress (Macdonald et al., in press).

In the authors' experience, this form of minimal parental involvement is most suited to work with older children, who are highly motivated, where the family is generally supportive and where there are no major family issues. The advantages of this approach are that it empowers the young person and allows them to be the focus of the work in a very simple way. This model involves using CBT in a way that is most closely analogous to CBT with adults.

7.2.2.2   Parent as co-therapist – child offered individual CBT with parent(s) present

Where parents take on a more active role in which they prompt, monitor and review the child's use of cognitive skills, they may be conceived of as taking on the role of co-therapist (Stallard, 2002b). This generally involves the parent joining the child for sessions. There is some evidence that greater parental involvement in CBT can lead to better outcomes, particularly for children referred for anxiety, and especially for younger children (under 11 years), and where parental anxiety is high (Fonagy *et al.*, 2002).

Toren and colleagues (2000) report a study where parent–child dyads and triads were seen for 10-weekly group sessions as a treatment for anxiety. Parents were encouraged to work with the child and reinforce them in planning and addressing problems. Although parents' own anxieties and issues were not addressed directly, and indeed there was no diminution in levels of anxiety among the parents, the study found a significant decrease in anxiety of the majority of children in the group, particularly in those with more anxious mothers.

Including parents in this way may help parents to prompt the use of cognitive behavioural techniques in real-life situations not accessible to the therapist, in order to make overlearning and generalization possible. Increased parental involvement in therapy may also help the parents learn new techniques themselves for dealing with the difficulties with which the child is struggling, although the lack of change in parental anxiety levels found by Toren *et al.* (2000) suggests this is not invariably the mechanism of change.

This approach seems to be particularly suitable for younger children, particularly those with anxiety related problems, and where there are parallel difficulties in the parents and child (e.g. both have high anxiety).

7.2.2.3   Parent as client – intervention offered direct to parents in some form

Parents can sometimes be viewed as clients in their own right. CBT programmes that involve teaching parents new skills, whether they focus primarily on coping with their child (e.g. behaviour management) or their own emotions (e.g. dealing with their own anxiety), may be seen as falling into this category. In the former category, Friedberg and McClure (2002) describe a 'playbook' of interventions to help parents shape their child's behaviour which includes giving parents knowledge of developmentally appropriate behaviour, encouraging realistic expectations, teaching parents how to reinforce positive behaviours and helping parents to ignore negative behaviour. In the latter category, Barrett and colleagues (1996) describe a programme aimed at tackling parental anxiety and faulty cognitions as well as providing them with improved techniques to shape their child's behaviour. Such training may take place with or without the child present and may be offered either individually or in groups.

Perhaps the most widespread use of parents as clients from a CBT perspective is the many parent-training programmes that focus on parents developing new ways of controlling and shaping their children's behaviour – e.g. the Webster–Stratton parenting groups and the Oregon Social Learning Program (Webster-Stratton and Herbert 1994; Fonagy et al., 2002). Parenting training groups without any child work have been shown to have very good outcomes, especially for children aged 10 and under. However, they have less good outcomes with older children, where there are other problems present, where the problems are severe, where there is socioeconomic disadvantage and where there is high parental discord and/or antisocial behaviour (Fonagy et al., 2002). It is also unclear how far parent training is appropriate across all cultural groups (Forehand and Kotchick, 1996).

For anxiety problems, there is also some research evidence for the effectiveness of parent-targeted interventions. Barrett and colleagues (Barrett et al., 1996) describe a systemic model to empower parents and children to form an 'expert team' in tackling childhood anxiety. During 'Family Anxiety Management' (FAM), parents are taught how to 'reward courageous behaviour and extinguish excessive anxiety' in the child, how to deal with their own emotional upsets and how to improve their communication and problem-solving skills. Cobham et al. (1998) describe a structured intervention that includes both child-focused CBT (ten sessions) to treat child anxiety and a programme designed to reduce parental anxiety (four sessions for parents). Parents are taught to recognize the effect of their own behaviour on the development and maintenance of their child's problems and how to address their own anxiety.

Although in both cases the inclusion of such parent-focused interventions has led to some improved outcomes, their effect long term is not clear. While the inclusion of FAM led to improved outcome initially, this was not maintained in all domains at 6-year follow-up (Barrett et al., 2001). Moreover, it is unclear whether the specific targeting of parental anxieties was more efficacious than the less resource-intensive intervention outlined by Toren and colleagues (2000), which included parents but remained child focused.

A further way in which parents may commonly be engaged as 'clients' when the initial family assessment reveals complex family issues is for the family either to be offered family work as a first approach or family work interspersed with individually focused CBT. While this combination is widespread in clinical practice, there is little research to investigate the effectiveness of this approach. Moreover, where family work has been offered, it has traditionally been seen as a separate treatment modality from CBT. However, there may be some scope for a specific form of family CBT – perhaps where case formulations are based on the thoughts, feelings and behaviour of both children and parents.

The above hierarchy represents a very tentative first attempt to try to pull out criteria for determining how best to involve parents in CBT for children and young people. There is still the need for much greater research into the differential effects on treatment outcome of each of these different forms of parental involvement.

7.2.3   Promoting genuine collaboration

Regardless of whether parents are perceived to have clinical issues in their own right, the aim remains to position them so that they can collaborate with both the therapist and the referred child in supporting the child's development and progress in therapy (see Table 7.1). The only exception arises if there are child protection issues that cannot be dealt with in a collaborative framework.

Many parents come into initial contact with mental health services viewing themselves as bringing a child they want 'fixed'. They often come feeling very worried that mental health professionals will hold them responsible for their child's difficulties and blame them for their problems. Therefore, they often come feeling defensive and hear any suggestion that they be included or directly involved in therapy as a reflection of this blaming stance (Wolpert, 2000). It may be important to address issues of responsibility and blame at the outset of therapy. The clinician should stress to families that suggesting family involvement does not mean that family members are 'to blame' for the difficulties but that their involvement may help the child and be part of the solution to the difficulties.

In order to promote genuine collaboration, the therapist needs to be sensitive to the cultural and ethnic background of both parents and children. In negotiating forms of parental involvement, it may be that different groups have different preferences in this regard, as with other aspects of child mental health provision (Forehand and Kotchick 1996; Friedberg and McClure 2002; Stein et al., 2003). This is clearly an area which requires much further research.

The authors suggest that it may be helpful to be as explicit as possible with parents about their role in therapy, and to try to make parents feel part of the solution not the problem. It is the authors' belief that both parents and children should be treated as collaborators wherever possible and given access to case formulation, and indeed invited to contribute to the process of reformulating the problem and its solutions during the course of the work. In addition, it is to be recommended that the therapist is as transparent in his/her practice as possible. Letters to other professionals concerning a given child or family should be routinely copied to parents and/or children where this is developmentally appropriate. Shared goals should be recorded in the case file and made open to family members. Where therapists routinely evaluate their work, they should make the outcomes of such evaluation as open as possible to all family members in appropriate forms.

7.3   Conclusion

Working with parents in providing CBT for children raises a range of challenges. Three key domains of ethical concern that need to be addressed in some way by clinicians seeking to use CBT with children have been identified. The authors acknowledge the current lack of a research base to guide clinicians as to how best to include parents and have argued for the need for further research in this important area. Drawing on what research there is (and on the authors' clinical experience where there is lack of research), the following has been argued.

In terms of *balancing different viewpoints*, clinicians need to recognize that there may be many different views as to what therapy is required and to what ends. Before embarking on CBT (or any other intervention), the clinician needs to be clear about who is providing consent for treatment. The clinician must continue to provide information to all interested parties in an appropriate form to allow for ongoing choices to be made during the course of treatment. It is suggested that the clinician draw on family therapy techniques such as reframing to help family members come to a shared view of the difficulties.

In terms of *addressing family issues*, initial assessments for individual CBT should start with a full family assessment. Such an assessment does not just serve to provide information for the clinician, but can also be used to develop a shared formulation of the difficulties that all family members can agree on. This formulation should not involve blaming the referred child or other family members, but should position all family members as collaborating to overcome the difficulties. If CBT is regarded as appropriate, the clinician should negotiate with the family as to the level and nature of parental involvement this will involve.

In terms of *promoting genuine collaboration*, it has been argued that it may be important to be explicit with parents about their role in therapy. Whether a parent is conceived at any given point as a facilitator, a co-therapist or client in

Table 7.3   Checklist for clinicians to help assessment of how far they are attempting to balance different view points, assessing family issues and promoting collaboration

Child	Parents
• Have you asked the child for their views of the referral and what they are hoping for from therapy?	• Have you asked parent(s) for their views of the referral and what they are hoping for from therapy?
• Have you provided information in a way that is appropriate for the child's developmental stage and cultural context?	• Have you provided information in a way that is appropriate for the parent's circumstances and cultural context?
• Have you explained directly to the child the process and content of any suggested intervention?	• Have you explained directly to the parent the process and content of any suggested intervention?
• What choices have you offered the child, if any?	• What choices have you offered the parent, if any?
• Where you have acted contrary to the views or wishes of the child, what is your rationale for this?	• Where you have acted contrary to the views or wishes of the parent, what is your rationale for this?
• How have you recorded the views of children in the case notes?	• How have you recorded the views of parent in the case notes?
• Have you addressed any ways the child may feel responsible or blamed for the difficulties?	• Have you addressed any ways the parent may feel responsible or blamed for the difficulties?
• Have you found a way of describing the problem that all family members can agree to?	• Have you found a way of describing the problem that all family members can agree to?
• Have you discussed with the child what role the parents are to take in therapy and offered a rationale for this?	• Have you discussed with the parents what role they are to take in therapy and offered a rationale for this?
• Have you copied any professional correspondence to the child?	• Have you copied any professional correspondence to the parents?
• Have you shared any evaluation of the therapy with the child?	• Have you shared any evaluation of therapy with the parents?

Adapted from Wolpert *et al.*, 2001.

their own right, and whether they are directly or indirectly involved in work with their child, the goal remains to establish a collaborative relationship. The clinician should act to enhance genuine collaboration by avoiding blaming formulations and by employing interviewing techniques such as reflexive questioning and externalizing conversations that help to position parents as part of the solution rather than part of the problem. Parents should be routinely copied into all professional correspondence and the results of any formal evaluations should be shared with family members.

7.3.1   Clinical checklist

Rather than present case examples, Table 7.3 provides a checklist that may be used to remind clinicians of some of the issues raised in this chapter. Not all the questions need invariably be answered in the affirmative, but the list is designed to help clinicians reflect on their own practice in the light of the issues that have been raised.

7.4   Acknowledgement

The authors would like to thank Peter Fuggle for his comments on an earlier version of this chapter. They would also like to acknowledge Peter Fuggle, Chrissie Verduyn and Vicki Curry for their contribution to the thinking behind this chapter in terms of their involvement in a workshop with the first author on the role of parents in CBT at the BABCP conference in London 2000.

7.5   REFERENCES

Angold, A., Weissman, M., Merikangas, J. K. *et al.* (1987). Parent and child reports of depressive symptoms in children at low and high risk of depression. *Journal of Child Psychology and Psychiatry*, **28**, 901–15.

Bainham, A. (1998). *Children: The Modern Law*, 2nd edn. Bristol: Family Law.

Barrett, P. M., Dadds, M. R. and Rapee, R. M. (1996). Family treatment of childhood anxiety: a controlled trial. *Journal of Consulting and Clinical Psychology*, **64**, 333–42.

Barrett, P. M., Duffy, A. L., Dadds, M. R. and Rapee, R. M. (2001). Cognitive behavioural treatment of anxiety disorders in children: long-term (6 years) follow-up. *Journal of Consulting and Clinical Psychology*, **69**, 135–41.

Beck, J. S. (1995). *Cognitive Therapy: Basics and Beyond*. New York: Guilford Press.

British Medical Association and Law Society. (1995). *Good Practice Guidelines*. London: British Medical Association.

Carr, A. (1999). *The Handbook of Child and Adolescent Clinical Psychology. A Contextual Approach*. London: Routledge.

Cobham, V. E., Dadds, M. R. and Spence, S. H. (1998). The role of parental anxiety in the treatment of childhood anxiety. *Journal of Consulting and Clinical Psychology*, **66**, 893–905.

FOCUS information sheet 3. (1999). Treatment decisions in young people (2) Practice Guidelines. London: Royal College of Psychiatrists' Research Unit.

Fonagy, P., Target, M., Cottrell, D., Phillips, J. and Kurtz, Z. (2002). *What Works for Whom? A Critical Review of Treatments for Children and Adolescents*. New York: Guilford Press.

Forehand, R. L. and Kotchick, B. A. (1996). Cultural diversity: a wake-up call for parent training, *Behavior Therapy*, **27**, 187–206.

Friedberg, R. D. and McClure, J. M. (2002). *Clinical Practice of Cognitive Therapy with Children and Adolescents: The Nuts and Bolts*. New York: Guilford Press.

Fuggle, P, Douglas, J. and Powell, R. (2001). *Practice Guidance on Consent for Clinical Psychologists Working with Children and Young People*, position paper of the Division of Clinical Psychology: Faculty for Children and Young People. Leicester: Division of Clinical Psychology, British Psychological Society.

Glaser, D. (1996). The voice of the child in mental health practice. In R. Davie, G. Upton and V. Varma (eds.), *The Voice of the Child: A Handbook for Professionals*. Falmer Press.

Hennessy, E. (1999). Children as service evaluators. *Child Psychology and Psychiatry Review*, **4**, 153–61.

Hoffman, L. (1981). *Foundations of Family Therapy – A Conceptual Framework for Systems Change*. USA: Basic Books.

Kazdin, A. E. (1995). Child, parent and family dysfunction as predictors of outcome in cognitive-behavioural treatment of antisocial children. *Behaviour Research and Therapy*, **33**, 271–81.

Kendall, P. C. (1994). Treating anxiety disorders in children: results of a randomized control trial. *Journal of Consulting and Clinical Psychology*, **62**, 100–10.

Kendall, P. C. and Morris, R. J. (1991). Child therapy: issues and recommendations. *Journal of Consulting and Clinical Psychology*, **59**, 777–84.

Klein, R. G. (1991). Parent child agreement in clinical assessment of anxiety and other psychopathology: a review. *Journal of Anxiety Disorders*, **5**, 187–98.

MacDonald, E., Chowdhury, U., Dabney, J., Wolpert, M. and Stein, S. (in press) A social skills group for children: the importance of liaison with parents, teachers and professionals. *Emotional and Behavioural Disorders*, **8**.

Maguire, P., Rowlands, A., Drinkwater, J. and Wolpert, M. (2001). *Promoting user participation in clinical psychology services for children and young people: how to hear the voice of the child*, position paper of the Division of Clinical Psychology: Faculty for Children and Young People. Leicester: Division of Clinical Psychology, British Psychological Society.

March, J. S. and Mulle, K. M. (1998). *OCD in Children and Adolescents. A Cognitive-Behavioural Treatment Manual*. New York: Guilford Press.

McGoldrick, M. (ed.) (1998). *Re-visioning Family Therapy: Race, Culture and Gender in Clinical Practice*. New York: Guilford Press.

Pearce, J. (1994). Consent to treatment during childhood. *British Journal of Psychiatry*, **165**, 713–16.

Pearce, W. B. and Cronen, V. E. (1980). *Communication, Action and Meaning: The Creation of Social Realities*. New York: Praeger.

Royal College of Psychiatrists (1997). *Behavioural and Cognitive Treatments: Guidance for Good Practice*, London Council Report CR 68. London: Royal College of Psychiatry.

Stallard, P. (2002a). *Think Good-Feel Good: A Cognitive Behaviour Therapy Workbook for Children and Young People*. Chichester: John Wiley and Sons.

(2002b). Cognitive behaviour therapy with children and young people: a selective review of key issues. *Behavioural and Cognitive Psychotherapy*, **30**, 297–309.

Stein, S., Christie, D., Shah, R., Dabney, J. and Wolpert, M. (2003). Knowledge of and attitudes to CAMHS: differences between white and Pakistani mothers. *Child and Adolescent Mental Health*, **8**, 29–34.

Tomm, K. (1987a). Interventive interviewing. I. Strategising as a fourth guideline for the therapist. *Family Process*, **26**, 3–13.

(1987b). Interventive interviewing. II. Reflexive questioning as a means to enable self-healing. *Family Process*, **26**, 167–83.

Toren. P., Wolmer, L., Rosental, B. *et al.* (2000). Case series: brief parent-child group therapy for childhood anxiety disorders using a manual based cognitive-behavioural technique. *Journal of the American Academy of Child and Adolescent Psychiatry*, **39**, 1309–12.

Watzlawick, P., Weakland, J. and Fish, R. (1974). *Change: Principle of Problem Formation and Problem Resolution*. New York: Random House.

Webster-Stratton, C. and Herbert, M. (1994). What really happens in parent training? *Behaviour Modification*, **17**, 407–56.

White, M. and Epston, D. (1990). *Narrative Means to Therapeutic Ends*. New York: Norton.

Wilkinson, I. (1998). *Child and Family Assessment – Clinical Guidelines for Practitioners*, 2nd edn. London: Routledge.

Wolpert, M. (2000). Is anyone to blame? Whom families and their therapists blame for the presenting problem. *Clinical Child Psychology and Psychiatry*, **5**, 115–31.

Wolpert, M., Maguire, P. and Rowland, A. (2001). Should children be seen and not heard? User Participation in Clinical Psychology Services for Children and Young People. *Clinical Psychology Forum*.

8

Cognitive behaviour therapy with prepubertal children

Paul Stallard

Royal United Hospital, Bath, UK

8.1 Introduction

Cognitive behaviour therapy (CBT) embraces a range of psychotherapeutic interventions that aim to ameliorate and/or reduce psychological distress and maladaptive behaviour by altering cognitive processes. CBT uses both behavioural and cognitive strategies and seeks to 'preserve the efficacy of behavioural techniques but within a less doctrinaire context that takes account of the child's cognitive interpretations and attributions about events' (Kendall and Hollon, 1979). Identifying, challenging and learning alternative skills to counter and replace the cognitive deficits and distortions assumed to underpin emotional and behavioural problems is the primary focus of CBT.

8.2 At what age are children able to engage in CBT?

The age at which children have sufficient cognitive development to engage in CBT has been the subject of debate. Some argue that CBT requires the ability to 'think about thinking' and that this meta-cognition allows children to reflect on their own behaviour and cognitive processes and to detect patterns and structures within them. This level of cognitive maturity and sophistication has led to a view that CBT is best suited for children of middle and later childhood. In a meta-review, Durlak *et al.* (1991) found that children aged 11–13 derived significantly more benefit from CBT than younger children. The influential sequential staged approach to cognitive development proposed by Piaget adds further support to the view that older children are better suited for CBT. Piaget suggested that more complex mental processes that allow the development of logical reasoning do not develop until the concrete operational stage, typically acquired at 7–8 years of age.

Cognitive Behaviour Therapy for Children and Families, ed. Philip J. Graham.
Published by Cambridge University Press. © Cambridge University Press 2004.

In practice, although CBT can involve sophisticated and complex cognitive tasks, the cognitive demands of most CBT programmes with children are quite limited. Many tasks require an ability to reason effectively about concrete matters and issues rather than higher order abstract and conceptual thinking (Harrington *et al.*, 1998). This has led some to suggest that the cognitive development of 7-year-old children is sufficient for many of the basic tasks of CBT. By the age of 7, children are reasonably able to competently reflect on their own cognitive processes (Salmon and Bryant, 2002).

While there is an emerging consensus that children as young as 7 years of age can engage in CBT, the question arises as to whether children below this age have sufficient cognitive skills to engage actively in a modified form of CBT. Support for this possibility comes from research exploring how children develop a representational understanding of mind, i.e. how they understand that people have internal mental states such as thoughts, beliefs and images that may represent or misrepresent the world (Wellman *et al.*, 1996). In a series of studies examining preschool children's understanding of thought bubbles, Wellman *et al.* (1996) showed that with preliminary training 3-year-old children could understand that thought bubbles represent what a person may think. In addition, their results suggest that children of this age can distinguish between thoughts and actions, can acknowledge that thoughts are subjective and thus that two people can have different thoughts about the same event and that thoughts can misrepresent an event. In terms of self-awareness and recognition of inner speech, Flavell *et al.* (2001) suggest that this is acquired during the first years at school. This implies that some children of 5 or 6 years of age are able to articulate their cognitions and understand the concept of 'talking to oneself', one of the most commonly used strategies in CBT programmes with children.

Further evidence supporting the possibility that younger children may be able to engage in some of the tasks of CBT has come from research evaluating Piaget's theory of cognitive development. Piaget's assumption that failure on particular cognitive tasks indicates the absence of a particular set of underlying cognitive skills has been challenged. Performance on similar cognitive tasks can vary depending on the specific way the task or information is presented and does not necessarily reflect the absence or presence of an assumed set of cognitive skills (Thornton 2002). Interest in a more process-orientated approach to the understanding of cognitive development has led to the questioning of another basic tenet of Piaget's theory – namely, the assumed link between a set of cognitive skills (i.e. logical processes) and their use (i.e. logical reasoning). Thornton (2002) argues, for example, that logical inferences may not necessarily reflect the use of logical cognitive processes. Cognitive reasoning may be based around information and meaning rather than rules of logical inference. Relevant information can, therefore, be used to construct a mental model, which in turn can be used to reach conclusions about the relationships between one event and another. Changes in knowledge can therefore create powerful new ways of reasoning leading Thornton (2002) to conclude that it is information not age that plays an important part in determining a child's performance on cognitive tasks.

These findings lead to the intriguing possibility that children as young as 5 or 6 years of age may be able to participate in some forms of CBT if sufficient attention is paid to the way tasks are structured and presented. Clinicians need to attend to the child's cognitive development to ensure that cognitive interventions and techniques are adapted and modified so they do not exceed the child's cognitive or emotional capabilities (Salmon and Bryant, 2002). How this essential task is achieved in clinical practice has received surprisingly little attention. Standardized CBT programmes, often spanning wide age ranges, seldom specify how they have been adapted for use with younger age groups. Many programmes appear to assume that the techniques and strategies are universally applicable to children of all ages (Barrett, 2000).

There are some helpful examples in the literature where clinicians have modified CBT to match the child's cognitive capabilities. Kane and Kendall (1989) for example found that, although younger children had problems identifying their own anxious cognitions, both in imaginal situations and *in vivo*, they could engage in a third party discussion about what might happen to another child in a similar situation. Williams *et al.* (2002) noted that, although young people often failed to report any cognitions spontaneously, a therapist-led guided approach could help the children discover possible thoughts associated with emotional reactions. Similarly, Spence *et al.* (2000) observed that, while younger children experienced difficulty with cognitive restructuring involving challenging and testing the evidence for their thoughts, they were able to use simpler cognitive strategies such as positive self-instruction.

These examples highlight how the cognitive processes and tasks of CBT can be adapted to match the capabilities of the child. This would suggest that younger children may be able to engage with less sophisticated, specific, concrete cognitive techniques such as developing positive coping self-talk. Providing specific and relevant information that would allow the development of cognitive models of reasoning appears to be important. The provision of such information may help the child to reach conclusions about specific problems even though they may be unable to recognize overarching rules, the cognitive processes they use or generalize their conclusions to other situations. Understanding the mechanisms by which change is achieved – e.g. that emotions are effected by particular cognitions – may not be possible for children under 5 years of age (Flavell *et al.*, 2001). The process of guided discovery which underpins CBT may therefore require a more active and direct therapeutic approach with younger children, with the therapist providing information and developing strategies for the child to use and test. The clinician's role with older children may be more facilitative as adolescents may be more able to develop and evaluate cognitive strategies for themselves. Working with higher order, more abstract and complex tasks such as identifying dysfunctional assumptions, evaluating evidence for and against beliefs or cognitive restructuring may not be appropriate until middle adolescence (Bailey, 2001).

8.3   How often is CBT used with children under the age of 12?

In a review of child psychotherapy research, Durlak *et al.* (1995) identified 101 studies that compared the use of CBT with a control group. Of these, the majority (79%) involved children under the age of 11 years, with 6% involving preschool children. Randomized controlled treatment trials reveal that prepubertal children are often involved in intervention studies addressing a wide range of problems including school refusal (King *et al.*, 1998), school phobia (Last *et al.*, 1998), recurrent abdominal pain (Sanders *et al.*, 1996), enuresis (Ronen *et al.*, 1995), anxiety disorders (Kendall, 1994; Barrett *et al.*, 1996; Kendall *et al.*, 1997; Mendlowitz *et al.*, 1999; Silverman *et al.*, 1999a), specific phobias (Silverman *et al.*, 1999b), social phobias (Spence *et al.*, 2000), sexual abuse (Cohen and Mannarino, 1996) and depression (Vostanis *et al.*, 1996; Wood *et al.*, 1996). Many of these studies have included children as young as 7 years of age and there are reports of CBT being undertaken with children even younger. Six-year-old children have been included in studies using CBT to treat anxiety disorders (Silverman *et al.*, 1999a) and encopresis (Ronen, 1993). King *et al.* (1998) used CBT with a 5-year-old with school refusal while Jackson and King (1981) reported the use of emotive imagery with a 5-year-old boy with darkness phobia. In terms of preschool children, cognitive behavioural programmes have been used with children who have been sexually abused, some being as young as 3 years of age (Cohen and Mannarino, 1996). The programme appears to involve cognitive interventions with both children and their parents as children are helped to explore their attributions regarding the abuse and encouraged to develop coping strategies such as mediated self-talk, thought stopping and positive imagery.

8.4   Is CBT with prepubertal children effective?

While CBT has been widely used with prepubertal children, the question arises as to whether CBT is efficacious with this age group. The results of randomized controlled trials that have included children under the age of 12 suggest that, when compared with waiting list controls, CBT results in significant improvements. The use of CBT has resulted in superior gains post-treatment and at follow-up in the treatment of generalized anxiety disorders (Kendall, 1994; Kendall *et al.*, 1997; Silverman *et al.*, 1999a), school refusal (King *et al.*, 1998) and specific phobias (Cornwall *et al.*, 1996).

When compared with other active interventions, the superiority of CBT is less marked. In the treatment of depression with children aged 8–17, Vostanis *et al.* (1996) found no significant differences between CBT and a non-focused intervention. Similarly, in a study with depressed children aged 9–17, Wood *et al.* (1996) found that, compared with relaxation training, CBT resulted in superior post-treatment improvements, although these differences were no longer significant at 6 months. In terms of phobias, Last *et al.* (1998) found no significant differences in the outcome of children aged 6–17 with school phobia who received CBT or an attention placebo condition. Similarly, Silverman *et al.* (1999b) found comparable improvements in children aged 6–16 with specific phobias who received CBT, contingency management or educational support. Finally, in terms of sexual abuse, although Cohen and Mannarino (1996) reported the superiority of CBT over non-directive supportive therapy, Berliner and Saunders (1996) found that CBT and traditional treatment both resulted in marked improvements in sexually abused children aged 4–13.

Although some studies have highlighted similar post-treatment improvements between CBT and other active interventions, some additional benefits of CBT have been noted at follow-up. Sanders *et al.* (1996) found that CBT and standard paediatric care resulted in comparable post-treatment improvements in children aged 7–14 with recurrent abdominal pain, although at follow-up the CBT group had lower relapse rates and less intense pain. Similarly, in terms of enuresis, Ronen *et al.* (1995) noted that children aged 7–12 with enuresis responded equally well to a token economy, bell and pad and CBT, although the gains with CBT were better maintained at 3 months.

8.5   Is CBT more or less effective with younger children?

The wide age range in many of the studies reported above raises the question as to whether CBT is more or less effective with younger children. Some researchers have noted a tendency for younger children to benefit more from CBT. Sanders *et al.* (1996) noted a non-significant trend for younger children with abdominal pain to respond better to CBT. Last *et al.* (1998) noted that better outcomes were obtained when the children were younger and had higher baseline rates of school attendance. Similarly, in a study with depressed children aged 10–17, Jayson *et al.* (1998) noted that younger and less severely impaired children responded better to CBT. Whether the additional improvements noted in these studies reflect earlier intervention, less severe problems or the superiority of cognitive behavioural interventions with a younger age group is unclear.

The results are not, however, consistent, since other researchers have found the outcome of CBT to be unaffected by the child's age (Vostanis *et al.*, 1996; Dadds *et al.*, 1997). Durlak *et al.* (1991) undertook the most extensive examination of the effect of age on the outcome of CBT. The authors undertook a meta-analysis of 64 CBT studies involving children under the age of 13. The average age of the children was 9 years (range 4.5–13) and an analysis of the effectiveness of CBT within three age bands – 5–7, 7–11 and 11–13 years – was undertaken. The average length of the interventions in the studies examined was 9.6 hours (12 sessions), and two-thirds were delivered in school settings and three-quarters used more than one treatment component (e.g. self-instruction, task-orientated problem-solving, etc.). Although the analysis revealed that CBT was effective with all age groups, the effect size for children at the formal operational stage (aged 11–13) was twice that obtained for younger children. This led the authors to suggest that children entering treatment at more advanced levels of cognitive functioning benefit more from CBT than younger children at less advanced levels. These authors acknowledge the limitations of this study and highlight how the child's cognitive development was not directly assessed but was assumed on the basis of their age. Thus, children were classified according to Piaget's cognitive stages, with 5–7-year-olds being assumed to function at the pre-operational stage, 7–11 at concrete operational stage and 11–13 at formal operational stage. Similarly, the premise that the child's level of cognitive maturity is related to outcome would suggest a linear relationship with age. The results did not support such a relationship since the 5–7-year-old group derived as much benefit as the 7–11 group.

8.6 cBt or CBT?

Attending to the child's cognitive processes is clearly important in the delivery of CBT. The cognitive demands of the intervention must not exceed the child's cognitive capacity. However, an examination of the treatment components of CBT programmes suggests that the cognitive demands of many are quite limited.

The cognitive component is often confined to developing one particular cognitive technique such as positive self-talk, a strategy which forms the backbone of programmes for obsessive compulsive disorder (OCD) and anxiety disorders. In the OCD programme, 'How I ran OCD off my land', children learn to 'boss back' their OCD by the use of constructive self-talk (March *et al.*, 1994). Replacing anxious self-talk with coping self-talk is the main cognitive component of the 'Coping Cat' programme for the treatment of anxiety disorders (Kendall, 1994). The major emphasis of these programmes is on more behavioural strategies such as emotional identification, anxiety management, graded exposure and positive reinforcement.

In terms of depression, cognitive restructuring forms the main cognitive component of the programmes that have been used with prepubertal children (Vostanis *et al.*, 1996; Wood *et al.*, 1996). These programmes devote two sessions to this cognitive element with the remaining six or seven focusing on emotional recognition and management, self-reinforcement and problem-solving. Given the limited cognitive focus of many CBT programmes, it would seem essential that treatment fidelity be assessed to ensure that the cognitive intervention had been delivered. Feehan and Vostanis (1996), for example, report that only 50% of their group actually attended the sessions on cognitive restructuring.

The wide variation in treatment components used in CBT programmes with prepubertal children was highlighted by Durlak *et al.* (1991) – the authors concluded that 'as currently practiced, CBT is an umbrella term for a non-standardised package of different treatment techniques that can be offered in many different sequences and permutations'. This wide variation in treatment components may in part explain why their analysis failed to substantiate the predicted association between changes in cognitive processes and behaviour. The authors speculate that it would be 'disconcerting to find that cognitive variables, which are emphasised in CBT, do not in some way relate to outcomes'. However, if the cognitive components of CBT programmes were limited, then the effect on cognitive outcome would not necessarily be significant.

In considering this issue, it is important to acknowledge that the cognitive components of treatment programmers may not have been fully described. It is also probable that 'non-cognitive' treatment sessions, focusing, for example, on emotional recognition or social problem-solving, would also have a cognitive element. Nonetheless, it does appear that CBT programmes with children are overwhelmingly behavioural in orientation with a direct focus on cognitions and cognitive processes being limited. This is in contrast to CBT undertaken with adults where increased emphasis is placed on identifying cognitions and understanding how events are appraised (see, for example, Salkovskis, 1999; Ehlers and Clark, 2000).

This brief overview highlights that the 'cognitive' component and focus of many CBT programmes with children is extremely limited. Typically, the cognitive element involves one strategy, with the most frequently used being the development of coping self-talk. The cognitive demands of many CBT programmes therefore appear quite limited, and as such would be within the capabilities of most prepubertal children.

8.7   Adapting CBT for use with younger children

In order for CBT to be effective, materials need to be adapted and presented at the right developmental level. Abstract concepts and strategies need to be translated into simple examples and metaphors from the child's everyday life, which can be accessed through age-appropriate media such as art or play. This theme is emphasized by Vostanis et al. (1996) who suggest that CBT needs to be modified for younger children by using fewer verbal and more visual techniques. The authors described how their therapeutic programme was adapted by using simpler language, age-appropriate examples and drawings of different emotions (Feehan and Vostanis, 1996).

Metaphors provide a helpful way for abstract concepts to be presented to children in concrete understandable ways. Barrett et al. (2000) describe unhelpful thoughts as 'thought invaders' which children are encouraged to destroy. Williams et al. (2002) used the analogy of an irritating tune that keeps popping into one's mind to explain intrusive thoughts. Stallard (2002) used the metaphor of an audiotape playing in the child's head to explain automatic thoughts, and videotape to understand intrusive repetitive images. The images can be developed to teach children how to control their thoughts and images by learning to turn their tape off or to turn the volume down. Similarly, children can be helped to identify, test and evaluate their thoughts and behaviour by the use of metaphors encouraging them to assume the role of a 'Private I' (Friedberg and McClure, 2002), 'social detective' (Spence, 1995) or the 'thought tracker' (Stallard, 2002). The metaphor of an anger volcano can be used to help children understand and visualize their anger build-up and to explore how the volcano can be helped to stop erupting. Finally, the use of positive coping imagery has been used with young children in order to counter unpleasant emotional reactions such as anxiety or anger. Jackson and King (1981), for example, used the fantasy hero Batman to help a 5-year-old boy overcome his fear of the dark. To be effective, images should be tailored to the age of the child and build on their existing interests.

The use of play and games to explain the core concepts of CBT provides a natural, non-threatening and entertaining way of working with young children. Ronen (1993) highlights how a 6-year-old boy with encopresis was able to engage with CBT once the therapist understood the child's 'way of thinking'. The concepts of automatic (i.e. doing something without thinking about it) and mediated (i.e. a command or order sent to the body from the brain) thoughts were highlighted through a game of soldiers. Mediated thoughts were explained as a commander (brain) sending orders to their soldiers (child's body). Barrett *et al.* (2000) provided another example of the use of games. The authors describe a task in which children are required to get a balloon from one side of a room to another as a way of teaching a structured approach to problem-solving. Similarly, dolls, puppets and toys can be used to act out difficult situations during which the child is encouraged to suggest what the toys may be thinking. However, Salmon and Bryant (2002) caution that preschool children experience difficulties if they are asked to use the doll to represent themselves. They have difficulties understanding that a doll can be both an object (toy) and a symbol (representation of themselves).

There is also a need to make CBT with younger children fun, interesting and engaging. The use of visual media such as black/white boards, flip charts and drawings is helpful. Quizzes provide a useful and entertaining way of accessing children's cognitions. Unfinished sentences can be used to identify thoughts related to specific situations and feelings (Friedberg and McClure, 2002). Sorting games can be used to help children distinguish between thoughts, feelings and actions (Stallard, 2002). Cartoons and thought bubbles can provide fun and helpful ways of accessing a child's thoughts; they can be used to generate alternative ways of thinking or to highlight that different people may have a range of thoughts about a particular event (Kendall, 1994; Stallard, 2002).

In terms of process, CBT with prepubertal children is less didactic than that with adults, with the therapist adopting a more active role within therapy sessions. If the child is reticent or unforthcoming, the therapist may adopt a rhetorical approach, guessing out loud what the child might be thinking. Similarly, the use of structured questioning and regular feedback can be used to help the child make links between thoughts and feelings or to discover important beliefs and assumptions. The therapist may work more as a 'thought catcher', identifying important cognitions when they occur and bringing them to the attention of the child (Turk, 1998). A further process issue is highlighted by Bailey (2001) who suggests the need to pay particular attention to issues of pacing, the content and speed of therapy. Treatment sessions may be shorter in order to reflect the child's attention span.

8.8   The role of the parent in CBT with prepubertal children

When undertaking CBT with prepubertal children, it is important to consider the role of parents in treatment and in the development and maintenance of their child's psychological problems. Viewing the child in isolation without recognizing or involving significant systemic influences, particularly the role of the family and peers, is inappropriate. In clinical practice, parents are often involved in CBT programmes, although developmentally appropriate theoretical models that inform the nature of this involvement are currently lacking. A notable exception is the work of Rapee (2001) who has described a model for generalized anxiety disorder that highlights the effect of parental cognitions and behaviour on the development and maintenance of the child's problems. In particular, parental overcontrol, overprotection, overly critical behaviour and reinforcement of avoidant behaviour have been identified as important factors that are associated with the development of anxiety disorders in children.

It is surprising that, despite their potential importance, the role of parents in CBT programmes, particularly with prepubertal children, has received such little attention. Programmes have involved parents in different ways, such as facilitators, co-therapists or as clients in their own right (Kendall, 1994; Barrett et al., 1996; Toren et al., 2000). The parent facilitator is the more limited role and is highlighted in the 'Coping Cat' programme (Kendall, 1994). The predominant focus of the intervention is on individual CBT with the child, with parents receiving one or two educational sessions designed to encourage their cooperation with treatment. As co-therapists, parents are more extensively involved in therapy sessions and are encouraged to monitor, prompt and reinforce their child's use of cognitive skills outside of treatment sessions (Mendlowitz et al., 1999; Toren et al., 2000). With the facilitator and co-therapist models, the child continues to remain the focus of the intervention, with the parents working towards reducing their child's psychological distress.

An alternative model is where both the child and parents are the subject of direct intervention. Children may, for example, engage in parallel child-focused CBT and participate in family sessions during which the family learns alternative ways of managing anxiety or problem-solving skills. Barrett (1998) describes such a model in which parents and children are empowered to form an 'expert team' to tackle anxiety. Therapy sessions involve parents and children, the open sharing of information is promoted and the content and process of therapy is jointly determined, with emphasis placed on identifying and reinforcing existing skills of family members. Cobham et al. (1998) described a similar model. The authors report an intervention that incorporates both child-focused CBT to treat child anxiety and a programme designed to reduce parental anxiety. Children received ten therapy sessions while their parents received four specifically designed sessions to help them recognize the effect of their own behaviour on the development and maintenance of their child's problems and how to address their own anxiety.

The final model, which has received less attention, is where child-focused concerns are indirectly addressed by cognitive work with parents. Parental attributions about the child's behaviour, beliefs about parenting or perceptions of parenting efficacy can be identified and reappraised via direct cognitive work with the parents. This model may be useful for working with preschool children or in preventive approaches. A recent example was described by Bugental et al. (2002) who found that parents of newly born infants who were encouraged to identify non-blaming causal attributions to explain their child's behaviour were less likely to engage in harsh or abusive parenting.

The focus, content and nature of these interventions are very different, thereby raising the question of what is the most effective way of involving parents in CBT with children. A number of researchers have suggested that parental involvement may enhance the effectiveness of CBT (King et al., 1998; Mendlowitz et al., 1999; Toren et al., 2000). More systematic attempts to evaluate the additional contribution of parental involvement have been undertaken in a series of studies with children with generalized anxiety disorders. Barrett et al. (1996) compared child-focused CBT with child-focused CBT plus family anxiety management and found that involving parents resulted in additional benefits, particularly for younger children. These improvements were maintained at 12 months, although, contrary to predictions, the addition of family anxiety management did not result in any additional gains when assessed at 6 years (Barrett et al., 2001). Similarly, Cobham et al. (1998) found that child-focused CBT was enhanced by the inclusion of parental anxiety management, but only for children with at least one anxious parent. These gains, however, became less evident at 6- and 12-month follow-up. The results are not, however, consistent with the findings of Spence et al. (2000) who failed to find any significant effects of parental participation in a CBT programme with children with social phobia at 12-month follow-up.

8.9   Conclusion

This chapter has attempted to highlight some of the many issues involved in undertaking CBT with young children. There is a general consensus that children of 7 years and above are able to participate in CBT. Younger children may be able to engage in some CBT programmes if the cognitive demands of the intervention are matched to the child's cognitive development. Although aware-ness of the need to adapt and modify CBT for use with prepubertal children is growing, comparatively few studies describe how this has been achieved. Pro-grammes currently span a comparatively wide age range and there are few reports of the use of CBT with children under the age of 7. Comparatively few randomized controlled trials have yet been reported and the issue of whether or not CBT is more or less effective with younger children has received little attention. Research evaluating the active treatment components and the bal-ance between the cognitive and behavioural elements has seldom been investi-gated. As highlighted by Bailey (2001), CBT with younger children will probably involve a higher proportion of behavioural to cognitive strategies; this raises the important definitional question of when behaviour therapy becomes CBT.

In terms of theoretical development, cognitive models to explain the onset and maintenance of psychological problems in children are notably absent. The unique developmental context of the child has rarely been considered as CBT models derived from research with adults have been downloaded and applied to children (Barrett *et al.*, 2000). Developmentally appropriate models that consider the child's age and the role of the family are not widely developed. Similarly, while parental involvement in CBT programmes, particularly with younger children, appears to be inherently logical, there is, as yet, no consistent evidence that effectiveness is enhanced by such involvement. Further work is required to develop theoretically sound models to explain the development and mainten-ance of dysfunctional cognitive processing in children that, in turn, will inform the most effective way of involving parents in CBT programmes with their children.

8.10   REFERENCES

Bailey, V. (2001). Cognitive-behavioural therapies for children and adolescents. *Advances in Psychi-atric Treatment*, 7, 224–32.

Barrett, P. M. (1998). Evaluation of cognitive-behavioural group treatments for childhood anxiety disorders. *Journal of Clinical Child Psychology*, **27**, 459–68.

(2000). Treatment of childhood anxiety: developmental aspects. *Clinical Psychology Review*, **20**, 479–94.

Barrett, P. M., Dadds, M. R. and Rapee, R. M. (1996). Family treatment of childhood anxiety: a controlled trial. *Journal of Consulting and Clinical Psychology*, **64**, 333–42.

Barrett, P. M., Duffy, A. L., Dadds, M. R. and Rapee, R. M. (2001). Cognitive-behavioural treatment of anxiety disorders in children: long-term (6 year) follow-up. *Journal of Consulting and Clinical Psychology*, **69**, 135–41.

Barrett, P., Webster, H. and Turner, C. (2000). *The FRIENDS Group Leader's Manual for Children*, edn 111. Australian Academic Press.

Berliner, L. and Saunders, B. E. (1996). Treating fear and anxiety in sexually abused children. Results of a controlled 2-year follow-up study. *Child Maltreatment*, **1**, 294–309.

Bugental, D. P., Ellerson, P. C., Lin, E. K., Rainey, B., Kokotovic, A. and O'Hara, N. (2002). A cognitive approach to child abuse prevention. *Journal of Family Psychology*, **16**, 243–58.

Cobham, V. E., Dadds, M. R. and Spence, S. H. (1998). The role of parental anxiety in the treatment of childhood anxiety. *Journal of Consulting and Clinical Psychology*, **66**, 893–905.

Cohen, J. A. and Mannarino, A. P. (1996). A treatment outcome study for sexually abused preschool children: initial findings. *Journal of the American Academy of Child and Adolescent Psychiatry*, **35**, 42–50.

Cornwall, E., Spence, S. H. and Schotte, D. (1996). The effectiveness of emotive imagery in the treatment of darkness phobia in children. *Behaviour Change*, **13**, 223–9.

Dadds, M. R., Spence, S. H., Holland, D. E., Barrett, P. M. and Laurens, K. R. (1997). Prevention and early intervention for anxiety disorders: a controlled trial. *Journal of Consulting and Clinical Psychology*, **65**, 627–35.

Durlak, J. A., Furnham, T. and Lampman, C. (1991). Effectiveness of cognitive-behaviour therapy for maladapting children: a meta-analysis. *Psychological Bulletin*, **110**, 204–14.

Durlak, J. A., Wells, A. M., Cotton, J. K. and Johnson, S. (1995). Analysis of selected methodological issues in child psychotherapy research. *Journal of Clinical Child Psychology*, **24**, 141–8.

Ehlers, A. and Clark, D. M. (2000). A cognitive model of posttraumatic stress disorder. *Behaviour Research and Therapy*, **38**, 319–45.

Feehan, C. J. and Vostanis, P. (1996). Cognitive-behavioural therapy for depressed children: children's and therapists' impressions. *Behavioural and Cognitive Psychotherapy*, **24**, 171–83.

Flavell, J. H., Flavell, E. R. and Green, F. L. (2001). Developments of children's understanding of connections between thinking and feeling. *Psychological Science*, **12**, 430–2.

Friedberg, R. D. and McClure, J. A. (2002). *Clinical Practice of Cognitive Therapy with Children and Adolescents: The Nuts and Bolts*. New York: Guilford Press.

Harrington, R., Wood, A. and Verduyn, C. (1998). Clinically depressed adolescents. In P. Graham (ed.). *Cognitive Behaviour Therapy for Children and Families*, 1st edn. Cambridge: Cambridge University Press.

Jackson, H. J. and King, N. J. (1981). The emotive imagery treatment of a child's trauma-induced phobia. *Journal of Behaviour Therapy and Experimental Psychiatry*, **12**, 325–8.

Jayson, D., Wood, A., Kroll, L., Fraser, J. and Harrington, R. (1998). Which depressed patients respond to cognitive-behavioural treatment? *Journal of the American Academy of Child and Adolescent Psychiatry*, **37**, 35–9.

Kane, M. T. and Kendall, P. C. (1989). Anxiety disorders in children: a multiple baseline evaluation of a cognitive behavioural treatment. *Behaviour Therapy*, **20**, 499–508.

Kendall, P. C. (1994), Treating anxiety disorders in children: results of a randomised clinical trial. *Journal of Consulting and Clinical Psychology*, **62**, 100–10.

Kendall, P. C. and Hollon, S. D. (eds.) (1979). *Cognitive-Behavioural Interventions: Theory, Research and Procedures*. New York: Academic Press.

Kendall, P. C., Flannery-Schroeder, E., Panichelli-Mindel, S. M., Sotham-Gerow, M., Henin, A. and Warman, M. (1997). Therapy with youths with anxiety disorders: a second randomized clinical trial. *Journal of Consulting and Clinical Psychology*, **65**, 366–80.

King, N. J., Tonge, B. J., Heyne, D. *et al.* (1998). Cognitive behavioral treatment of school-refusing children: a controlled evaluation. *Journal of the American Academy of Child and Adolescent Psychiatry*, **37**, 395–403.

Last, C. J., Hansen, C. and Franco, N. (1998). Cognitive-behavioural treatment of school phobia. *Journal of the American Academy of Child and Adolescent Psychiatry*, **37**, 404–11.

March, J. S., Mulle, K. and Herbel, B. (1994). Behavioral psychotherapy for children and adolescents with obsessive-compulsive disorder: an open clinical trial of a new protocol-driven treatment package. *Journal of the American Academy of Child and Adolescent Psychiatry*, **33**, 333–41.

Mendlowitz, S. L., Manassis, M. D., Bradley, S., Scapillato, D., Miezitis, S. and Shaw, B. F. (1999). Cognitive behavior group treatments in childhood anxiety disorders: the role of parental involvement. *Journal of the American Academy of Child and Adolescent Psychiatry*, **38**, 1223–9.

Rapee, R. M. (2001). The development of generalised anxiety disorder. In M. W. Vasey and M. R. Dadds (eds.), *The Development of Psychopathology in Anxiety*. New York: Oxford University Press.

Ronen, T. (1993). Intervention package for treating encopresis in a 6 year old boy: a case study. *Behavioral Psychotherapy*, **21**, 127–35.

Ronen, T., Rahav, G. and Wozner, Y. (1995). Self-control and enuresis. *Journal of Cognitive Psychotherapy*, **9**, 249–58.

Salkovskis, P. (1999). Understanding and treating obsessive-compulsive disorder. *Behaviour Research and Therapy*, **37**, 29–52.

Salmon, K. and Bryant, R. A. (2002). Posttraumatic stress disorder in children: the influence of developmental factors. *Clinical Psychology Review*, **22**, 163–88.

Sanders, M. R., Cleghorn, G., Shepherd, R. W. and Patrick, M. (1996). Predictors of clinical improvement in children with recurrent abdominal pain. *Behavioural and Cognitive Psychotherapy*, **24**, 27–38.

Silverman, W. K., Kurtines, W. M., Ginsburg, G. S., Weems, C. F., Lumpkin, P. W. and Carmichael, D. H. (1999a). Treating anxiety disorders in children with group cognitive behavioral therapy: a randomized clinical trial. *Journal of Consulting and Clinical Psychology*, **67**, 995–1003.

Silverman, W. K., Kurtines, W. M., Ginsburg, G. S., Weems, C. F., Rabian, B. and Setafini, L. T. (1999b). Contingency management, self control and education support in the treatment of childhood phobic disorders a randomized clinical trial. *Journal of Consulting and Clinical Psychology*, **67**, 675–87.

Spence, S. H. (1995). *Social Skills Training: Enhancing Social Competence with Children and Adolescents*. Windsor: NFER.

Spence, S. H., Donovan, C. and Brechman-Toussaint, M. (2000). The treatment of childhood social phobia: the effectiveness of a social skills training-based cognitive behavioural intervention with and without parental involvement. *Journal of Child Psychology and Psychiatry*, **41**, 713–26.

Stallard, P. (2002). *Think Good Feel Good: A Cognitive Behaviour Therapy Workbook for Children and Young People*. Winchester: John Wiley.

Thornton, S. (2002). *Growing Minds: An Introduction to Cognitive Development*. Hampshire: Palgrave Macmillan.

Toren, P., Wolmer, L., Rosental, B. *et al.* (2000). Case series: brief parent-child group therapy for childhood anxiety disorders using a manual based cognitive-behavioral technique. *Journal of the American Academy of Child and Adolescent Psychiatry*, **39**, 1309–12.

Turk, J. (1998). Children with learning difficulties and their parents. In P. Graham (ed.), *Cognitive Behaviour Therapy for Children and Families*, 1st edn. Cambridge: Cambridge University Press.

Vostanis, P., Feehan, C., Grattan, E. and Bickerton, W. (1996). Treatment for children and adolescents with depression: lessons from a controlled trial. *Clinical Child Psychology and Psychiatry*, **1**, 199–212.

Wellman, H. M., Hollander, M. and Schult, C. A. (1996). Young children's understanding of thought bubbles and thoughts. *Child Development*, **67**, 768–88.

Williams, T. I., Salkovskis, P. M., Forrester, E. A. and Allsopp, M. A. (2002). Changes in symptoms of OCD and appraisal of responsibility during cognitive behavioural treatment: a pilot study. *Behavioural and Cognitive Psychotherapy*, **30**, 69–78.

Wood, A., Harrington, R. and Moore, A. (1996). Controlled trial of a brief cognitive-behavioural intervention in adolescent patients with depressive disorders. *Journal of Child Psychology and Psychiatry*, **37**, 736–46.

9

Cognitive behaviour therapy in inpatient environments

Jonathan Green

Booth Hall Children's Hospital, Manchester, UK

9.1 Introduction

Children and adolescents treated within inpatient child and adolescent psychiatry units form a heterogeneous population in terms of age, functional difficulties and diagnosis. Adaptation of cognitive behaviour therapy (CBT) for use within these units therefore needs to take into account their varied characteristics. It also needs to consider the particular features of an inpatient unit as a treatment environment. Consequently, this chapter will begin by reviewing each of these two areas – the patient group and the treatment environment – before going on to consider the role of CBT as a treatment within the inpatient setting.

9.2 Characteristics of child and adolescent inpatients

9.2.1 Diagnostic pattern

Recent national UK survey data (O'Herlihy *et al.*, 2001) have provided a comprehensive cross-sectional picture of the current diagnostic composition of inpatient practice in the UK (Table 9.1). Surveys from other countries have shown similar patterns of morbidity (Sourander and Turunen, 1999).

The census reflects some key diagnostic patterns in inpatient populations:

- Eating disorders represent a high percentage of female admissions in both child and adolescent groups.
- Acute psychosis is an important cause of admission in adolescence but is not at all negligible in children.
- Despite often being thought of as contraindications for admission, conduct disorder and other externalizing problems are highly prevalent in child admissions, especially in younger boys.

Cognitive Behaviour Therapy for Children and Families, ed. Philip J. Graham.
Published by Cambridge University Press. © Cambridge University Press 2004.

Table 9.1 Clinician-reported diagnosis of patients at a day census of 71 UK child and adolescent inpatient units (Sept 2000). Groups reported by gender and age – results as a proportion within each group

	Male under 13 ($n = 91$) (%)	Female under 13 ($n = 65$) (%)	Male over 13 ($n = 162$) (%)	Female over 13 ($n = 287$) (%)
Organic brain disorder	2.2	2.9	1.2	1.0
Substance misuse-related disorder	2.2	2.9	2.3	1.7
Psychotic disorder	4.4	8.8	33.3	13.8
Mood disorder	9.7	4.4	21.1	18.1
Anxiety disorder	8.6	5.9	4.1	3.4
Acute stress reaction	3.2	2.9	2.9	7.4
Pervasive developmental disorder	3.2	0	2.9	0.3
Hyperkinetic disorder	12.9	4.4	1.8	0.3
Conduct disorder/mixed conduct and emotional disorder	22.6	5.9	4.7	1.7
Elimination disorder	3.2	7.4	0.6	0
Eating disorders	3.2	30.9	4.7	32.2
Sleep disorder	0	1.5	0	0
Somatizing/somatoform disorder	1.1	2.9	0.6	2.3
Personality disorder	0	0	3.5	6.0
Others	16.1	13.2	9.4	7.4

Reproduced with permission from O'Herlihy *et al.*, 2001.

- Pervasive developmental disorders and other neuropsychiatric conditions are most common in child units.
- Mood disorders are an important component of both adolescent and child populations.

9.2.2   Functional impairment

Diagnosis alone, however, is not the main predictor of outcome or need in this population (Green *et al.*, 2001; Green, 2002). Functional assessments such as the Children's Global Assessment Scale (CGAS; Shaffer *et al.*, 1983) and the Health of the Nation Outcome Scales for Children and Adolescents (HoNOSCA; Gowers *et al.*, 1999) allow relatively simple weighting of case complexity and functional impairment. A recent UK prospective study showed that these measures are a good marker of health gains made during admission (Green *et al.*, 2001).

Table 9.2 Percentage of patients with health needs unmet or persisting despite intervention on admission to child and adolescent units

Domain	% needs, child units ($n = 76$)	% needs, adolescent units ($n = 74$)
Self-care	29	34
Physical illness/mental impairment	13	28
Leisure problems	32	63
School attendance	32	71
Educational performance	71	70
Social relationships	79	51
Family relationships	63	40
Destructive behaviour	67	24
Hostile behaviour	84	36
Oppositional/disruptive behaviour	85	31
Deliberate self-harm	28	51
Mood problems	47	75
Hallucinations/delusions	7	33
Hyperactivity	68	13
Anxiety/PTSD	57	65
Eating disorders	11	24
Obsessive compulsive disorder/tics	39	22
Pervasive developmental disorder	27	5
Elimination disorders	28	0
Cultural/racial identity	—	8

From Green J. M. *et al.* (2001) with permission.

9.2.3 Health needs

'Health need' refers to a situation in which: (1) there is symptomatology above a predetermined threshold in a specific area; (2) there is a desire on the part of the sufferer to receive help for this; and (3) an appropriate treatment exists but is not being given. Health needs methodology rates such needs from multiple perspectives, with emphasis on the views of users and carers, and in domains wider than the purely psychopathological – such as leisure activities, educational progress, friendships, self-care and family relationships (Kroll *et al.*, 1999). Preliminary data on inpatient health needs from a representative subsample of the current UK Children and Young Persons Inpatient Evaluation (CHYPIE) Study are summarized in Table 9.2. This method serves to amplify the picture that we have of this client group.

Child units show particularly high levels of unmet need in areas of:

(1) Social and family relationships – over 50% of admissions show difficulties in these areas: imminent family breakdown is a common factor in requesting admission (see below).

(2) Externalizing behaviours – nearly 90% of admissions show hostility and oppositional destructive behaviour and 70% show overactivity. These behavioural difficulties (reflecting also the preponderance of boys on child units) may be the main presentation or may be comorbid with other difficulties.

In the adolescent group, there are high unmet needs in:

(1) Mood problems, psychotic-type disorders and specific anxiety disorders.

(2) Educational problems and social activities outside the home (leisure activities). These overall difficulties in social functioning in a broad sense reflect major issues for inpatients that will be considered further below.

9.2.4   Case severity and complexity

The needs data highlight the complexity and multifaceted nature of inpatient cases, often including both developmental and psychosocial symptoms. Strategic targeting of treatment goals (Shaw, 1998) can help to clarify treatment direction within this complexity and this is an essential component of modern inpatient practice. But, however useful, goal setting cannot remove the reality of the complexity and interdependence of the various domains of difficulty in many cases – factors that often act to undermine progress.

9.2.5   Comorbidity

Comorbidity is an aspect of case complexity. Multiple comorbidity in inpatients is the rule. This matters in treatment design when the fact that a difficulty is associated with one kind of problem may undermine proposed treatments for another. For example, covert pervasive developmental disorder, commonly not recognized in complex outpatient cases, may undermine a child's ability to make use of psychological treatments of all kinds unless the treatments are adapted (see case vignette, Section 9.4.2.2.7). Admitted children commonly have unrecognized neurodevelopmental vulnerabilities, which have contributed to their problems of being treatment resistant in outpatient settings. Comorbidity has a major influence on treatment design.

9.2.6   Social and developmental impairments

The needs analysis suggests that general impairments in social functioning are a notable feature of admissions. Two other studies support this view. Widespread social difficulties were found in 58 consecutive general admissions in New

Zealand, combined with moderate to severe language handicap in 40% of cases (Paterson *et al.*, 1997). A US study of 126 hospitalized children and adolescents (Luthar *et al.*, 1995) similarly found severe impairments on Vineland social competency scores in patients admitted with externalizing and mixed internalizing/ externalizing disorders, associated specifically with reduced specific reading retardation. Treatments targeting such social impairments are a priority for consideration.

9.2.7   Family breakdown

As the needs data suggests, functional breakdown in family care is a common reason for the request for admission. This does not necessarily imply that the family is a primary aetiological agent in the disorder. Indeed, cases where family failure is the primary element, such as neglect and abuse, will often need social care rather than inpatient psychiatric provision. However, there are many other cases where the impact of the child's mental illness on the family overwhelms their resources and the interaction between family process and the child's development and mental illness becomes negative and escalating. It is usually in these conditions that psychiatric admission is useful. This fact influences treatment choices during admission: family-focused work is essential if treatment gains are to be maintained following discharge (Green, 1994).

9.2.8   Involvement of multiple agencies

A UK thematic review of child mental health services (National Health Service Health Advisory Service, 1995) provides a persuasive model of how, as patients move through successive 'tiers' of specialized care, it is increasingly likely that they will be involved with multiple agencies in addition to health, particularly social services and education. Population-based epidemiological studies (Kurtz, 1994) point to the same conclusion. To be successful, inpatient treatment design therefore needs to be multimodal and involve links with other agencies.

9.2.9   Treatment resistance, consent and therapeutic alliance

The inpatient treatment will often be seen as the 'last resort' by families or professionals following failed outpatient treatments – but not uncommonly by the patient as a 'punishment' or rejection. Surveys suggest that children rarely feel involved or in agreement with the decision to admit. However, the therapeutic alliance with the child – marked by the child's positive adjustment to the ward environment and active participation in treatment programming – has been found to be one of the best predictors of symptom change during admission

(Green *et al.*, 2001); in contrast, the alliance with parents did not predict. This emphasizes the great importance of pre-admission preparation and intensive child-/adolescent-focused work. These are not easy cases and the initial task will often be to foster motivation and hope. Any individual treatment needs to be seen in the context of the overall child alliance to the unit and their individual consent and motivation (Green, 2002).

9.3 Characteristics of the inpatient treatment environment

Inpatient child and adolescent units are examples of low-volume, high-intensity specialist environments. They may be administratively free standing, part of and sited within the campus of a general children's hospital (child units) or part of and sited within adult mental health services. Staffing typically involves multi-professional teams comprising ward staff (usually mental health-trained or children's trained nurses and play specialists), psychiatrists and a variable range of allied professionals including clinical psychologists, social workers, occupational therapists, family therapists, psychotherapists and speech and language therapists. Within the UK and US contexts, guidance has been set down as to the quantity and range of professionals that should be expected to constitute the inpatient team (American Academy of Child and Adolescent Psychiatry, 1990; Royal College of Psychiatrists, 1999). In practice, the composition of teams often falls far short of these standards (Green and Jacobs, 1998a) and the application of CBT needs to take such reality into account.

Patients are typically resident for 5 or 7 days. Time is often structured around a conventional school day in a specialized school unit attached to the ward or a more generic school environment nearby. Non-school time will be structured partly according to basic care provision (thus, there will be regular mealtimes, playtimes, leisure time, etc.) and also by the provision of structured therapeutic ward activities.

9.3.1 Principles of therapeutic care

Inpatient treatment offers a complex mix of therapeutic opportunities:

- There is the very fact of admission; in other words, the removal of the young person from the home environment of family, school and community into a specialized social and educational setting. For some types of problem, removal itself can bring about rapid gains for the patient (Green *et al.*, 2001; Green, 2002).
- Many patients admitted to inpatient units have overt or covert developmental difficulties, specific learning difficulties, social impairments and a history of school failure. The specialized and intensive setting of the inpatient environment,

combining social and educational environments, can produce rapid gains in these areas as well as in self-esteem.

- The ward environment allows many opportunities for various forms of 'social therapy'. These can include therapeutic groups, activities of daily living and the oversight of basic issues such as, for example, food intake in an eating disorder.

- There are additional opportunities for specialized treatment programmes, which can be conducted within the ward environment or by removal to 'office-based' environments. Examples of the former might be programmes where intensive supervision is necessary, such as response prevention. Examples of the latter will be treatments conducted in a more conventional outpatient-type format such as various forms of psychological therapy including CBT, oversight of medication and family therapy.

The multidisciplinary nature of this undertaking means that if treatments are to be delivered on the ward then this must be done using a whole team approach with shared protocols. When 'office-based' treatments are used, there is still the issue of integrating this with the ward-based programme. Ward work and individualized work may conflict – for instance, the patient group being aware that one person is getting one sort of therapy while others are getting other forms. Such problems have been discussed in relation to the dynamic psychotherapeutic treatments that have historically predominated in inpatient environments (Leibenluft et al., 1993; Magagna, 1998). The use of CBT in inpatient care will need to address the same systemic issues.

The nature of the ward environment also affects measurement of outcome and progress. Since treatment within the inpatient environment is multimodal, it is often hard to target which element of treatment is affecting particular symptoms and thus adjust treatments accordingly. Design of treatment programmes and their monitoring has to take this fact into account.

9.4   Adapting CBT treatment to inpatient practice

9.4.1   Adapting to the treatment environment

9.4.1.1   CBT and multidisciplinary working

Everyday contact with patients is largely with the nursing and other members of the ward team. Behavioural aspects of CBT such as programmes to reduce aggressive behaviours, response prevention for obsessive compulsive disorders and programmes to modify eating behaviour thus all need to be mediated by ward staff. Cognitive components may also be undertaken by members of the ward staff or other members of the multidisciplinary team. Coordinating such a large and diverse team to deliver consistent treatments well is a major challenge, which is particular to inpatient practice. Complex treatments need to be operationalized for front-line shift staff and therapy programmes must be clearly defined and flexible enough to adapt to this team environment. A number of characteristics of CBT are well adapted to this:

(1) The emphasis on explicit treatment contracting helps clarify complex therapeutic relationships with numerous team members.

(2) The explicit goal focus of CBT practice and its relatively structured procedures can help generate team goal setting with shared explicit and understandable aims.

(3) Baseline measurement and systematic recording of therapeutic outcome is helpful in focusing team efforts and monitoring complex disorders.

(4) The process-orientated time-limited framework of much CBT is helpful for organizing complex treatments within short admission stays.

9.4.1.2   CBT and unit ethos

The CBT approach is consistent with the core ethos of much of modern Child and Adolescent Mental Health Services (CAMHS) and fits in well with many current inpatient treatment environments; it is characterized by relatively short stays, an orientation towards evaluation and measurement and treatment plans that are constructed from specific aims and treatment objectives. Wever (1998) gives an excellent example of this approach. It is crucial that the underlying unit ethos is compatible with CBT methods – otherwise, systemic tensions will inevitably impact on unit coherence and good patient care (Green and Burke, 1998).

Many units and their staff have a leaning towards psychodynamic ideas and treatments and a synthesis of approaches often needs to be engendered for the ward environment to be coherent. A number of typical features of psychodynamic approaches remain invaluable in assessment and formulation: the emphasis on careful listening and observation; the response to the 'whole patient'; and the view that behavioural and emotional problems may have important underlying causes that are not immediately obvious but need to be tackled before further progress can be made. These values inform good comprehensive assessment and are a valuable precursor to the application of CBT, which current evidence suggests is more likely than psychodynamic psychotherapy to bring about focused behavioural change in many situations.

Similarly, the ongoing therapeutic environment of the ward needs to be sufficiently structured to bring a sense of order to the lives of children whose home lives are often chaotic, but also sufficiently flexible and permissive to encourage the expression of emotions and difficulties that might illuminate the

psychopathology where this is not immediately apparent. This presents a challenging, but not impossible, task to the staff of inpatient units, especially those
engaged in day-to-day interactions with children.

9.4.2   Adaptations to the client group

9.4.2.1   General issues

9.4.2.1.1   *Case complexity*

One of the challenges for any treatment modality practised within the inpatient
environment is the complexity of presentations. As has already been seen, the
patients often have a mixture of diagnoses along with developmental vulnerabilities or impairments. CBT delivered on an outpatient basis typically targets
specific single diagnoses or behaviours, such as specific anxiety disorders, obsessive compulsive disorder, uncontrolled anger or depression. It is sometimes suggested that CBT can and should only be applied in situations where the disorder
is tractable and motivation good. However, this view is not always sustainable
in inpatient units that have a mandate to manage complexity and that are often
the treatment location of last resort. Ingenuity and effort therefore have to be
applied to framing complex cases in a manner that opens the way to helpful
treatment approaches. Core CBT techniques such as behavioural analysis can
be very valuable here.

9.4.2.1.2   *Behavioural management*

Children are often admitted in the hope that intensive inpatient assessment will
clarify complex or treatment-resistant disorders. To some extent, this expectation is reasonable, particularly in relation to more intrinsic, environmentally
stable aspects of child behaviour such as social impairments or attention difficulties. However, the patterns of behavioural reinforcers and relationships
on the ward will be different from those at home and it is hardly surprising
that behavioural symptoms are often modified by admission, especially early
on. This 'honeymoon period' can cause false negative ascertainment in short
admissions.

The CBT approach focuses on baseline observations and functional analysis;
the inpatient environment allows precise event recording, duration recording,
time sampling and interval recording of behaviours (Jacobs, 1998a). It is important to have systematic means of recording that are consistent across ward staff
shift changes. The assessment should also focus on analysing a child's positive
features and strengths and on likely social and material reinforcers appropriate
for use in future behavioural programmes. Useful reinforcers within the inpatient environment must be within the therapist's control and specific to the

treatment (sweets and crisps are examples of poorly effective reinforcers because they are dispensed freely by visitors). They must be used in a graded and practical way – the inpatient environment allows them to be used immediately after the occurrence of required behaviour. They should be agreed with parents and Jacobs (1998a) makes the important point that it is counterproductive to introduce a behavioural management programme on the inpatient unit that is too complex to be generalized to home following discharge.

Some negative reinforcers are usefully incorporated into behavioural programmes. These include ignoring unwanted behaviours, distraction onto other activities or 'time out' methods. Here, the dynamics of the patient group affect strategies. Ignoring unwanted behaviours within a group context is often ineffective and can threaten group escalation. The group is often sensitive to different responses being applied to different patients. Much staff training, supervision and support needs to be applied to this area: it is one of difficulty and one which staff stress in the front line inpatient work. A staff group that is mutually supportive, well informed by coherent theory and supported by other members of the team such as clinical psychologists and psychiatrists will find the management of the group much more tolerable. Group dynamics can, however, powerfully promote change when positive expectations become the dominant feature of the ward culture.

Some form of 'time out' is commonly practised within inpatient environments, particularly in children's units, but the exact details of how this is applied vary considerably (Green and Jacobs, 1998b). Child, staff and parents must understand that the purpose is not to punish the child but to remove him from things that are 'working him up' and to give him a chance to 'calm down'. Removal of the child must be done confidently and with a minimum of ambivalence or fuss (any staff uncertainty is immediately picked up by the child). The period in a time out room should be short and specified. The room itself must be an adequate non-stimulating space – units have tended to move away from an austere featureless room prevalent in the past to a more comforting but quiet environment. Teams also now have to be extremely sensitive to issues of coercion and restriction of liberty while undertaking time out. Old practices of locking the room or extended periods in seclusion are not now acceptable except in explicit circumstances for which consent has been specifically obtained.

Time out procedures will be available when needed but will not be the main focus of behaviour management in well-functioning units – which generally have a predominant emphasis on promoting positive pro-social behaviours and expectations. In contrast, a sensitive sign of a staff team that is becoming overwhelmed or dysfunctional is a predominant focus on crisis management and on decreasing unwanted behaviours through various forms of punishment or control of the child (Green and Jacobs, 1998b). Most units will experience both extremes at times. A high level of resilience and skill is expected from inpatient staff. Appropriate contemporary emphasis on child rights and avoidance of coercion must be kept in mind while staff are faced with managing a group of behaviourally disturbed young people. Maintaining a coherent set of positive contingencies within the ward culture is a sustained task that needs constant input and support from the whole staff team, a high level of sophisticated treatment planning and confident positive leadership. The transparency of behavioural analysis and the practical nature of behavioural techniques can be a helpful unifying focus for the team in this context.

9.4.2.1.3   Social skills

As described above, around 80% of young people admitted to inpatient units have problems with social functioning. They may have social cognitive *deficits* – a relative lack of ability to process social information effectively or to respond appropriately – or there may be social cognitive *distortions* – a tendency to misconstrue ambiguous situations particularly in relation to hostile intent (Crick and Dodge, 1994). Perhaps because it is not readily identifiable with specific diagnosis or symptoms, social skills training is an under-utilized treatment in the inpatient environment. Various forms of CBT for enhancing social competence have been well described elsewhere (see Chapter 23) and should be a central mainstay of inpatient CBT treatment both at an individual and group level. The advantage of the inpatient environment for this work, as with behavioural modification, is the 24-hour environment, which allows a potentially constant opportunity to enhance and practise new social skills within the peer group setting.

A reciprocal potential disadvantage of the inpatient environment is that usually all the peer group are also disturbed and do not provide either easy partners in social change or positive role models for normality. This concentration of disturbance is voiced as a frequent concern about inpatient practice. It is true that a poorly functioning peer group environment can be at best unhelpful and at worst destructive. However, the peer environment offers an opportunity for interaction with children with similar problems, creates a sense of shared difficulty and is an opportunity for enhanced self-esteem. Children who are failures outside may become successes in the inpatient group. With careful decisions on case mix, it is usually possible for staff to maximize the potential benefits of inpatient treatment and minimize its deficits. At the very least, the admission can clarify the problems and make a start on their improvement – linking with external agencies to promote appropriate placement and further change following discharge.

9.4.2.1.4   *Desensitization and response prevention*

The inpatient unit can be a powerful location for graded desensitization and response prevention techniques. These are usually used in the context of anxiety and obsessive compulsive disorders (see Chapter 18). Graded exposure to an increasing hierarchy of feared situations, previously established with the child, is a powerful treatment for various forms of specific anxiety. Similarly, programmes of response prevention for children with severe compulsive behaviours can sometimes be more effectively undertaken with the greater control available in the inpatient setting; Wever (1998) usefully discusses the indications for this.

9.4.2.1.5   *Therapeutic alliance and motivational interviewing*

Therapeutic alliance between child and the unit as a whole provides one of the best predictors of health gain during the inpatient treatment stay (Green *et al.*, 2001). Motivational interviewing (see Chapter 5) linked to the use of CBT is particularly well suited to achieve a therapeutic alliance in complex situations, where the child may not have been the main decision maker for admission.

9.4.2.2   Specific disorders

9.4.2.2.1   *Conduct and hyperkinetic disorders*

Conduct and oppositional behaviours are prevalent in units (Tables 9.1 and 9.2) but admitting such children has been controversial since they can be disruptive to the milieu and are often thought to have poor outcome (although this reflects the general view about outcome for the disorder in any setting). However, there are some positive indications for admission. In one study (Green *et al.*, 2001), conduct disorder patients who developed a positive therapeutic alliance seemed to do as well as other cases – suggesting that it is not the diagnosis *per se* but the engagement into useful treatment that is the key factor. This finding was independent of overall symptom severity. (Poor alliance and poor outcome was nevertheless the rule – and particularly associated with high levels of aggression.) Admission can allow the detailed analysis of aetiological and comorbid factors in resistant cases and the opportunity for intensive group work (Jacobs, 1998b). The effective use of CBT techniques in oppositional and conduct disorders in the outpatient or community setting is described in Chapters 13 and 25; similar principles can be applied to the ward setting. A ward milieu combining positive and explicit behavioural expectations with labelled praise and an emphasis on pro-social activities in the group can be a powerful corrective learning experience for the child. Anger management techniques can be applied individually in an office-based fashion or within a ward milieu context. Ward-based therapeutic groups that combine social problem-solving, social emotional awareness and anger management techniques are an important component and can be informed by outpatient programmes such as Webster–Stratton's dinosaur school (Webster-Stratton and Hammond, 1997). A strength of inpatient treatment is that the 'homework' expected of children between such group sessions is done within the inpatient setting as part of a coordinated behaviour management programme. When school-based behavioural programmes on the unit are effectively combined with ward-based therapeutic groups and active staff management can remain consistent over time, the child can benefit from a very powerful total learning environment. Cotton (1993) gives an excellent indication of these possibilities.

9.4.2.2.2   Adjustment disorders including abuse and trauma

There is surprisingly little systematic evidence on the prevalence of past experience of abuse and trauma in inpatient populations. However, clinical experience suggests that the rates are high. New disclosures of abuse are not uncommon during admission, and these can then finally make sense of a perplexing presentation. A number of studies have shown the advantages of CBT interventions for abuse over non-directive supporting treatment or standard community treatment (Brent *et al.*, 2002; see also Chapter 10).

9.4.2.2.3   Mood disorders

It has been seen that mood disorders are common presentations in inpatient units and cognitive therapy is now well established as a first-line treatment in adolescent affective disorder (Harrington *et al.*, 1998; see also Chapter 16). CBT in the inpatient setting will be conducted in a similar fashion to the outpatient context. Useful additions within the inpatient environment will be additional behavioural measures such as the use of time structuring and peer therapy groups to enhance interpersonal contact.

9.4.2.2.4   Eating disorders

Eating disorders form a substantial proportion of adolescent inpatient admissions (see above). Admission is very widely used for weight restoration and the stabilization of eating behaviours, although there is currently lively debate about the specific value of this over outpatient management (Green, 2002). Weight restoration programmes are essentially based on operant conditioning. Today, these will be embedded in other approaches including cognitive work with the young person as well as family therapy. In eating disorders such as bulimia nervosa, when normal weight is preserved, there has been emphasis recently on outpatient rather than inpatient treatment although hospitalization is still recommended on occasion as a way of breaking through the vicious cycle of starvation, bingeing and vomiting (Steinhausen, 2002).

9.4.2.2.5 *Psychosis*

The incidence of schizophrenia rises steadily through adolescence and the disorder forms an important component to admissions to adolescent units (Table 9.1). CBT of schizophrenia in adults has been used to reduce the impact of treatment-resistant positive symptoms (Tarrier *et al.*, 1993). There has been increasing interest recently in the use of such methods for younger patients. However, there is currently no evidence base for this approach. The use of CBT for psychosis is likely to be more applied to family interventions in the context of reducing expressed emotion. How relevant this is to early-onset schizophrenia in adolescence is as yet unclear since families of children and adolescents with schizophrenia tend to express lower levels of criticism and hostility than parents of adult-onset patients (Asarnow *et al.*, 1994). Hollis (2002) considers that family interventions in adolescence aiming to reduce high expressed emotion do not, at the present time, have a strong evidence base to support them.

9.4.2.2.6 *Personality disorders*

'Personality disorder' is diagnosed in a high proportion of girls admitted to adolescent units (see Table 9.1). The concept is contentious in adolescence. Hill (2002) points out that the use of the term is often essentially used to signify a set of related ongoing problems lying beyond an episodic illness, such as difficulties in wider areas of social adjustment. The needs analysis on adolescent inpatient units (Table 9.2) shows just how prevalent such social difficulties are. Following relevant assessment, CBT can be useful in targeting these through social skills training, by a specific focus on mood disorder or by treatment for traumatic memories.

9.4.2.2.7 *Case vignette*

This case illustrates the case complexity of many admissions, assessment and treatment planning and the successful use of modified CBT alongside other treatments. Sarah was a 7-year-old girl referred from specialist colleagues for further assessment. She had presented with a severe oppositional disorder at school and at home, beginning at 3 years, which had led to exclusion from a number of primary schools. Sarah had more recently expressed abnormal beliefs and anxieties: for instance, that a boy in the neighbourhood, whom she did not know, was trying to poison her. She had a number of obsessional routines, which dominated other family members – forcing them to enact episodes of a TV soap opera for hours a day and controlling the way her parents ate because of her sensitivity to chewing sounds. When aroused, she would develop a frenzy of agitation, with fragmented, distractible and aggressive behaviour, and could hardly be settled. Her play reflected her high arousal, apparently delusional states and intense fears of objects and people. She had been a day patient for 7 months and had attracted a number of different diagnoses including attention deficit disorder, conduct disorder and psychosis. There had also been concern about the possibility of sexual abuse.

Sarah had been a long-awaited child: an early adoption after many miscarriages. At the time of admission, both parents were at breaking point and said there were times when they screamed and shouted and hit Sarah, in order to try and keep in control. They were, though, devoted to her care and in their attempts to find some understanding of her problems. Detailed developmental history showed the early emergence of resistance to change, unusual use of language, overactivity and poor social relating.

On admission, Sarah was an extremely difficult management problem, but gradually her arousal levels reduced, her thinking became clearer and her fragmented behaviour lessened. The ward team were initially perplexed by her presentation and unsure how to proceed. Clinically, she could at times be behaviourally almost appropriate for her age but at other times of high arousal showed the emergence of abnormal ideas, possible auditory hallucinations and bizarre behaviour. She played out extreme and sadistic fantasies in relation to her family but her heightened feeling towards her parents waxed and waned and there was no convincing evidence to support a notion of abuse. She began to engage on the unit and developed close positive ties with many of the staff (as well as intense aversions to others).

Assessment on WISC showed Full-Scale IQ of 86 with no Verbal Performance discrepancy. Assessment on structured assessments for autism (Autism Diagnostic Interview (ADI), Autism Diagnostic Observation Schedule (ADOS), Childhood Autism Rating Scale (CARS)) suggested a subtle atypical autistic development. Language assessment showed no semantic deficits in language but significant deficits in the pragmatic use of language and higher order perceptual processing. Occupational therapy assessment showed significant dyspraxic and visuo-perceptual deficits – confirmed on neurodevelopmental examination. Chromosomes, computer tomography and biochemical screens were normal.

This presentation of atypical autistic disorder with high arousal states linked to episodic abnormal quasi-psychotic thinking led to a diagnostic formulation of 'multiplex developmental disorder' (Towbin *et al.*, 1993). The use of a low-dose neuroleptic, initially combined with stimulants, improved her cognitive functioning, lowered her activity levels and had some benefit on social rapport. In this improved state, cognitive treatments were begun, using play materials but focused around structured cognitive tasks. The aims were: (1) to engage her in trying to make sense of her experience and (2) to help her structure her thinking and orientation and counter her cognitive disorganization. In this latter goal, an ABC (antecedents, behaviour, consequences) schema was used to organize her thinking:

Nurse: 'All right Sarah, I can see that you are very angry. Now tell me what happened. What happened first? What did you see? What did you feel? What did you think? Then what did you do? Then what happened next? Let's make a picture of this . . .'

By using drawn visual stimuli, sitting alongside her (rather than face to face, in order to decrease social overload) and writing down what happened in such an ABC scheme, arousal reduction was attempted and alternative behaviours proposed. What she had written or drawn could be used to help her orientation and reinforce cognitive strategies in new situations. Cognitive methods to 'externalize' and master delusional and hallucinatory thinking were also introduced.

Regular occupational therapy focused on sensory integration techniques with similar positive benefit on her behavioural organization. Increasingly, the staff were able to develop more normal capacities in her behaviour and thinking. By the time of her discharge, she had made immense progress, both socially and at school, even though the pervasive developmental problems remained. Intensive work was undertaken with the family to help their understanding and to reduce expressed emotion. She was placed in a weekly residential school, where she remains stable and generally well functioning on low-dose neuroleptic treatment several years after discharge. Attempts to reduce medication too far have led to acute deterioration.

9.4.2.3   Potential contraindications or disadvantages of CBT treatments

A number of these have already been mentioned. There are areas where CBT practice may not be appropriate for the inpatient environment or where considerable adaptation is necessary before it is likely to be useful:

(1)   In some cases of case complexity, it may not be possible to formulate clear treatment goals.

(2)   Too rapid a closure on CBT or treatment goal planning without review may close the team's minds to other emerging aetiologies and problems.

(3)   The CBT approach may not be appropriate for some disorders. For some patients, broader and less well-defined treatment goals may be necessary. It will be one among a range of treatments available on the inpatient unit.

9.4.2.4   Staffing and training implications

Use of CBT effectively in the inpatient unit is only possible if there is leadership from practitioners skilled in the treatment. At a minimum, an experienced clinical psychologist, psychiatrist or senior nurse trained in CBT methods needs to be available to oversee the design and delivery of CBT treatments in this complex environment. Their role will involve both face-to-face interactions with patients and consultation and supervision to other ward staff. Staffing for modern inpatient units should include such professionals (American Academy of Child and Adolescent Psychiatry, 1990; Royal College of Psychiatrists, 1999).

It is also a great advantage if other members of the ward team, including trainees who are psychology graduates, have specific CBT training in order to give strength and depth to the skill mix of the team.

9.5   REFERENCES

American Academy of Child and Adolescent Psychiatry (1990). *Model for Minimum Staffing Patterns for Hospitals Providing Acute Inpatient Treatment for Children and Adolescents with Psychiatric Illnesses*. Washington DC: American Academy of Child and Adolescent Psychiatry.

Asarnow, J. R., Thompson, M. C., Hamilton, E. B., Goldstein, M. J. and Guthrie, D. (1994). Family expressed emotion childhood onset depression and childhood onset schizophrenic spectrum disorders: is expressed emotion a non-specific correlate of psychopathology or a specific risk factor for depression? *Journal of Abnormal Psychology*, **22**, 129–46.

Brent, D. A., Gaynor, S. T. and Weersing, V. R. (2002). Cognitive behavioural approaches to the treatment of depression and anxiety. In M. Rutter and E. Taylor (eds.), *Child and Adolescent Psychiatry*, 4th edn. Oxford: Blackwells, pp. 921–37.

Cotton, N. S. (1993). *Lessons from the Lion's Den: Therapeutic Management of Children in Psychiatric Hospitals and Treatment Centres*. San Francisco, CA: Jossey-Bass.

Crick, N. R. and Dodge, K. A. (1994). A review and reformulation of social information process mechanisms in children's social adjustment. *Psychological Bulletin*, **115**, 74–101.

Gowers, S. G., Harrington, R. C., Whitton, A. *et al.* (1999). A brief scale for measuring the outcomes of emotional and behavioural disorders in children: the Health of the Nation Outcome Scales for children and adolescents (HoNOSCA). *British Journal of Psychiatry*, **174**, 413–16.

Green, J. M. (1994). Child in-patient treatment and family relationships. *Psychiatric Bulletin*, **18**, 744–7.

(2002). Provision of intensive treatment: inpatient units, day units and intensive outreach. In M. Rutter and E. Taylor (eds.), *Child and Adolescent Psychiatry: Modern Approaches*, 4th edn. Oxford: Blackwells, pp. 1038–50.

Green, J. M. and Burke, M. (1998). The ward as a therapeutic agent. In J. M. Green and B. W. Jacobs (eds.), *Inpatient Child Psychiatry. Modern Practice Research and the Future*. London: Routledge, pp. 93–110.

Green, J. M. and Jacobs, B. W. (1998a). Current practice: a questionnaire survey of inpatient child psychiatry in the United Kingdom. In J. M. Green and B. W. Jacobs (eds.), *Inpatient Child Psychiatry. Modern Practice Research and the Future*. London: Routledge, pp. 9–22.

(1998b). Team dynamics in different phases of admission. In *Inpatient Child Psychiatry. Modern Practice Research and the Future* (eds J. M. Green and B. W. Jacobs). pp. 170–82. Routledge. London.

Green, J. M., Kroll, L., Imre, D. *et al.* (2001). Health gain and predictors of outcome in inpatient and daypatient child psychiatry treatment. *Journal of the American Academy of Child and Adolescent Psychiatry*, **40**, 325–32.

Harrington, R. C. Whittaker, J. Shoebridge, P. and Campbell, F. (1998). Systematic review of cognitive behaviour therapies in child and adolescent depressive disorder. *British Medical Journal*, **316**, 1559–63.

Hill, J. (2002). Disorders of personality. In M. Rutter and E. Taylor (eds.), *Child and Adolescent Psychiatry*, 4th edn. Oxford: Blackwells, pp. 723–36.

Hollis, C. (2002). Schizophrenia and allied disorders. In M. Rutter and E. Taylor (eds.), *Child and Adolescent Psychiatry*, 4th edn. Oxford: Blackwells, pp. 612–35.

Jacobs, B. W. (1998a). Behavioural and cognitive therapies. In J. M. Green and B. W. Jacobs (eds.), *Inpatient Child Psychiatry: Modern Practice Research and the Future*. London: Routledge, pp. 110–24.

(1998b). Externalising disorders: conduct disorder and hyperkinetic disorder. In J. M. Green and B. W. Jacobs (eds.), *Inpatient Child Psychiatry: Modern Practice Research and the Future*. London: Routledge, pp. 220–32.

Kroll, L. Woodham, A. Rothwell, J. *et al.* (1999). Reliability of the Salford Needs Assessment Schedule for Adolescents. *Psychological Medicine*, **29**, 891–902.

Kurtz, Z. (1994). *Treating Children Well*. London: Mental Health Foundation.

Leibenluft, E., Tasman, A. and Green, S. A. (1993) (eds.). *Less Time to Do More: Psychotherapy on the Short-Term Inpatient Unit*. Washington DC: American Psychiatric Press.

Luthar, S. S. Woolston. J. L. Sparrow. S. S. and Zimmerman. L. D. (1995). Adaptive behaviours among psychiatrically hospitalised children: the role of intelligence and related attributes. *Journal of Clinical Child Psychology*, **24**, 98–108.

Magagna, J. (1998). Psychodynamic psychotherapy. In J. M. Green and B. W. Jacobs (eds.), *Inpatient Child Psychiatry: Modern Practice Research and the Future*. London: Routledge, pp. 124–43.

National Health Service Health Advisory Service (1995). *Thematic Review – Together We Stand. The Commissioning Role and Management of Child and Adolescent Mental Health Services*. London: HMSO.

O'Herlihy, A., Worrall, A., Banerjee, S. *et al.* (2001). *National In-Patient Child and Adolescent Psychiatry Study.* (Report submitted to the Department of Health, May 2001.) London: Royal College of Psychiatrists' Research Unit.

Paterson, R. Bauer, P. McDonald, C. A. and McDermott, B. (1997). A profile of children and adolescents in a psychiatric unit: multidomain impairment and research implications. *Australian and New Zealand Journal of Psychiatry*, **31**, 682–90.

Royal College of Psychiatrists (1999). *Guidance for the Staffing of Child and Adolescent Inpatient Units. Council Report 62.* London: Royal College of Psychiatrists.

Shaffer, D. Gould, M. S. Brasic, J. *et al.* (1983). A children's global assessment scale (CGAS). *Archives of General Psychiatry*, **40**: 1228–31.

Shaw, M. (1998). Goal setting. In J. M. Green and B. W. Jacobs (eds.), *Inpatient Child Psychiatry. Modern Practice Research and the Future.* London: Routledge, pp. 51–6.

Sourander, A. and Turunen, M. M. (1999). Psychiatric hospital care among children and adolescents in Finland: a nationwide register study. *Social Psychiatry and Psychiatric Epidemiology*, **34**, 105–10.

Steinhausen (2002). Anorexia and Bulimia Nervosa. In M. Rutter and E. Taylor (eds.), *Child and Adolescent Psychiatry*, 4th edn. Oxford: Blackwells, pp. 555–70.

Tarrier, N. Beckett, R. Harwood, S. Baker, A. Yusupoff L. and Ugartebur I. (1993). A trial of two cognitive behaviour matters of treating drug resistant residual symptoms of schizophrenic patients. *British Journal of Psychiatry*, **162**, 524–32.

Towbin, K. E., Dykens, E. M., Pearson, G. S. and Cohen, D. J. (1993). Conceptualising 'borderline syndrome of childhood' and 'childhood schizophrenia' as a developmental disorder. *Journal of the Academy of Child and Adolescent Psychiatry*, **32**, 775–82.

Webster-Stratton, C. and Hammond, M. (1997). Treating children with early onset conduct problems: a comparison of child and parent training interventions. *Journal of Counselling and Clinical Psychology*, **65**, 93–109.

Wever, C. (1998) Obsessive compulsive disorder. In J. M. Green and B. W. Jacobs (eds.), *Inpatient Child Psychiatry. Modern Practice Research and the Future.* London: Routledge, pp. 247–58.

Part IV

Applications in psychosocial adversity

10

Cognitive behavioural treatment of the emotional and behavioural consequences of sexual abuse

Bruce Tonge

Centre for Developmental Psychiatry, Clayton, Victoria, Australia

Neville King

Monash University, Clayton, Victoria, Australia

Child sexual abuse has been defined as 'the involvement of dependent, developmentally immature children and adolescents in sexual activities that they do not fully comprehend, are unable to give their informed consent to and that violate the social taboos of family roles' (Schechter and Roberge, 1976). Recent research across a number of different countries has shown a consistently high prevalence of child sexual abuse. For example, using a random sample of adult women in San Francisco, Russell (1983) showed that 12% of women recalled at least one experience of extrafamilial abuse before the age of 14 with 28% recalling either intrafamilial or extrafamilial sexual abuse before the age of 14. Twenty-eight per cent recalled either intrafamilial or extrafamilial sexual abuse before that age. A survey from the UK found that 12% of females and 8% of males reported that they had been sexually abused before the age of 16 (Baker and Duncan, 1985), while an Australian study of almost 1000 tertiary students found that 13% recalled sexual experiences with an adult before the age of 12 (Goldman and Goldman, 1986). In a New Zealand investigation of 3000 women, Anderson *et al.* (1993) found that nearly one woman in three reported having one or more unwanted sexual experiences before the age of 16. Although methodological problems and inconsistencies are acknowledged with these studies, it is clear that child sexual abuse has a high prevalence.

Child sexual abuse can have a devastating impact on the development of the child. The immediate and short-term responses to child sexual abuse include distress, anxiety, nightmares, increased hostility, shame, guilt, depression and

Cognitive Behaviour Therapy for Children and Families, ed. Philip J. Graham.
Published by Cambridge University Press. © Cambridge University Press 2004.

inappropriate sexual behaviour (Browne and Finkelhor, 1986). These responses can seriously disrupt the child's relationships with parent figures and peers as well as adversely affecting their social, interpersonal, sexual and education progress and development. Although the acute distress occasioned by sexual abuse often settles, there is an increased risk of long-term adverse consequences. Mullen *et al.* (1988, 1994) have shown that, in adult life, those giving a history of child sexual abuse are more likely to suffer depressive disorders, eating disorders, behave in self-damaging and suicidal ways, to have difficulty forming and sustaining an intimate relationship, to have sexual problems, higher rates of divorce and separation and to appear to fail to fulfil their potential in both education and work. Effective management of the immediate emotional disturbances and disruptions occasioned by child sexual abuse should significantly reduce the risk of long-term negative outcomes for victims.

The successful treatment of the emotional and behavioural consequences of sexual abuse in children is crucial if these young people are to be relieved of their suffering and to steer them back onto a normal developmental trajectory and limit the risk of long-term adverse mental health outcomes (Wolfe and Birt, 1995; King *et al.*, 2003). There is now empirical evidence for the efficacy of manual-based, cognitive behavioural treatment (CBT) for sexually abused young people experiencing severe psychopathology. The applicability of CBT in community and primary care settings and its cost-effectiveness justify CBT as the treatment of first choice in the evidence-based clinical care pathway for the management of the mental health problems of sexually abused children (Farrell *et al.*, 1998; King *et al.*, 2000).

What might be the explanation for the effectiveness of CBT? Cognitive behavioural approaches are superior in the treatment of anxiety and phobic disorders in children (King *et al.*, 2000; Ollendick and King, 2000). The emotional and behavioural responses of children to sexual abuse can also be conceptualized as an anxiety response, often taking the form of post-traumatic stress disorder (PTSD) (see Chapter 20). Sexually abused children usually experience at least some symptoms, which fulfil criteria for PTSD as defined in the Diagnostic and Statistical Manual of Mental Disorders IV (American Psychiatric Association, 1994). For example, a study of 92 sexually abused children found that 85% had symptoms of re-experiencing behaviours, 52% had three or more avoidance behaviours, 72% had symptoms of autonomic hyper-reactions and nearly 50% met all the criteria for PTSD (McLeer *et al.*, 1992). Another study of 36 sexually abused children referred for treatment found that all had some symptoms of PTSD and 75% had a primary diagnosis of PTSD with complete diagnostic agreement by an independent clinician on a random sample of 12 cases

(King *et al.*, 2000). The majority of these cases (92%) also had other comorbid disorders particularly other anxiety disorders, depression and externalizing disorders. There are a number of risk factors which contribute to the development of PTSD in sexually abused children, such as female gender, self-deprecatory attributional style, pre-existing child psychopathology, more intrusive and persistent abuse, the perpetrator being known and trusted by the child, overprotective parenting and parental psychopathology (Browne and Finkelhor, 1986; Mennen, 1993). Therefore, the primacy of anxiety-based psychopathology together with the likelihood of self-deprecatory cognition suggest that a cognitive behavioural approach to treatment is justified. An additional rationale is the potential value of exposure in which the child is helped to confront the abuse-related thoughts in order to overcome associated anxiety, shame and guilt (Marks, 1987). Other aspects of CBT that are also likely to contribute to therapeutic effectiveness are non-specific aspects of the therapist–child relationship, education about child abuse, and social and communication skills training (Barlow, 1988; Heyne *et al.*, 2002).

What is the evidence for the effectiveness of CBT in the treatment of the mental health consequences of child sexual abuse? A number of controlled studies of CBT have produced evidence of superior efficacy (Berliner and Saunders, 1996; Cohen and Mannarino, 1996; Deblinger and Heflin, 1996; Cohen and Mannarino, 1997; Farrell *et al.*, 1998; King *et al.*, 2000). For example, a study of the treatment of emotional and behavioural disorder in sexually abused preschool children found that CBT was more effective than non-directive supportive therapy (Cohen and Mannarino, 1996). To date, evidence for the effectiveness of CBT for the psychopathology associated with child sexual abuse has focused on treatment of individual children and families. Comparative studies of group versus individual CBT need to be conducted.

The necessity to involve parents in the psychological treatment of children has been emphasized (Kendall *et al.*, 1992). This might be especially important in the treatment of sexually abused children where parents often react and shield the child from any discussion or experiences that might remind the child of the abuse. This overprotective parental response, although understandable, can act to prevent emotional recovery (Mennen, 1993).

Evidence for the value of inclusion of the parent in CBT for sexually abused children has been examined in several studies. Deblinger *et al.* (1996) in a study of the effectiveness of CBT in the treatment of PTSD associated with child sexual abuse randomly assigned families to a child-only treatment, a non-offending mother-only intervention, a combined child and mother treatment or a community care control group. The child therapy consisted of education, gradual exposure and coping and prevention skills training. The mothers received education and training in communication and behaviour management skills. All of the interventions were of therapeutic benefit relative to the community care control group. There were also some differential outcome effects between the treatment conditions. Inclusion of the child in therapy, with or without the parent, was associated with significantly better recovery from PTSD symptoms. Involvement of the mother in therapy, with or without the child, was associated with a significant improvement in parenting skills and a greater reduction in the child's level of externalizing behavioural disturbance.

In a study conducted by the authors and colleagues (King *et al.*, 2000), 36 sexually abused young people aged 5–17 years were randomly allocated to child-alone CBT, family CBT or a waiting list control group. The 20-session, manual-based, child-focused CBT was based on the protocol used by Deblinger and colleagues (Deblinger and Heflin, 1996; Deblinger *et al.*, 1996) and comprised education and goal setting, coping and relaxation skills, cognitive restructuring, graded exposure, relapse prevention and safe behaviours. The family CBT used the same 20-session programme for the child. In addition, the non-offending mother and the father or stepfather, if he was not the offender and was involved in the care of the child, received 20 sessions of education and parenting skills training. The sessions comprised education on child sexual abuse, communication, problem-solving and child behaviour management skills, and training and monitoring their own anxiety and emotional distress. In comparison with the children in the waiting list control group, those who received treatment experienced significant improvement in their symptoms of PTSD and were less fearful and anxious. Although the therapists in this study reported that they found the family CBT to be more clinically satisfying and that it was well received by the parents, there was no evidence that parental involvement in the treatment significantly improved outcome. The only significant differential finding was that family CBT was associated with greater improvement in child-rated fearfulness compared with child-alone CBT. A relatively small sample size ($n = 36$) might account for the inability of this study to demonstrate a similar differential effect for parent involvement found by Deblinger *et al.* (1996) who had 90 participants. Parent involvement in both these studies is focused on understanding and managing the child. However, in the authors' study (King *et al.*, 2000), the parents, particularly the mothers, frequently reported that they also suffered from stress and a range of emotional problems such as anxiety and depression. Nearly one-half of the mothers also reported that they had been sexually abused during childhood, although most had never received any professional help for any adverse emotional consequences. Therefore, it is possible that the addition of specific CBT sessions focused on treatment of the parents' own mental health problems might further improve outcomes for both the child and parents. Clearly, further research is required on the relative benefits of parent involvement in treatment and what might be the most effective treatment protocol.

Treatment manuals help therapists in several major ways including the provision of a theory-based treatment plan, structured sessions and worksheets for use with clients. Moreover, they are conducive to objective assessments of treatment 'adherence' on the part of therapists in a controlled trial (King and Ollendick, 1998, 2000). In the authors' study (King et al., 2000), a third of the therapy sessions were videotaped and checked for treatment adherence by an independent clinician. This revealed a concordance of 95% between the treatment manual and session content. However, it is emphasized that the manual contains a variety of age-appropriate activities and resources to ensure that each session is appropriate to the developmental level of the child. In clinical practice, the use of a manual-based CBT programme provides a structure for therapy but nevertheless allows flexibility to respond to individual and contextual issues for the child and family (Deblinger and Heflin, 1996).

The structure, emphasis and form of the child component of current CBT approaches to the treatment of psychopathology associated with child sexual abuse may vary but they all have a broad similarity in content. The authors now provide a broad outline of a typical CBT programme for young people suffering the emotional and behavioural consequences of sexual abuse, which has empirical support (King et al., 2000). This programme comprises modules, the content of which can be introduced in a different order to how they are listed and some may take a greater or lesser number of sessions depending on the individual needs and developmental level of the child.

10.1 An individual CBT programme for sexually abused children aged 6–18 years

10.1.1 General considerations

- The therapist provides positive reinforcement for commencing therapy and attempts to establish a therapeutic alliance.
- Homework tasks are essential and provide the opportunity to develop skills.
- Homework is reviewed at the start of each session. Impediments to homework tasks form the basis of subsequent communication and problem-solving activities and success is reinforced.
- The therapist models confidence and calmness when discussing abuse-related material.
- Focus on the child's strengths and model behavioural and cognitive coping skills.

10.1.2   Module A: groundwork (one to two sessions)

10.1.2.1   Purpose

To establish rapport and help the child feel safe. The overall plan for the treatment is explained. Information on sexual abuse and sexual terminology is provided, in order to desensitize the child to embarrassment or uncertainty with the topic. The child will develop goals for the therapy and begin to build hope for a positive outcome.

10.1.2.2   Activities

The child is introduced to the therapy process and how she/he will learn skills to cope with negative feelings, face what has happened and learn about the link between thoughts, feelings and behaviour. The child is given the opportunity to ask questions and express uncertainty about the treatment.

Age-appropriate education about sexual abuse includes hand-outs and discussion on the prevalence and nature of abuse and the short- and long-term problems and post-traumatic emotional and behavioural symptoms it can cause. Information on why perpetrators sexually abuse young people might also be provided. Information on the effectiveness of the treatment programme and how it can change thoughts, feelings and behaviour is discussed.

Within an age-appropriate framework, there is discussion and activity, such as the use of body part pictures, that explore the child's terminology for body parts and sexual acts. The therapist provides education regarding 'appropriate' terminology and a consensus is developed on the terminology to be used during therapy.

An activities and worksheet folder is introduced and the child/adolescent is encouraged to identify their goals for treatment and general areas for change such as making friends and specific goals such as making one friend at school. Discussion of the positive outcomes that would follow from achieving these goals builds hope.

10.1.3   Module B: addressing feelings (two sessions)

10.1.3.1   Purpose

To teach the child/adolescent to recognize and express appropriately a range of emotions, especially abuse-related feelings.

10.1.3.2   Activities

Emphasize both positive and negative emotions and link them to thoughts, bodily experiences and behaviour. The concept of fear as a feeling response to danger is introduced and explained.

Printed and multimedia material on feelings are used as a stimulus to generate the listing of different feelings. The child/adolescent is encouraged to give examples of situations which produce both positive and negative feelings. Discussion about the various ways of expressing feelings is used to reinforce acceptable and appropriate outlets for emotions.

The notion of fear as a normal response to danger is discussed and the young person produces a list of situations which might produce fear, such as thunder. Fear is automatic and produces three responses: fight, flight or freeze. Examples of personal experience of these responses are elicited or picture prompts are used to imagine potential responses. Role plays or story writing can further reinforce understanding.

Fear is expressed as feelings, thoughts and actions, and the child is encouraged to generate lists of possible reactions in the three categories of 'feel, think and do'. The child is then encouraged to add fear reactions to their abuse experience.

Explain that sometimes fear responses occur even when there is no actual danger, such as when there are reminders of their abuse experience. The child is asked to identify reminders of their abuse which trigger feelings of fear, preferably making a list using words or pictures. Many of the tasks in this session can be reinforced with homework. These sessions end in an optimistic and positive manner.

10.1.4   Module C: learning coping skills (six to eight sessions)

10.1.4.1   Purpose

To teach cognitive and behavioural coping strategies preparatory to exposure to memories of the abuse experience. This includes training in progressive relaxation and the generalization of relaxation coping skills; learning to restructure cognitions especially in relation to correcting negative attributions associated with the abuse; and learning specific mental and behavioural rehearsal skills for coping with stressful situations and integrating these strategies to handle situations that produce fear and anxiety.

10.1.4.2   Activities

The therapist outlines the cognitive behavioural coping model that addresses manifestations of fear in three categories of feel, think and do. Existing positive coping strategies already used by the young person are identified. Progressive relaxation training is introduced, modified for age, using scripts or audio- or videotapes. Feelings associated with relaxation are identified and contrasted with those of fear and anxiety. Word or visual relaxation cues are developed which facilitate relaxation in real life settings. Relaxation exercises become a regular homework activity helped by the provision of a personalized relaxation tape made by the therapist.

The therapist explains how feelings of distress can be due to unhelpful thoughts or self-talk. The use of cartoons and drawings are used to identify unhelpful self-talk and the link to feelings and behaviours. A link is made to the abuse situation and the young person identifies her/his specific negative self-attributions and how these may have adversely affected their self-esteem and behaviour. These unhelpful beliefs and self-statements are challenged collaboratively with the aim of converting these into a list of positive self-statements. The thought stopping technique is explained, demonstrated and practised by the young person. Positive qualities of the young person and examples of situations that were handled well are identified. Positive self-talk and self esteem role play or writing exercises are used. Homework tasks involve recording self-talk thoughts, feelings and positive events.

The skills required to monitor feelings and 'play the detective' are taught and practised to enable the child to attend to and evaluate realistically their feelings.

The process of covert or mental rehearsal is explained. The child identifies a situation of a distressing nature and with eyes closed is encouraged to describe the situation until anxious feelings are evoked. The young person is then encouraged to continue to imagine themselves in that situation, but to picture themselves feeling calmer and overcoming the situation. Relaxation and positive self-statement skills are used.

The young person then learns about behavioural rehearsal. The young person identifies a real life situation of difficulty with another person such as a parent or friend. The young person then role plays the situation with the therapist and is encouraged to be verbally and non-verbally assertive. The therapist provides feedback and with praise and encouragement coaches the young person to become proficient and confident.

The various coping strategies of rehearsal, relaxation and cognitive procedures are applied to some fear-producing situations identified by the young person which are not related to abuse and may be further practised in homework tasks.

10.1.5   Module D: exposure to memories of the abuse experience (four to six sessions)

10.1.5.1   Purpose

To help the young person recall and describe the abuse experience and experience the associated emotional responses to that experience, but in a supportive environment using the coping skills he or she has learned to manage negative affect.

10.1.5.2　Activities

Review what the young person has learned about abuse-related feelings and thoughts, the specific reminders of abuse which trigger fear and their newly acquired coping skills. Now that the young person has better ways of handling fear, it is time to work on developing a detailed account of the abuse experience. The young person is led to imagine the abuse experience. This might require writing notes, using doll play, drawing, singing, writing poetry or making an audiotape. These are all imaginal techniques and usually involve the construction of a hierarchy of events from least stressful to most stressful. This imaginal approach to systematic desensitization is linked to the progressive application of relaxation, cognitive and rehearsal coping strategies. On occasions, when there is an unrealistic avoidance and anxious response to aspects of daily life, it may be necessary to use a process of *in vivo* systematic desensitization to a hierarchy of situations such as approaching a park, entering the park, taking the path to the bandstand and so on.

The child usually needs to work through their memory of the abuse on several occasions.

10.1.6　Module E: dealing with disclosure (one to two sessions)

10.1.6.1　Purpose

To teach the young person how to anticipate and manage situations related to disclosure about the abuse experience.

10.1.6.2　Activities

The young person is asked to identify events since the abuse that may have caused distress, such as undergoing a medical examination or talking to the police, and, if possible, to write a story or draw a picture about this event. Explain how these situations may also generate negative feelings, thoughts and behaviours. Cognitive restructuring or systematic desensitization with the application of coping strategies is used to overcome the negative affect associated with these remembered experiences.

These sessions might also lead to identifying feelings related to the offender. These feelings are often complex and may be both positive and negative. It is helpful for the child to generate a list, draw a picture, write a letter or speak about all of the feelings they may have towards the offender. Emphasize that feelings of fear are reminders of the abuse experience, but do not necessarily mean that they are currently in real danger. Discuss the importance of distinguishing between actual danger and abuse reminders of past experiences. Generate examples of actual danger such as being alone with the offender, as opposed to an abuse reminder such as seeing someone who looked like the offender. Help the child to identify safety factors in their situation at home, school and their neighbourhood such as vigilant teachers, having a mobile phone and the existence of a restraining order. Homework tasks may involve the application of their coping skills, such as using calming statements and relaxation exercises, when they have thoughts about the offender.

10.1.7   Module F: body awareness and sexuality (one to two sessions)

10.1.7.1   Purpose

To enhance an accurate and positive view of the physical self and explore sexual knowledge, values and feelings in an age-appropriate fashion. To use cognitive restructuring as a method to identify and correct negative thoughts about the body and sexuality.

10.1.7.2   Activities

Ask the young person to generate a list of questions about bodies and sexuality including what they imagine sexually abused young people might worry about in relation to their body. Identify any negative body and sexual development thoughts. Challenge these thoughts and develop positive self-statements. Use written or multimedia information at an age-appropriate level to illustrate normal sexual development, identify the child's own stage of development and comfortably describe the function of body parts including the genitals. Identify, perhaps through the use of life-size tracing, the parts of the body that the young person likes most.

Use written or multimedia material to discuss appropriate sexual values and behaviour including the concepts of maturity, consent and mutuality. Identify fears or worries the young person may have about sexuality. Provide information and apply cognitive and behavioural methods to cope with troublesome thoughts such as cognitive restructuring for thoughts of not wanting to grow up. Use modelling or behavioural rehearsal to teach acceptable behaviour such as neutral touching. Homework may include a review of reading and multimedia material on sexuality and appropriate behaviour.

10.1.8   Module G: prevention training and termination (one to two sessions)

10.1.8.1   Purpose

To review the knowledge gained in the programme, to work on prevention concepts, reinforce the young person's sense of self-efficacy and reinforce self-protective behaviours and identify a support system.

10.1.8.2 Activities

The child is asked to recapitulate what they have learnt particularly about fear and coping strategies. Use a worksheet to identify dangerous and safe situations with other people, identify behaviours and strategies that can help deal with a difficult or dangerous situation. Recapitulate on the difference between actual danger and abuse reminders. Use behavioural rehearsal or role-playing techniques to practice protective behaviours.

Develop the use of a diary, which encourages planning and the identification of cues that signal the need to use coping skills and the daily use of strategies such as positive self-statements and relaxation exercise. The diary might also include useful community resources and contact numbers of trusted people who can help with problems.

The sessions end on a positive note with the presentation of a reward such as a bound copy of important printed material from the sessions, or a gift that emphasizes the qualities of the young person or the presentation of a graduation or 'bravery' certificate.

10.2 Conclusions

A manual-based structured CBT programme for young people suffering the emotional and behavioural effects of child sexual abuse encourages them to confront their abusive experiences and provides a number of coping skills to enable them to deal with their disturbed emotions. The follow-up of sexually abused children who have been treated with CBT indicates that therapeutic gains are maintained, although long-term follow-up studies are required to determine if the long-term adverse mental health consequences of childhood sexual abuse in adults are to be prevented (King *et al.*, 2000). However, current evidence suggests that CBT should be the first treatment offered to young people suffering the emotional and behavioural consequences of sexual abuse.

10.3 REFERENCES

American Psychiatric Association (1994). *Diagnostic and Statistical Manual of Mental Disorders,* 4th edn. Washington, DC: American Psychiatric Association.

Anderson, J., Martin, J., Mullen, P., Romans, S. and Herbison, P. (1993). Prevalence of childhood sexual abuse experiences in a community sample of women. *Journal of the American Academy of Child and Adolescent Psychiatry,* **32,** 911–19.

Baker, A. W. and Duncan, S. P. (1985). Child sexual abuse: a study of prevalence in Great Britain. *Child Abuse and Neglect,* **9,** 457–67.

Barlow, D. A. (1988). *Anxiety and Its Disorders. The Nature and Treatment of Anxiety and Panic.* New York: Guilford Press.

Berliner, L. and Saunders, B. E. (1996). Treating fear and anxiety in sexually abused children: results of a controlled 2-year followup study. *Child Maltreatment,* **1**, 294–309.

Browne, A. and Finkelhor, D. (1986). Impact of child sexual abuse: a review of the research. *Psychological Bulletin,* **99**, 66–77.

Cohen, J. A. and Mannarino, A. P. (1996). A treatment outcome study for sexually abused preschool children: initial findings. *Journal of the American Academy of Child and Adolescent Psychiatry,* **35**, 42–50.

(1997). A treatment study for sexually abused children: outcome during a one-year follow-up. *Journal of the American Academy of Child and Adolescent Psychiatry,* **36**, 1228–35.

Deblinger, E. and Heflin, A. E. (1996). *Treating Sexually Abused Children and Their Nonoffending Parents.* Thousand Oaks, CA: Sage.

Deblinger, E., Lippmann, J. and Steer, R. (1996). Sexually abused children suffering posttraumatic stress symptoms. Initial treatment outcome findings. *Child Maltreatment,* **1**, 310–21.

Farrell, S. P., Hains, A. A. and Davies, W. H. (1998). Cognitive behavioral interventions for sexually abused children exhibiting PTSD symptomatology. *Behaviour Therapy,* **29**, 241–55.

Goldman, R. and Goldman, J. (1986). Australian children's sexual experiences within the family. *Sixth International Congress on Child Abuse and Neglect,* Sydney. Abstract No. 7, p. 69.

Heyne, D., Rollings, S., King, N. and Tonge, B. (2002). *Parent, Adolescent and Child Training Skills 2: School Refusal.* Oxford: Blackwell.

Kendall, P. C., Chansky, T. E., Kane, M. T. *et al.* (1992). *Anxiety Disorders in Youth. Cognitive-Behavioral Interventions.* Boston: Allyn and Bacon.

King, N. J. and Ollendick, T. H. (1998). Empirically validated treatments in clinical psychology. *Australian Psychologist,* **33**, 89–95.

(2000). In defence of empirically supported psychological interventions and the scientist-practitioner model: a response to Andrews (2000). *Australian Psychologist,* **35**, 64–7.

King, N. J., Heyne, D., Tonge, B., Mullen, P., Rollings, S. and Ollendick, T. H. (2003). Sexually abused children suffering from posttraumatic stress disorder: assessment and treatment strategies. *Cognitive Behaviour Therapy,* **32**, 2–12.

King, N. J., Tonge, B. J., Mullen, P. *et al.* (2000). Treating sexually abused children with posttraumatic stress symptoms: a randomized clinical trial. *Journal of the American Academy of Child and Adolescent Psychiatry,* **39**, 1347–55.

Marks, I. M. (1987). *Fears, Phobias and Rituals. Panic, Anxiety and Their Disorders.* New York: Oxford University Press.

McLeer, S. V., Deblinger, E., Henry, D. and Orvashel, H. (1992). Sexually abused children at high risk for post-traumatic stress disorder. *Journal of the American Academy of Child and Adolescent Psychiatry,* **31**, 875–9.

Mennen, F. E. (1993). Evaluation of risk factors in childhood sexual abuse. *Journal of the American Academy of Child and Adolescent Psychiatry,* **32**, 934–9.

Mullen, P. E., Martin, J., Anderson, J. C., Romans, S. E. and Herbison, G. P. (1994). The effect of child sexual abuse on social, interpersonal and sexual function in adult life. *British Journal of Psychiatry,* **165**, 35–47.

Mullen, P. E., Romans-Clarkson, S. E., Walton, V. and Herbison, P. (1988). Impact of sexual and physical abuse on women's mental health. *Lancet*, **1**, 841–6.

Ollendick, T. H. and King, N. K. (2000). Empirically supported treatments for children and adolescents. In P. C. Kendall (ed.), *Child and Adolescent Therapy. Cognitive-Behavioral Procedures*, 2nd edn. New York: Guilford Press, pp. 386–425.

Russell, D. E. H. (1983). The incidence and prevalence of intrafamilial and extrafamilial sexual abuse of female children. *Child Abuse and Neglect*, **7**, 147–53.

Schecter, M. D. and Roberge, L. (1976). Sexual exploitation. In R. E. Helfer and C.H. Kempe (eds.), *Child Abuse and Neglect: The Family and the Community*. Cambridge, MA: Ballinger, pp. 66–77.

Wolfe, V. V. and Birt, J. (1995). The psychological sequelae of child sexual abuse. In T. H. Ollendick and R. J. Prinz (eds.), *Advances in Clinical Child Psychology*, **17**. New York: Plenum Press, pp. 233–63.

11

Adjustment to parental separation and divorce

Martin Herbert

University of Exeter, Exeter, UK

11.1 Introduction

The terms 'adjustment', 'separation' and 'divorce' are not as straightforward as they might appear at first sight. Adjustment is a multidimensional concept and requires contextual and operational definitions to be clinically useful. Divorces are diverse in their manifestation, and multifactorial in their origins, pathways and outcomes. The adjustment of adults, children and adolescents to the impact of divorce and separation can be measured in various ways (e.g. Munsinger and Kaslow, 1996), as is the case with the rating of the acrimony accompanying the break-up (e.g. Kurdek, 1987; Emery, 1992). Adjustment may refer to adaptation to trauma, itself a matter of degree, in any or all of several domains: emotional, behavioural, cognitive or social. These reactions may be concurrent, brief in duration, long term or delayed ('sleeper effects'). The adaptation required may not necessarily be to a life event perceived as traumatic, but rather to one experienced as a happy release from maltreatment (Browne and Herbert, 1997).

Increasingly, it is not a marriage that is ending in separation, but a cohabiting relationship that has failed. In the early 1960s, some 90% of children and teenagers were raised in homes with two married birth parents; today, the figures are around 59% in the UK and 40% in the USA. This marked reduction in numbers is due to the dramatic increase in divorces and separations. It can hardly be claimed, given a statistically high base rate for divorce of around 40%, that it represents an aberrant or necessarily stigmatizing incident in the lives of today's children. It may be a common shared experience in the West, but like attendance at the dentist that does not necessarily make it painless. Divorce is a decree that affects all members of the family, not only the marriage partners. It is the life event that receives the second highest stress rating out of 43 potentially traumatic

Cognitive Behaviour Therapy for Children and Families, ed. Philip J. Graham.
Published by Cambridge University Press. © Cambridge University Press 2004.

circumstances listed in the *Social Readjustment Scale* (Holmes and Rahe, 1967). What all the statistics indicate is that an increasing number of children, some 40%, spend periods of their childhood and teenage years in homes with divorced, remarried, single parents, step-parents and with step- or half-siblings.

11.1.1   Reconstituted families

Reconstituted families, in which one or both partners are combining two families into one, are currently another common phenomenon. Following divorce, most children (84%) reside with their mother in a single parent home, although this is quite likely to be a temporary arrangement. Remarriages are popular as are repeat cohabitation partnerships, for those who choose to live with someone but not to remarry. In approximately one out of every three marriages, one or both parents have been married before. The difficulties of being a stepchild or step-parent are legendary. Research has confirmed these legends. There is, for example, an increased risk of psychological problems in children whose parents remarry, especially where it is the parent of the same sex as the child who finds a new spouse. As divorce rates are higher in remarriages than first marriages, the need to adjust to separation and loss is often not a one-off ordeal. Children who are exposed to such multiple marital transitions are subject to the most adverse outcomes (Capaldi and Patterson, 1991). A self-perpetuating cycle of disadvantage is at work here, with a long-term association between parental divorce and divorce and depression in the next generation (O'Connor *et al.*, 1999). However, what is encouraging is that the number of children being brought up in unbroken families has reached a plateau in the last decade and it is clear that a majority of children who suffer parental separation do not go on to develop psychiatric disorders.

11.2   Assessment and formulation

A professional faced with a referral involving the serious disruption of individuals in the throes or aftermath of a divorce has a many-sided problem to assess: whether their needs are for any or all of the services of conciliation, support of various kinds or a therapeutic intervention. If the latter, what form of treatment is likely to be most effective? The dissolution of a marriage or long-term cohabitation is not a time-limited isolated event. The main and side effects are cumulative and possibly unremitting. In addition, the diversity of reactions to divorce is a function of the interaction of many risk and protective factors, ranging from individual attributes of the child and parents to dynamic features of the family's lifestyle and history.

Whether the consequences are benign (for some, divorce means an escape from a partner's abuse of the children, domestic violence, addiction or criminal activities) or malignant depends on a host of moderating influences: predisposing, precipitating or maintaining variables (e.g. Amato and Booth, 1997). Among the important changes that beset custodial parents (usually mothers) are the following:

(1)   adjusting to being single after being one of a couple;
(2)   becoming the solitary head of a single-parent family with the main, and often sole, responsibility for decisions, discipline, caring and providing for the children;
(3)   coping with children's grief, bewilderment and (not unusually) with their emotional and behavioural problems;
(4)   frequently having to leave the family home to set up house in an unfamiliar neighbourhood;
(5)   having to make new friends, while sometimes losing old ones;
(6)   having (in many cases) to deal with some degree of impoverishment;
(7)   having to cope with the disorganization and disruption of family life;
(8)   experiencing corrosive emotions such as jealousy, anger, bitterness and loss of self-confidence; and
(9)   later, perhaps, adjusting to the strains of reconstituted family life.
        Numbers (4)–(9) are difficulties also experienced by the children.

11.3   Transitions

A 'transition' constitutes a discontinuity in a person's life flow. The crucial point about major transitions is that no matter what life crisis an individual faces (the disintegration of a family, life in a new family or substantial changes in attachments and relationships) successful adaptation depends on the child and/or adult discovering new adaptive behaviours (different tactical and strategic responses) to meet changed and changing circumstances. Therapists' understanding and explication of the typical reactions of children of different ages to transitional events should help them to create new 'stories' (reframing/cognitive restructuring) about themselves and their lives, and about the processes of change 'submerging' them during these unsettling times. The successful treatment of children relies on a choice of interventions that are congruent with the child's stage of development and on the commitment of support from the family. In the Wallerstein and Kelly studies of the 1970s and early 1980s, it was clear that children responded to divorce in different ways, related to their ages (Wallerstein and Kelly, 1975, 1980). An examination of the characteristic reactions and behavioural changes revealed that typically:

(1)   young preschool children (aged $2\frac{1}{2}$–$3\frac{1}{4}$ years) tended to manifest regressive behaviour;

(2)   middle preschool children (aged $3\frac{3}{4}$–$4\frac{3}{4}$) showed irritability, aggressive behaviour, self-blame and bewilderment;

(3)   older preschool children (aged 5–6 years) displayed increased anxiety and aggressive behaviour;

(4)   younger latency-aged children (aged 7–8 years) reacted with sadness, grieving, fear, fantasies of responsibility and reconciliation, plus anger and loyalty towards both parents;

(5)   older latency-aged children (aged 9–10 years) demonstrated feelings of loss, rejection, helplessness, loneliness, shame, anger and loyalty conflicts; and

(6)   adolescents (aged 11 years and over) portrayed sadness, shame, embarrassment, anxiety about their future and about marriage, worry, individualization and independence from parents and withdrawal.

Additionally, Wallerstein and Kelly (1980) found that somatic symptoms such as headaches and stomach-aches were reported by children in the 9–12-year-old group, with chronic asthma sufferers experiencing intensified and more frequent attacks.

Adolescents are clearly not immune to suffering when their parents separate. The results of a 2-year study by Sun (2001) of more than 10 000 American adolescents (798 children of divorce) revealed that negative effects on every indicator of psychological functioning examined – well-being, school attendance, behavioural disturbance and drug and alcohol abuse – were evident at least 1 year before the marriage ended. These consequences were accompanied by a decline in parental interest in and commitment to their offspring.

A 20-year longitudinal study of 2000 couples and 200 of their children who had reached 19 years of age (Amato, 1993) revealed that 40% had divorced by the previous year. A small majority appeared to be 'very good' marriages. Children were more harmed by parents who argue rarely and then divorce unexpectedly than by those whose parents confronted each other bitterly and frequently prior to breaking up. Forty per cent of divorces involved marriages in which the child's parents were in constant and violent conflict, but did not separate. Theirs was the worst plight of all.

As with other investigations, there was evidence that children benefit from the ending of violent, disharmonious partnerships, although they suffer grave disadvantages from the actual 'sound and fury' of the break-up itself. Children report a sense of relief when the conflict between the parents ends. Nevertheless, one likely result of marital separation is children's reappraising their own relationships with their parents and, indeed, questioning the nature of all social and intimate relationships. For younger children in particular, there is the painful realization that some family relationships may not last forever. Many childish reactions at such a time are expressions of the fear of being abandoned by one or both parents. Such fears are likely to be most acute if contact has been lost with a parent. If relationships between parents and child remain intact, and supportive, these fears are lessened (Neugebauer, 1988/89).

Children who consider themselves most damaged are (e.g. Walczak, 1984): (1) those whose parents are not able to talk to them about divorce (apart from blaming their ex-spouse); (2) those who do not get on well with at least one parent after separation; and (3) those who are dissatisfied with custody and access arrangements. Among teenage and adult populations of females, parental divorce has been associated with lower self-esteem, precocious sexual activity, delinquent behaviour and more difficulty establishing gratifying, lasting adult heterosexual relationships (e.g. Capaldi and Patterson, 1991; Hetherington *et al.*, 1998; Hetherington and Stanley-Hagen, 1999). Following a divorce, decreased financial resources are the fate of children from all social classes. However, children from low-income families are quite likely to experience real poverty, particularly where their mothers lack employable skills. Children from upper-income families may experience the greatest relative reduction in resources and lifestyle (Furstenberg and Cherlin, 1991).

Divorced and single-parent mothers are most likely to be the custodial parents, and are confronted not only with financial losses but also employment and career worries, plus constant care-giving demands. Young children need special attention and nurturance but the parent may have little choice but to seek employment. Finding satisfactory substitute caregivers can be both difficult and expensive. Housing is also a common and costly problem. Many unresolved difficulties may deplete the last emotional resources of the mother or father left to cope with a family alone.

11.4   Interventions

When families present themselves with post-separation adjustment difficulties, a multimodal, systemic intervention package based on a thorough assessment and treatment plan is a necessary course of action. An intervention may not only involve therapy. The man or woman alone will need financial, practical and personal help. Another need is for good, accurate information about their children's ongoing development given these fraught circumstances.

Multilevel programmes may involve work with the previous and new family systems, including the original and reconstituted families, new partners and their children. It may also include an intervention with a variety of subsystems, including individual family members. There are many therapeutic programmes for the clinician to choose from, including: psychodynamic psychotherapy, narrative- and solution-focused therapy, no-talk therapy, cognitive and non-cognitive play therapy, conflict resolution approaches and cognitive behaviour therapy (CBT) (e.g. Stuart and Abt, 1981; Rossiter, 1988; Webster-Stratton, 1999). There is a paucity of evaluative research on most of these treatment models. Nevertheless, reviews of group-based, child-focused and adult interventions suggest that some of them, notably CBT, achieve significant improvements in personal and family adjustment. Reviews by Lee *et al.*, 1994 and Fonagy *et al.*, 2002 are particularly valuable as they suggest which therapies are effective for what, which do not work and which as yet lack validation.

Family-based interventions (e.g. behavioural and non-behavioural family therapy, parent skills training and counselling) have been strongly recommended as ways of helping family members adjust to their new roles, child management difficulties and other problems of the kind listed earlier. The most common divorce-related adjustment problems in children include: disturbances of conduct in early childhood (see Chapter 13); anxiety problems (see Chapter 18); depressive reactions (see Chapter 16); and delinquent activities in adolescence (see Chapter 25).

In most of the other problems of adjustment following separation and divorce, there is a role for CBT, behavioural family therapy or parent training (see Herbert, 2002). These problems include:

- marital conflict (Cummings and Davies, 2002);
- bereavement (Herbert, 1996);
- deterioration of academic performance (Bisnaire *et al.*, 1990);
- drug and alcohol abuse (Sun, 2001);
- relationship difficulties with step-family members (Bray, 1995);
- diminished self-concepts (self-esteem, self-confidence) (Parish, 1987);
- self-injurious behaviour (Bogolob, 1995);
- truancy (Blagg and Yule, 1994);
- divided loyalties (triangulation by parents) (Herbert and Harper-Dorton, 2003);
- access by non-custodial parent difficulties (Parish, 1987); and
- developmental problems (Herbert, 2003).

11.5   Parent training and counselling

A broad spectrum of pre- and post-divorce difficulties such as child management problems and issues such as loss of self-esteem and self-confidence can be addressed with a high degree of success in parent counselling/training groups which combine several theoretical components. The concept of self-empowerment is at the centre of what seem to be the most effective approaches to issues of the kind raised by divorce and its after-effects. They might, at a theoretical level, be said to incorporate a convergence of relational factors (humanist core conditions), cognitive processes (e.g. constructs, attributions and self-evaluations) and problem-solving ideas from skilled-based counselling theory (Egan, 1986).

These approaches generate curricula content for interventions, but also, importantly, involve subtle relationship processes that facilitate change. Webster-Stratton and Herbert (1994) emphasize the melding of *content* and *process*, the latter being embodied in a collaborative style of working with clients. The authors attempt to empower parents using a three-pronged approach: (1) giving them a knowledge base concerning children's developmental needs, behaviour management principles and individual temperamental differences, plus an understanding of how these affect social and intimate relationships; (2) helping them learn the important skills involved in communicating, initiating and maintaining social relationships, problem-solving and tactical/strategic thinking about their offspring; and (3) accepting and respecting their values and beliefs and exploring how these impact on their family lives, rules and relationships.

Wallerstein and Blakeslee (1989) provide data that are worth noting when the curriculum of a group programme is being constructed. They reported a 10-year follow-up of their original sample from the 1970s in their book entitled *Second Chances*. The study illustrated the psychological tasks facing adults and children at the time of the divorce. Divorce sets two major tasks for the adults: (1) to rebuild their lives as adults so as to make good use of the second chance that the divorce provides and (2) to parent the children after divorce, protecting them from the crossfire between the former partners and nurturing them as they grow up. The psychological tasks are as follows:

(1)   ending the marriage;
(2)   mourning the loss;
(3)   reclaiming oneself;
(4)   resolving or containing passions;
(5)   rebuilding; and
(6)   helping the children through preschool, the early school years (5–8 years), the later school years (9–12 years) and adolescence.

Once the decision to divorce was made, the following were perceived as important as means of helping children:

(1)   the expression of sadness, because it gave children permission to cry and mourn without having to hide their feelings of loss from the adults or from themselves;
(2)   rationality, because it contributed to the child's moral development;
(3)   clarity, so that children would not be encouraged to undertake any efforts at reconciliation;

(4) reluctance, because children needed to feel that parents were aware of how profoundly upset the children would be;

(5) preparing children for what lay ahead in as much specific detail as possible;

(6) reassuring children by giving them the assurance that they would be kept informed of all major developments;

(7) because children felt so completely powerless in the divorce situation, inviting them to make suggestions that the adults would seriously consider;

(8) needing to tell children over and over again that the divorce did not weaken the bond between non-custodial parent and child, despite the fact that they would now live apart;

(9) parents needing to give the children permission to love both parents freely and openly;

(10) avoiding the complications that arise when parents 'cling' to their children, overcompensating their loss of their partners by requiring them to grow up prematurely with adult responsibilities ('parentification'), by overindulging and 'spoiling' them or creating a 'claustrophobic' emotional intimacy (e.g. ignoring adult boundaries) that is inappropriate and potentially abusive; and

(11) considering conciliation/mediation (see below).

Wallerstein and Blakeslee (1989) concluded that the psychological tasks for the children are:

(1) Understanding the divorce.

(2) Strategic withdrawal – children and adolescents need to return to living their own lives as soon as possible after the divorce. It is important for them to recommence their usual activities at school and at play, and to return both physically and emotionally to the normal tasks of growing up.

(3) Dealing with loss.

(4) Dealing with anger.

(5) Working through and resolving guilt.

(6) Accepting the permanence of divorce.

(7) Avoiding feeling unlovable or culpable because of the divorce. They should be encouraged to accept realistically that they can both love and be loved, and convinced that they bear no responsibility for the break-up of an adult relationship.

11.6　A counselling and cognitive behaviour management course

An example of a multimodal counselling, life skills and cognitive course, designed for divorced and separated individuals by Joy Edelstein and the present author is the programme entitled *Separation and Divorce: A Collaborative Training and Counselling Course* (Edelstein, 1996). The life skills component draws on suggestions and examples from the work of Hopson and Scally (1980). These authors suggest that 'self-empowerment' is essentially the belief that there are choices and alternatives available in any situation. The skill is being able to select, and then to act on one of the choices, on the basis of personal values, priorities and commitments. Edelstein (1996) was able to demonstrate (in a doctoral research evaluation of the programme) that this cognitive behavioural counselling and life skills training programme for divorced mothers facilitates a significant degree of recovery from the adverse effects of the separation. Further, it improved maternal coping, increased understanding of children's attributions and behaviour, and served to alleviate, in some measure, the damaging effects of divorce evidenced by their post-separation emotional and behaviour problems. The programme on child management made use of parent training methods from the *Child Wise Behaviour Management Manual* (Herbert and Wookey, 2004).

11.6.1   The collaborative training and counselling programme

Outlined below is an abbreviated account of some of the themes in the programme.

11.6.1.1   Orientation

The participants are introduced to each other and to the programme facilitator/s. The approach adopted by the group leader/s stresses that divorce is a major life event that is transitional in nature. It is possible to help clients collaboratively to cope more effectively with such transitions in their lives. And because children are the parents of tomorrow, it is of the utmost importance to alleviate divorce-related emotional and other worries that disturb them.

11.6.1.2   Reassurance for the children

This session focuses on ways parents can reassure their children. It details the attributions and reactions of children in the throes and aftermath of a divorce, and the defence mechanisms such as denial, 'acting-out' behaviour and aggression they employ, to stave off the hurt and resentment they feel. Methods for managing the working through or acting-out behaviours that children frequently display following the trauma of divorce are shared, discussed and debated at this session.

11.6.1.3   Reassurance for the divorced person

This session focuses on providing reassurance for the participants themselves. It includes a description of common (immediate and delayed) reactions to the break-up and emphasizes that such reactions are normal, although they may feel 'abnormal'. It also recognizes the possible need in some cases to 'mourn' a lost marriage. There are suggestions on how to cope with the loneliness that follows a divorce and on ways of handling self-doubt. This session stresses the importance of combating the resentment and bitterness that stem from a broken marriage and outlines (with the help of brainstorming and discussion) constructive ways that participants can help themselves face the future on their own.

11.6.1.4   Looking after yourself and confronting some thorny issues

The ideas of supportive self-talk and the expression of feelings are introduced, and the concept of 'appropriateness' is explained. Skills for managing emotions are described, as are criteria for adequate self-care. Group members participate in a relaxation exercise. The thorny issues of custody, maintenance and access are confronted and ways of dealing with frustrating access problems are discussed and debated.

11.6.1.5   Letting go of the past and hints for managing difficult childhood behaviours

Pointers are given for explaining divorce to children. The essential step of 'letting go' of the past once the grief of a broken marriage is 'worked through' to a more manageable level. This step is underlined as a fundamental element of emotional recovery. The irrational beliefs and attributions that people harbour are examined and techniques for venting anger constructively, discussed and brainstormed again. Parents are helped to pinpoint, observe and record unwanted childhood behaviours in terms of the problem-solving ABC formulation of cognitive behavioural methodology (Herbert, 1987). This is discussed and role played – one of several important 'digressions' to the main adult agenda.

11.6.1.6   'Know yourself' and more hints for managing difficult childhood behaviours

The important self-knowledge questions: (1) 'Would I have chosen for this to have happened?' and (2) 'Do I know what I want from this new situation?' are posed and debated. The first two questions leave the individual with three possible options – namely, accept and put up with the situation, refuse to accept the situation or accept the situation and try to benefit from it. The effects of these options are carefully examined and the usefulness of a follow-up question (3) 'What is the worst that can happen?' explored. The fourth question, 'Do I know what I want from this new situation?', is used to introduce the technique of *values clarification* as a means of distilling needs and values. Differing consequences of proactive and reactive behaviour at times of stress are discussed. Stress management techniques are described and practised.

11.6.1.7 'Loose ends'

More hints for managing difficult childhood behaviours are given, along with ideas for managing the longer term consequences of divorce (see Webster-Stratton and Herbert, 1994). In addition, effective ways of using rewards and penalties, and encouraging pro-social and attending behaviour, are illustrated and discussed. There is, as usual, an opportunity to ask questions and raise issues for debate.

11.6.1.8 Farewells/final session

Participants are invited to comment on aspects of the Course that were helpful and/or unhelpful. A general reprise of the course is given, and principles/ strategies suggested by participants and facilitators remembered and written up on the much-used flip chart. Farewells are said and arrangements made for keeping in contact, if needed, and for 'refresher/booster sessions'.

11.7 Conclusions

We learn from the testimony of adults who have lived through divorce as children, grew up, married and raised their own families that, contrary to received wisdom, divorce can have a *lifelong* impact. Divorce does not easily recede into the memories of children as they enter adulthood (Hetherington, *et al.*, 1998). Wallerstein and Blakeslee (1989) report that divorce continues to occupy a central emotional position in the lives of many adults, 10–15 years after the event. Both men and women told them that the stress of being a single parent never lessens and the fear of being alone never ceases. Wallerstein and Blakeslee (1989, p. 60) conclude their review of the literature as follows:

> We wanted to believe that time would lessen the feelings of hurt and anger, that time itself heals all wounds and that people by nature are resilient. But there is no evidence that time automatically diminishes feelings or memories; that hurt and depression are overcome; that jealousy, anger and outrage will vanish. Some experiences are just as painful ten years later; some memories haunt us for a lifetime.

Nor were the continuing effects of divorce restricted to the adults alone. Wallerstein and Blakeslee (1989) found that after 10 years the children of the broken homes maintained that growing up was harder for them as children of divorce than it was for children from intact families. They felt that their lives had been overshadowed by their parents' divorce, and they felt deprived of a broad range of economic and psychological supports. Many of the children entered adolescence and young adulthood with deep reservoirs of unresolved feelings, particularly anger about how their parents had behaved during their marriage. Bitterness was another feeling typically expressed. No factors were identified that predicted the long-term effects of divorce on children (or adults) from how they react at the outset.

Hetherington and Stanley-Hagan (1999) also conclude, at the end of an important review of the literature, that divorce can have a lifelong impact. They add that the consequences are not always negative or regressive ones. Many children who grow up in the aftermath of a divorce overcome the trauma and go on to contribute to, rather than rebel against, society. Although children in divorced families, in comparison with those in non-divorced families, are at risk of developing more social, emotional, behavioural, and academic problems, most eventually emerge as competent, well-functioning individuals. Inevitably, there will be those who are quite happy with their present lives and who have no regrets about their divorce. This was true of about one-half of the men and women in the Wallerstein and Kelly (1980) sample when interviewed some 10 years later by Wallerstein and Blakeslee (1989).

As always, it is necessary to take individual differences into account. In attempting to explain the origins and nature of a child's 'maladjustment' following divorce, clinicians ignore moderating variables at their peril. Formulations positing a linear relationship between a single heterogenous precursor such as the 'breakdown of a family' and the later development of adverse reactions could miss the impact on the child's development of other experiences that determine his or her vulnerability or resistance to stressful life events.

In 1996, the Family Law Act was passed in the UK, requiring all those seeking divorce to first attend an information meeting to apprise them of the consequences of divorce, including the impact on children, the likely costs and the legal and welfare services (notably *mediation/conciliation*) available (Fisher, 1990). A mandatory period of reflection and consideration was stipulated before there could be formal acceptance that the marriage had broken down irretrievably (James, 2002). Beyond this point, as has been seen, there are various forms of help (preventive and remedial) available, in which CBT alone, or in combination with other methods within multimodal group programmes, have proved most effective.

11.8   REFERENCES

Amato, P. R. (1993). Children's adjustment to divorce. Theories, hypotheses, and empirical support. *Journal of Marriage and the Family,* **55**, 23–38.

Amato, P. R. and Booth, A. (1997). *A Generation at Risk: Growing Up in an Era of Family Upheaval.* Cambridge, MA: Harvard University Press.

Bisnaire, L., Firestone, P. and Rynard, D. (1990). Factors associated with academic achievement in children following parental separation. *American Journal of Orthopsychiatry*, **60**, 67–76.

Blagg, J. and Yule, W. (1994). School refusal. In T. H. Ollendick, N. J. King and W. Yule (eds.), *International Handbook of Phobic and Anxiety Disorders in Children and Adolescents*. New York: Plenum Press, pp. 169–86.

Bogolub, E. B. (1995). *Helping Families through Divorce*. New York: Springer Publishing Company.

Bray, J. (1995). Systems oriented therapy with stepfamilies. In R. Mikesell, D. Lusterman and S. McDaniel (eds.), *Integrating Family Therapy: Handbook of Family Psychology and Systems Theory*. Washington, DC: American Psychiatric Association.

Browne, K. and Herbert, M. (1997). *Preventing Family Violence*. Chichester: Wiley.

Capaldi, D. M. and Patterson, G. R. (1991). Relationship of parental transmissions to boys' adjustment problems. *Developmental Psychology*, **27**, 489–504.

Cummings, M. and Davies, P. T. (2002). Effects of marital conflict on children: recent advances and emerging themes in process-oriented research. *Journal of Child Psychology and Psychiatry*, **43**, 31–64.

Edelstein, J. (1996). *Psycho-social Consequences of Divorce: A Group Counselling Programme of Prevention*. Unpublished Ph.D. thesis, University of Leicester.

Egan, G. (1986). *The Skilled Helper*. Monterey, CA: Brooks/Cole.

Emery, R. (1992). Interparental conflict and the children of discord and divorce. *Psychological Bulletin*, **92**, 310–30.

Fisher, T. (ed.) (1990). *Family Conciliation within the UK: Policy and Practice*. Bristol: Family Law.

Fonagy, P; Target, M., Cottrell, D. *et al.* (2002). *What Works for Whom? A Critical Review of Treatments for Children and Adolescents*. London: Guilford Press.

Furstenberg, F. and Cherlin, A. (1991). *Divided Families: What Happens When Parents Part?* Cambridge, MA: Harvard University Press.

Herbert, M. (1987). *Behavioural Treatment of Children with Problems*, 2nd edn. London: Academic Press.

(1996). *Supporting Bereaved and Dying Children and Their Parents*. Leicester: BPS-Blackwell Pacts Series.

(2002). Behavioural therapies. In M. Rutter and E. Taylor (eds.), *Child and Adolescent Psychiatry*, 4th edn. Oxford: Blackwell Scientific.

(2003). *Typical and Atypical Development: From Conception to Adolescence*. Oxford: BPS-Blackwell.

Herbert, M. and Harper-Dorton, K. V. (2003). *Working with Children, Adolescents and their Families*. Oxford: BPS-Blackwell.

Herbert, M. and Wookey, J. (2004). *The Management of Children's Disruptive Disorders: The Child-Wise Parenting Skills Approach*. Chichester: Wiley.

Hetherington, E. M., Bridges, M. and Insabella, G. M. (1998). What matters? What does not? Five perspectives on the association between marital transitions and children's adjustment. *American Psychologist*, **53**, 167–84.

Hetherington, E. M. and Stanley-Hagan, M. (1999). Adjustment of children with divorced parents: a risk and resiliency perspective. *Journal of Child Psychology and Psychiatry*, **40**, 120–40.

Holmes, T. H. and Rahe, R. (1967). The Social Readjustment Rating Scale. *Journal of Psychosomatic Research*, **11**, 213–18.

Hopson, B. and Scally, M. (1980). *Lifeskills Teaching: Education for Self-Empowerment*. New York: McGraw-Hill.

James, A. L. (2002). Social work, divorce and the family courts. In M. Davies (ed.), *The Blackwell Companion to Social Work*. Oxford: Blackwell Publishing.

Kurdek, L. (1987). Children's beliefs about parental divorce scale: psychometric characteristics and concurrent validity. *Journal of Consulting and Clinical Psychology*, **55**, 712–18.

Lee, C., Picard, M. and Blain, M. (1994). A methodological and substantive review of intervention outcome studies for families undergoing divorce. *Journal of Family Psychology*, **8**, 3–15.

Munsinger, H. and Kaslow, K. (1996). *Uniform Child Custody Evaluation System*. Odessa, FI: Psychological Assessment Resources.

Neugebauer, R. (1988/89). Divorce, custody, and visitation: the child's point of view. *Journal of Divorce*, **12**, 153–68.

O'Connor, T. G., Thorpe, K., Dunn, J. and Golding, J. (1999). Parental divorce and adjustment in adulthood: findings from a community sample. *Journal of Child Psychology and Psychiatry*, **40**, 777–89.

Parish, T. S. (1987). Children's self concepts: are they affected by parental divorce and remarriage? *Journal of Social Behavior and Personality*, **2**, 559–62.

Rossiter, A. B. (1988). A model for group intervention with pre-school children experiencing separation and divorce. *American Journal of Orthopsychiatry*, **3**, 387–96.

Stuart, I. R. and Abt, L. E. (1981). *Children of Separation and Divorce: Management and Treatment*. New York: Van Nostrand and Reinhold.

Sun, Y.-M. (2001). Family environment and adolescents' well-being before and after parents' marital disruptions : A longitudinal analysis. *Journal of Marriage and Family*, **63**, 697–713.

Walczak, Y. (1984). Divorce: the kid's stories. *Social Work Today*, 18 June, pp. 12–13.

Wallerstein, J. and Blakeslee, S. (1989). *Second Chances*. New York: Ticknor and Fields.

Wallerstein, J. S. and Kelly, J. B. (1975) The effects of parental divorce: experiences of the pre-school child. *Journal of the American Academy of Child Psychiatry*, **14**, 600–16.

   (1980). *Surviving the Breakup: How Children and Parents Cope with Divorce*. New York: Basic Books.

Webster-Stratton, C. (1999). Marital conflict management skills, parenting style and early-onset conduct problems: processes and pathways. *Journal of Child Psychology and Psychiatry*, **40**, 917–27.

Webster-Stratton, C. and Herbert, M. (1994). *Troubled Families: Problem Children*. Chichester: Wiley.

Part V

Applications in specific child and adolescent psychiatric disorders

12

Behavioural approaches to eating and sleeping problems in young children

Jo Douglas

Rickmansworth, Hertfordshire, UK

When working with young children who have eating or sleeping problems, there are a range of therapeutic approaches that are utilized to tailor the treatment to the particular needs of the child and parents. Cognitive behavioural therapy (CBT) is one part of the armoury and, when the child is preschool age, this therapy is often directed at the parents rather than at the child. The fact that CBT has been lifted from the adult arena of treatment techniques and applied to the complex set of relationships of children in families means that our use of CBT has to widen to include not just 'individual' work with children but also with their parents and carers (Barrett, 2000). The behavioural and emotional problems of young children, in particular, make us rethink who is in treatment and how those treatment goals are best implemented. Helping parents change their behaviour towards their child can have a positive impact on the child's problems. This process will often involve the parents changing their cognitions and feelings about their child and his behaviour.

CBT programmes directed at parents are valid forms of treatment for children (Bugental and Johnston, 2000; Rapee, 2001), but they do raise the question: 'what is the goal of treatment?' There is an assumption of a mediating role of change for parental cognitions that produces change in their behaviour, which in turn affects their child's behaviour. There may be uncertainty whether, in these circumstances, change in the child's cognitions occurs before behaviour changes. The challenge of assessing cognitive change in young children as an indicator of outcome has received little attention and is an area for research that requires development of appropriate and methodologically robust methods of assessment (see Chapter 8).

As in other areas of behaviour, developmental issues play an important role in understanding the eating and sleeping problems of childhood. Younger children

Cognitive Behaviour Therapy for Children and Families, ed. Philip J. Graham.
Published by Cambridge University Press. © Cambridge University Press 2004.

can show a different range of fears and anxieties compared with older children (Barrett, 2000): they are developmentally immature in their cognitions and they are particularly vulnerable to the influences of parental cognitions (Stallard, 2002). These features of the cognitions of young children must be considered when trying to understand the impact of interventions to change their behaviour.

12.1   Eating problems in young children

Eating problems in young children present in a variety of forms including difficulties with eating age-appropriate textures, ranges and amounts of food. Children will cry and scream when food is presented to them, turn their heads away, spit, gag, dawdle excessively, vomit, throw food, run away from the table, refuse to open their mouths, refuse to self-feed or eat selectively. These problems may be associated with significant weight loss or failure to thrive.

Parents often feel that they are failing as parents when they cannot encourage their children to eat normally for their age. The aetiology of these problems is often varied and so treatment approaches may also need to involve several different components. Useful psychological models of aetiology include both behavioural and cognitive learning theory.

12.1.1   Behavioural learning theories help us understand the effect of prior learning experiences on present behaviour in both children and parents

12.1.1.1   Classical conditioning in children

When children pair unpleasant physical feelings of nausea, vomiting, allergic reactions or pain with eating they can start to refuse to eat. The stimuli associated with the presentation of food can acquire the ability to elicit the anxiety normally associated with the physical reaction (Linscheid et al., 1995). Even when the initial unpleasant physical symptoms have stopped, the child still avoids food because of the prior establishment of a conditioned response. Medical disorders including gastrointestinal, metabolic, neurological, cardiac and renal disorders will all affect a child's appetite, taste sensations and the quantity that can be eaten (Harris et al., 2000). More frequently than is generally realized, poor or delayed development of oral motor skills (so-called oral motor dysfunction) can be the basis of choking and gagging experiences (Mathisen et al., 1989).

Physical or emotional abuse from parents or carers, threats of physical violence or abandonment, parental anger and temper outbursts while the child is feeding can produce intense levels of anxiety and fear. This results in a conditioned avoidance of food based on the aversive experience.

12.1.1.2 Classical conditioning in parents

When parents witness their child's adverse physical reaction to food, the intense anxiety generated results in them avoiding offering the food that produced the problem. This can lead to a continued and unnecessary restriction in the range, texture or amount of foods offered by the parent, and may continue until long after the original problem has resolved. Repeated experiences of the child refusing food can make parents feel very anxious or depressed so that they start to dread meal times. Their consequent emotional reaction during the meal can also adversely affect the child.

12.1.1.3 Operant conditioning in children

Children can learn that, by refusing to eat non-preferred foods or textures, they are frequently offered more of their preferred food, which can lead to a restriction in what they will eat. They also learn that by running away from the table, spitting, throwing food or crying and making a scene the parent will stop offering them non-preferred food.

12.1.1.4 Operant conditioning in parents

Parents generally feel highly reinforced when their child eats. To maintain this pleasurable experience, parents will offer their children their preferred foods or textures leading to a restriction in what the child will eat. Efforts to widen the child's diet are met with opposition and distress by the child and avoidance of eating, so attempts by the parents to extend the child's diet are rapidly extinguished.

Parents learn from the child's reaction when they have had enough and if the child provides the wrong signals, is distractible or prefers to play then the parents may not provide sufficient nutrition (Chatoor *et al.*, 1998).

12.1.1.5 Parental management techniques

Poor child management techniques can result in: children drinking excessive amounts of milk or juice instead of eating, grazing throughout the day on snacks instead of eating meals at routine times, unpredictable and chaotic mealtimes and inappropriate expectations of the amount of food that a child can eat (Douglas and Bryon, 1996). A poor ability to set limits and boundaries to the child's behaviour can result in a wide range of eating difficulties (Frank and Drotar, 1994).

12.1.2   Cognitive learning theory can help us understand the distorted parental and child cognitions that can lead to and maintain problem behaviours

12.1.2.1   Misperception of the child's eating behaviour

Parents may think that their child's refusal to eat is due to naughtiness and bad behaviour, when in fact the child is ill or cannot eat for a physical reason (Harris et al., 2000). This can lead to pressure, force-feeding, anger and punishment, which results in the child being more avoidant and emotionally distressed.

12.1.2.2   Absent or distorted perceptions about their child's developmental and emotional needs when eating

Some parents are unaware of their child's needs for help with eating either because they are preoccupied with their own emotional difficulties or because they do not have sufficient knowledge about child development. They may offer inappropriate textures, quantities or ranges of foods and can seem inadvertently or deliberately neglectful (Drotar, 1995). Not providing the child with physical help to access food and support with eating, if needed, may result in the child being severely underfed (Batchelor, 1999). Parents who have attachment difficulties with their infants often show very poor observation of the infant's communication patterns around feeding (Chatoor et al., 1998).

12.1.2.3   Irrational or distorted parental cognitions about food

These can lead to parents restricting their child's diet due to distorted information from the media, fear of infection from the food, fear of additives, fear of illness or allergy, personal cognitions and beliefs in relation to religious or animal welfare considerations, and inappropriate expectations of the child's developmental ability to eat textures or quantity (Pugiliese et al., 1987).

12.1.2.4   Distorted parental cognitions and anxiety about cleanliness

Anxiety about hygiene, mess and cleanliness can be transmitted so that the child becomes reluctant to touch food and continually demands to have their hands and face wiped while eating. This can develop into concern about cleanliness of cutlery and crockery in older preschool children, concerns about contamination of one food touching another on the plate and a reluctance to eat off anything except their own plate in their own home.

12.1.2.5   Loss of parental confidence about parenting

Poor decision making in relation to feeding the child can occur when a young child has been ill or the parent has been undermined by another family member or by information from others in 'authority'. A child's illness in the first year of life – e.g. gastro-oesophageal reflux – can severely undermine parents' confidence in how to cope. Parental uncertainty may remain long after the physical problem has resolved (Douglas and Harris, 2001).

12.1.2.6   Parental overprotectiveness and difficulties with separation

Distorted cognitions of perceived threat can result in an inability to help the child move forwards developmentally, learn to self-feed or eat appropriate textures and foods for their age. Maternal overprotection conveys to the child the continual presence of threat and danger and also restricts the child's opportunities to develop successful coping strategies (Rapee, 1997). Parents may strive to keep the child at a younger developmental age than they are, encouraging dependence and more infantile patterns of behaviour.

12.1.2.7   Parental poor self-esteem

Poor self-esteem can lead to depression and affect some mothers' abilities to cope with their children's demands to be fed. There can be a build-up in negative attribution about the child, a sense of not being able to cope and of being a bad mother. The more the child refuses to eat, the more the mother's core belief of being a poor mother is reinforced, and her depression continues. She does not recognize the child's needs and cannot reciprocate or reinforce positively the child's attempts to eat (Batchelor, 1999).

12.1.2.8   Children's anxiety and misperception of threat

Parents can transmit their anxiety to their child, which results in the child's excessive and unnecessary avoidance of certain foods for fear of an adverse physical reaction – e.g. fear of anaphylactic shock, vomiting or choking. Children also gain information from their environment and may have observed another person experiencing an adverse reaction. In anxious children, this can be enough to trigger a severe avoidance reaction. They may develop a sense of incompetence or helplessness in the face of challenges – they overestimate the threat and underestimate their ability to cope (Roth and Dadds, 1999).

12.1.2.9   Children's distorted perceptions of food

Some young children will emphatically say that they cannot eat certain foods even when it is clear that they can manage the texture. They do not know why and the difference between 'cannot' and 'will not' is not apparent to them. They have no motivation to change and usually this is because they cannot think how to change. If forced to eat the new food, they will gag and try to vomit even without previous adverse experience of the food; they think that they cannot eat it (Douglas, 2000b).

12.2   Treatment approaches

Treatment of young children's eating problems requires integrative treatment including behavioural and cognitive behavioural approaches that meet the needs of each case.

In many cases, cognitive therapy with the parents is the first stage of treatment before some of the behavioural strategies of managing the child can be learned.

12.2.1   Treatment of parental cognitions and behaviour

12.2.1.1   Correct misperceptions about the child's illness, behaviour, emotional and developmental level

Parents' cognitions need to be understood in order to correct misperceptions or provide accurate knowledge. The provision of factual information about diet, calories, textures and what foods to try is a practical and pragmatic educational approach that can correct much misunderstanding and provide valuable knowledge.

Information about the developmental stages of children's eating will help parents set clearer and more appropriate expectations (Harris, 2000). Recognizing their child's fear or lack of ability to cope can help regulate the parents' emotional reactions.

12.2.1.2   Regulate the impact of parental emotional state on their ability to manage their child's eating

Parents' anxiety or depression distorts their ability to problem-solve and to observe their child's behaviour accurately (Hutchings et al., 2002). They require help and guidance in how to approach the child's eating problem more effectively. Depression can lead to a sense of 'learned helplessness' which will impair the parents' ability to cope with their child's problems. Building up a sense of competence with clear guidelines about how to manage the problem in small steps can help parents feel more effective. Structured parent training with repeated practise and experience of success is one of the most effective antidotes to depression. Providing cognitive approaches to managing their own anxiety and depression can be valuable. Helping volatile parents to recognize that the child is not misbehaving deliberately to upset them can defuse the anger and irritation, but they also need to learn how to set limits without losing their tempers.

12.2.1.3   Correct misattribution of blame or guilt

Many mothers feel blamed for their child's eating problem and then feel helpless to change. Understanding how the problem has evolved can provide perspective, but they also need reassurance that they reacted in a way meant to help their child rather than to exacerbate the problem. Blame and guilt are destructive feelings that prevent parents from changing. Unless this is addressed early in treatment, many parents will attribute therapeutic suggestions of how they could change as criticisms and may be uncooperative or become more depressed or anxious (Douglas, 2002a).

12.2.1.4 Enhance parental self-confidence

Parents need positive feedback about their efforts to change and how they are managing their child. Criticism or pointing out problems will demotivate them and undermine their self-confidence to change (Dadds and Barrett, 2001). Empathic support as well as precise guidance on how to cope will make them feel more confident and effective. A partnership between the therapist and parents allows a constructive and positive attitude to develop where the parent can start to identify the small steps of positive change. Any success should be attributed to their efforts.

12.2.1.5 Enhance problem-solving skills in relation to child management

As the parents grow in self-confidence and start to see success, they can be encouraged to generate their own solutions to problems presented by their child. This process of generalization involves creative and flexible thinking which is possible once parental emotional problems and self-esteem are being improved.

12.2.2 Treatment of the child's cognitions and behaviour

Although most of the child's behaviour is managed by the parents changing how they react to the child's eating pattern, there are some instances in which direct work on the child's cognitions can be helpful.

12.2.2.1 Correct misperception of self as a non-eater or of an inability to eat certain foods

Rehearsal of positive self-statements – e.g. 'I can eat . . .' and 'If my friend can eat it so can I' – helps build up a positive attitude. Understanding and agreement with a reward programme contingent on compliant behaviour can help the child to make the first steps in trying an agreed new food or eating a larger quantity of food.

12.2.2.2 Enhancing the child's strengths and self-confidence

A scrapbook of all of the foods that the child can eat enhances the child's view of himself as an eater, and pictures or labels of new foods can be added to the scrapbook once a defined amount has been eaten. Looking at the scrapbook helps to reinforce the child's memory and is a record of achievement. Star charts can have the same effect and help children feel positive about their efforts, providing a concrete record of change.

12.2.2.3   Reducing anxiety by setting small goals of change

Many children do not realize that they will not be asked to eat a large plateful of non-preferred or a new textured food once adults start to talk about change. They need help in understanding what will be expected and reassurance that they will be able to manage each step of change. Keeping the child calm is an essential part of treatment and their self-confidence will increase once they experience a little success.

12.2.3   Behavioural management of children's eating problems

12.2.3.1   Desensitization

Children who are anxious about food due to previous adverse experiences associated with eating require containment of their anxiety while being gradually exposed to the frightening food. Graded introduction of new foods, new textures and larger quantities enables the child to learn success in small stages without having a major confrontation. It requires patience, planning and consistency by the parent while progressing through a sequence of new behaviour with the child (Douglas, 2000b). Some children require desensitization of the fear of mess and touching food, while others need help with desensitizing their faces and mouths to being touched and textures or temperatures of foods (Wolf and Glass, 1992; Johnson and Babbitt, 1993; Schauster and Dwyer, 1996). Graded exposure to the feared object is the main ingredient of all attempts to overcome childhood phobias and fears (King and Ollendick, 1997).

12.2.3.2   Teaching parents behavioural management skills

Parents often report that they do not know how to change what is happening and that what they do does not work. They may feel uncertain about being more assertive with their child as they feel anxious about upsetting their child or worry that they will lose their tempers. Learning to establish clear and realistic goals of change using positive reinforcement approaches and setting gradual steps of change will enhance the parents' ability to manage their child's eating more effectively. Modelling, shaping and reinforcement approaches are all positive approaches to child management that parents can use (Douglas and Harris, 2001; Douglas, 2002a, b). Parents can model enjoyment of touching and eating food and praise their children for small steps of change. Using rewards and star charts for trying a taste of a new food or texture, or for eating a certain amount, can help children and parents recognize that progress is being made even though it may be slow. Ignoring inappropriate behaviour at meal times and attending to appropriate behaviour is effective in managing change (Hampton, 1996). Encouraging age-appropriate independence in eating can be an important step to reducing the parents' anxiety and their overinvolvement in meal times (Douglas, 2000a).

12.2.3.3   Case illustration

Suzie, aged 5 years, had become very anxious about food containing nuts, had severely restricted her diet and would continually ask for reassurance from her mother. Her anxiety had started to generalize to not having her food cooked in the same dish as the rest of the family, so that her food did not touch others', and concern about cleanliness of cutlery. She would not eat at friends' houses, parties or in restaurants. The family was unable to go away on holiday because of her food refusal.

A year previously, Suzie had had a mild anaphylactic reaction to eating nuts and her mother had been given an epi-pen for emergency use. Her mother had become a member of a parent support group for children with nut allergies and had become very knowledgeable. Suzie had become terrified of the epi-pen and would not even hold it, after having observed it being used on her older sister, who had an unexpected anaphylactic reaction during a nut challenge test in hospital. Suzie heard the pen click and saw her sister gasping and crying which frightened her. Suzie's anxiety increased markedly after this episode and her restriction on foods increased as she was terrified of the epi-pen and did not see it as a reassurance.

The treatment plan included: (1) helping Susie gain control of her anxiety by teaching her relaxation and breathing; (2) reducing any reinforcement for worrying statements by asking her mother not to reply to her continual requests for reassurance but to have a 10 minute 'worry time' at 6 pm each evening when Suzie could ask what she wanted to know; (3) to restrict any reinforcement of her anxiety by not allowing her to choose her cutlery; and (4) providing reinforcement via a star chart for accepting and trusting her mother to give her nut-free food at mealtimes. She agreed and planned to earn stars towards a bean baby. Her mother required help in learning not to respond to Suzie's worries, to be firmer in her management style, not to let Suzie take control at meals and to stay calm if Suzie panicked. It was clear that her mother was also a worrier and she tended to react to her children's demands rather than setting clear boundaries. She recognized that she needed to be clearer and firmer with all of them.

Once these first stages of change were achieved, the next plan was to reduce Suzie's anxiety in relation to the epi-pen. A desensitization programme of learning to hold the pen and then operate a trainer pen on a plastic doll was successful.

This allowed Suzie to feel more secure and she was able to take it to a friend's house at tea-time. Once this was achieved, it was possible to start increasing Suzie's range of foods to include foods that she had restricted for no good reason. Her mother needed to take charge of meals and decide what to cook rather than ask Suzie what she wanted to eat. Her confidence in deciding which foods to give Suzie required enhancing and then it was possible for her to start using foods that had 'may contain traces of nut' on the label. The aim was to move towards a situation where Suzie could be admitted to hospital for a nut challenge without panicking, as her blood tests had all been normal. Her mother realized how uncertain she had become with Suzie's demands and worries, and that this had led Suzie to stop trusting her and taking control at home. As her mother gained in confidence and control, Suzie became more relaxed and allowed her mother to take charge again.

12.3   Sleeping problems in young children

Sleeping problems in young children present in a variety of forms:
- problems about settling to sleep at bedtime;
- waking in the middle of the night;
- early waking in the morning;
- nightmares, night terrors and sleep walking; and
- a combination of these.

Children may cry or get up when put to bed, cry or get up in the middle of the night, demand bottles, breast-feeds or dummies, want to sleep in their parents' bed and need rocking to sleep.

12.3.1   Behavioural learning theories help us understand the effect of prior learning experiences on the present behaviour

12.3.1.1   Classical conditioning in the child

When a child has repeatedly experienced the pairing of falling asleep with sucking on the breast or bottle, or with being rocked or stroked, they become dependent on this soothing stimulation and are unable to fall asleep without these events occurring. When they go to bed or wake in the night, they need to suck or be rocked or stroked in order to fall asleep again. Parents also learn that these strategies were associated with the child falling asleep and so continue to use them until well after the age at which they were required.

12.3.1.2   Classical conditioning in the parent

Parents who are very anxious about their infant can establish patterns of soothing that are very dependent on their presence. These mothers will often carry their children around all day, have difficulty encouraging them to sleep alone and have problems reducing breast-feeding unless the child decides to stop. The pairing of the child sleeping or calming during the occurrence of these behaviours can create a powerful learning paradigm that parents find difficult to change. Anxious parents will respond very rapidly to their infant's cries and will often interfere with or prevent the infant from learning how to self-soothe (Burnham *et al.*, 2002).

12.3.1.3   Operant conditioning in the child

Children rapidly learn that a parent will go and comfort them, give them a feed, take them into their bed or let them stay up if they persist in crying. Their refusal to go to bed or go to sleep is reinforced by the parents' responses. Parental attention, cuddles, drinks, more playtime and watching more TV are all positive reinforcers for children staying awake. Intermittent reinforcement schedules are also very important as children will persevere in their disruptive behaviour as parents may have given in intermittently previously. Erratic or non-existent routines at bedtime, and inconsistent management of the child at night, will intermittently reinforce the child's attempts to get his own way, stay up late or sleep with the parents.

12.3.1.4   Operant conditioning in the parent

Parents often feel very anxious and distressed when their child cries and so any behaviour that stops the crying becomes rapidly learned. Some interestingly idiosyncratic behaviours can develop. Parents will learn that certain methods of settling their child to sleep have worked in the past and so sometimes will progress through a series or four or five different responses to find the one that will work again. It is highly reinforcing for the parent to see their child calmly fall asleep, so there is often a pattern of one-trial learning.

12.3.2   Cognitive learning theory can also help us understand parents' distorted cognitions that can reinforce the problem behaviour

Parents try to understand the reasons for their child's crying at night and make many suppositions, some of which are inaccurate and others which are more related to the parent's own emotional state and self-esteem than to an accurate observation of the child's behaviour.

12.3.2.1   Misperception of the child's behaviour

Children's cries can evoke intense stress in some parents whose own emotional state may lead them to misperceive the cries as attacks on them and so make them angry or they may think that the child is in severe distress and not recognize the cry as a method for gaining their own way. Their misperception of the reason for the child's cries reinforces their own anxiety or depression and they often react in ways to perpetuate the cycle.

12.3.2.2   Irrational or distorted parental cognitions and beliefs

These may lead parents to think that their child cannot manage to get through the night without a feed, or that the child will feel rejected or abandoned if made to sleep in their own bed (Wolfson, 1998). Some mothers feel that they should always be available to their child 24 hours a day and so are unable to create a sense of personal space and privacy for themselves. Parents may feel that they should not have to say 'no' to their child and that the child will come to their own best decision. Parents may have inappropriate expectations about how much a child will sleep.

12.3.2.3   Loss of parental confidence in making decisions about the child's sleeping pattern

Poor decision making about the child's sleep pattern can occur when a child has been ill or the parent has been undermined by another family member or by information from 'others' in authority. Father may want the child kept quiet so that he is not disturbed at night because of work. Grandparents may criticize mother's behaviour and newspapers, magazines and books all have different information to provide.

12.3.2.4   Distorted parental cognitions and anxiety

Anxiety may have been caused by concern about illness or disorder – e.g. parents thinking that asthmatic children, physically disabled children, learning disabled children or those with heart problems should not be allowed to get upset. A sense of guilt or intense compassion may lead to overprotectiveness and over-responsiveness. There are much higher rates of sleeping problems in these groups of children and part of the problem is the parental anxiety, which adversely affects how they manage their children at night (Clements *et al.*, 1986).

12.3.2.5   Parental poor self-esteem

Parental depression may have been caused by a sense of poor self-esteem as a result of their own early childhood experiences or broken adult relationships. The disturbed mood can make some parents unable to cope with their child's demands at night. An erratic pattern of responding with poor boundaries and unclear signals can confuse the child. Parents may erupt into uncontrollable rages or give in unpredictably. Exhaustion and poor routines lead to a cycle of irritable demanding behaviour by the child, which is matched by erratically volatile or passive responses from the parent (Wolfson *et al.*, 1992).

12.4   Treatment approaches

The combination of cognitive and behavioural approaches helps the parents make a clear decision about how best to tackle the sleep problem. Many health professionals find that just instructing parents in the behavioural methods alone will not work until the parents have worked out how they feel and made a clear commitment about what they want to do in partnership with the clinician.

12.4.1   Cognitive behavioural approaches to treatment

12.4.1.1   Correct parental misperceptions and distorted cognitions about the child's crying

Some parents require help in recognizing that their child's cries are often not due to distress but due to wanting company and obtaining their own desires. An opportunity to discuss the needs of all members of the family can help parents recognize that they also need sleep and peace in order to provide continued care and attention for their children during the day. Listing the number of excuses a child has for calling their parents into their room can often help parents recognize the humorous side of what is happening. Establishing limits and teaching the child boundaries to their night-time demands is a reasonable expectation when parents are becoming exhausted and irritable. Parents can be helped to understand this in the context of other boundaries that they readily set – e.g. wearing a car seat belt or not eating three bars of chocolate before lunch. Giving them permission to be firmer at night about sleep patterns will often provide the confidence for them to change their management style and this can also have a positive effect on the child's daytime behaviour (Minde *et al.*, 1994). Burnham *et al.* (2002) found that children of parents who wait longer to respond to their children's wakening at 3 months are more likely to encourage self-soothing behaviours in the children by 12 months of age. Being able to wait and see if the child can settle down alone requires a sense of confidence and calmness that there is nothing the matter.

12.4.1.2   Correcting parents' irrational beliefs and anxieties

Some mothers need help in recognizing that their child does not require feeds during the night once they have a good balanced diet in the day. Continued breast or bottle feeding at night is not needed for nutrition but is usually a comfort and soothing habit that helps the child go to sleep. Feeding and falling asleep have become confused and the parent needs to realize that the child can learn to fall asleep without sucking. If parents are concerned about the child needing a drink then they can be encouraged to leave out a bottle or a teacher beaker of water that the child can reach. Once parents recognize that their child will not accept water they understand that the child is not in fact thirsty. Behavioural strategies are then used to help parents decide whether they can use an extinction approach or a more graded approach to the management of drinks at night.

Very anxious parents, who are concerned and overprotective, may have irrational fears about their child at night – e.g. the child feeling rejected, fear of cot death and worry about temperature control. Firm reassurance and an opportunity to express their concerns and realize that they are irrational can help parents feel confident and more decisive about what to do.

12.4.1.3   Increasing parental confidence in decision making about their child's sleep

Including both parents in the consultation can often improve the likelihood of an agreement and decision to implement a treatment plan. Taking the problem seriously and engaging both parents in the discussion can increase the level of support that they provide for each other and increase their confidence. This prevents splits or undermining of authority and enables them to be firmer in their decisions. Follow-up sessions for them to report progress are important in maintaining motivation and compliance in treatment plans. Parents report that knowing that there are several ways of tackling any sleep problem helps them realize that if they are unsuccessful in one approach then they can try another. A realistic appraisal of the speed and success of different approaches is necessary to help them make the best decision about which approach to use. Treatment should be a partnership about the best treatment approach for any particular parent, taking into account their emotional state and any environmental- or child-based limitations.

Concerns about a child crying at night and the effect on siblings or neighbours should be addressed pragmatically. Sending siblings to relatives for a weekend and warning close neighbours that a couple of nights of crying may be possible during the implementation of an extinction sleep programme can set the scene for rapid change. Helping parents solve practical issues will increase their confidence in implementing change.

12.4.1.4   Improving parental emotional state

Parents need to recognize how their own emotional state affects how they react to their child. Self-regulation, containment of anger, consistency of response and firmness of resolve can all be taught and learned in the context of managing sleep patterns. Recognizing how exhaustion through lack of sleep can exacerbate parents' volatile emotional reactions can help them realize how important it is to solve the problem. Learning how to stay calm and ignore the child's demands without losing their temper is an important skill. Realizing that giving in to the child's demands on the tenth request or after an hour makes the whole problem worse and that they are teaching their child to persevere even harder is a necessary lesson to learn. Minde *et al.* (1993) found that one-half of their sample of poor sleepers had mothers who were anxious and depressed. These mothers were extraordinarily sensitive to the minimal cues of their children and would carry them around until they fell asleep. This had the effect of preventing the children learning how to fall asleep on their own or how to settle themselves if they awoke during the night. The mothers were trying to protect their children against any possible life stress. Support for this is evident in work by Benoit *et al.* (1992) which indicates secure attachment relationships between mother and child are related to better sleeping patterns in the children. Securely attached mothers will let their children cope on their own more and the children have no fear of abandonment.

Sleep diaries are not just a record of the child's sleep pattern but a record of the parents' reactions to the child's waking and can help parents maintain a treatment plan (Douglas and Richman, 1984). Star charts for children are also a way of showing parents how they have managed to change and are a reflection of their good management skills. Giving parents a sense of success and attributing the change to them can bolster their self-confidence and their emotional state.

12.4.2   Behavioural learning theory provides a number of strategies for managing children's sleep problems (Douglas, 2002b)

Minde *et al.* (1993) identified that all young children wake during the night but those defined as poor sleepers by their parents find it difficult to settle back to sleep again without parental presence and so wake up their parents. The task of treatment, therefore, is to teach the children to settle to sleep on their own at bedtime and after any night wakings, so that parents are not disturbed.

12.4.2.1   Extinction

Removal of positive consequences for the child's demands at night or at bedtime can rapidly extinguish the child's crying. In most cases, the child is being reinforced by parental presence and attention (Wolfson, 1998). Cuddles, drinks, going into the parent's bed, staying up longer, playing or the parent going into the child's bed are all highly reinforcing events for most children. Parents therefore need to analyse that what they are doing may be maintaining the child's waking. Once they stop responding to the child's waking, it is possible that the child's behaviour may temporarily become worse for a short period until the child learns the new pattern. They will try harder to get the parent to respond before they give up. Parents also need to learn that if they give in to the child's demands, then the child will rapidly learn what works and repeat the same behaviour again (Douglas and Richman, 1984). This approach is often called 'leaving to cry'. It works rapidly within 3–4 nights if parents are consistent in their approach. If parents are very anxious or find it very difficult to hear their child crying and not go into them then this is not an appropriate strategy. Many parents find that the incentive of a very short time to achieve change is a strong motivator. The most important feature of this approach is ensuring that the parents allow their child to fall asleep on their own after they have been crying and that they do not give in.

Extinction can be used for stopping bottles, breast-feeding or dummies at night if they have become a problem and children need to suck before they fall asleep. They will rapidly learn to fall asleep without this comfort habit if it is no longer provided.

12.4.2.2   Shaping

Some parents prefer to use a strategy that teaches their child the desired behaviour in several stages that avoids crying. They can use their presence while the child falls asleep as a reinforcer and gradually withdraw physical contact in defined stages thereby teaching their child that they can fall asleep without the previously high levels of contact. The number of stages of separation can be tailored to individual cases, but the aim is to reduce physical contact and proximity progressively so that the child learns to settle to sleep alone. Similarly, late bedtimes can be gradually made earlier by moving the bedtime routine earlier every few nights. But the child needs initially to learn that the bedtime routine ends in going to bed and falling asleep even if this all occurs at 10 pm.

12.4.2.3   Reinforcement

It is helpful to provide an incentive for the child to comply with a new routine. Star charts can be used very successfully with children over the age of 3 years. These are particularly useful when trying to stop a child going into the parent's bed during the night. They provide an incentive for cooperation and, when paired with an extinction approach, can be highly successful. Children feel happy despite not sleeping with their parents.

12.4.3   Case illustration

David, a $2^1/_2$-year-old boy, had severe sleeping difficulties and his mother had sought treatment from many different professionals. He was receiving sedative medication that did not work reliably. He had always woken on most nights and, more recently, since he had been moved out of his cot, had started to get out of bed, wander around the house and go into his mother's or the nanny's bed, but take some time to settle to sleep again.

He was adopted at the age of 3 months after being in a good foster home. He was the middle of three boys, but his brothers were not adopted. He had a good bedtime routine and could fall asleep on his own at 7.30 pm. He was a very strong willed little boy, who was very active and demanding during the day. Mother admitted that she was having some problems with managing his daytime behaviour as well as that of his older brother. The siblings argued and fought and a negative spiral would often develop with mother becoming angry. The nanny was very indulgent of him and they had a very close relationship with him.

Mother was exhausted and David's waking was wearing her out. She had tried previously to take him back to his bed and sit with him until he fell asleep but it had taken 2 hours and she could not manage sitting there for that length of time. She was also concerned about leaving him to cry as he would get out of bed by himself and wander around. He had a history of crying for up to 3 hours in his cot when younger. She was lacking in confidence about how to manage him and wondered whether it was due to being adopted.

The regular use of sedatives was stopped, as he was clearly used to them and they were having no effect. A plan of action between mother and nanny was agreed and they both decided not to let him into their beds but to take him back to his bed if he came in. Mother was concerned about his safety as he would wander around the house if not attended, and he could climb over a stair gate across his doorway. He could also open a closed door, so she agreed to locking the door if he came out. If he stayed in his room, it would not be locked. She was very concerned about the idea of locking the door but realized that it was her only option if she was going to achieve a fast change in his behaviour. Rapid learning was necessary and it was anticipated that the door would need to be locked only a few times until he learned the new pattern.

During the first week, he was taken back to his room and locked in four times in the middle of the night, but in the next month he was only locked in four times. He learned more rapidly than his mother expected and although he cried for up to $1^1/_2$ hours the first few nights he soon settled and learned that it would not work. As mother gained confidence in managing him at night, she was able to be clearer in her limit setting during the day and his behaviour started to improve generally. She no longer felt that there was something different about him.

12.5   REFERENCES

Barrett, P. M. (2000). Treatment of childhood anxiety: developmental aspects. *Clinical Psychology Review*, **20**, 479–94.

Batchelor, J. A. (1999). *Failure to Thrive in Young Children*. London: The Children's Society.

Benoit, D., Zeanah, C., Boucher, C. and Minde, K. (1992). Sleep disorders in early childhood: association with insecure maternal attachment. *Journal of the American Academy of Child and Adolescent Psychiatry*, **31**, 86–93.

Bugental, D. B. and Johnston, C. (2000). Prenatal and child cognition in the context of the family. *Annual Review of Psychology*, **51**, 315–44.

Burnham, M. M., Goodlin-Jones, B. L., Gaylor, E. E. and Anders, T. F. (2002). Nighttime sleep-wake patterns and self soothing from birth to one year of age: a longitudinal intervention study. *Journal of Child Psychology and Psychiatry*, **43**, 713–25.

Chatoor, I., Ganiban, J., Colin, V., Plummer, N. and Harmon, R. J. (1998). Attachment and feeding problems: a reexamination of non-organic failure to thrive and attachment insecurity. *Journal of the American Academy of Child and Adolescent Psychiatry*, **37**, 1217–24.

Clements, J., Wing, L. and Dunn, G. (1986). Sleep problems in handicapped children: a preliminary study. *Journal of Child Psychology and Psychiatry*, **27**, 399–407.

Dadds, M. R. and Barrett, P. M. (2001). Psychological management of anxiety disorders in childhood. *Journal of Child Psychology and Psychiatry*, **42**, 999–1011.

Douglas, J. E. (2000a). Behavioural approaches to the assessment and management of feeding problem in young children. In A. Southall and A. Schwartz (eds.), *Feeding Problems in Children*. Oxford: Radcliffe Medical Press, pp. 41–59.

   (2000b). The management of selective eating in young children. In A. Southall and A. Schwartz (eds.), *Feeding Problems in Young Children*. Oxford: Radcliffe Medical Press, pp. 141–53.

   (2002a). Psychological treatment of food refusal in young children. *Child and Adolescent Mental Health*, **7**, 173–81.

   (2002b). *Toddler Troubles: Coping with your under 5s*. Chichester: Wiley and Sons.

Douglas, J. E. and Bryon, M. (1996). Interview data on severe behavioural eating difficulties in young children. *Archives of Diseases in Childhood*, **75**, 304–8.

Douglas, J. and Harris, B. (2001). Description and evaluation of a day-centre based behavioural feeding programme for young children and their parents. *Clinical Child Psychology and Psychiatry*, **6**, 241–56.

Douglas, J. and Richman, N. (1984). *My Child Won't Sleep*. Harmondsworth: Penguin.

Drotar, D. (1995). Failure to thrive (growth deficiency). In M. C. Roberts (ed.), *Handbook of Pediatric Psychology*, 2nd edn. New York: Guilford Press, pp. 516–37.

Frank, D. A. and Drotar, D. (1994). Failure to thrive. In M. R. Reece (ed.), *Child Abuse: Medical diagnosis and Management*. Philadelphia: Lea and Febiger, pp. 298–325.

Hampton, D. (1996). Resolving the feeding difficulties associated with non-organic failure to thrive. *Child, Care, Health and Development*, **22**, 261–71.

Harris, G. (2000). Developmental, regulatory and cognitive aspects of feeding disorders. In A. Southall and A. Schwartz (eds.), *Feeding Problems in Children: A Practical Guide*. Oxford, Radcliffe Medical Press, pp. 77–89.

Harris, G., Blisset, J. and Johnson, R. (2000). Food refusal associated with illness. *Child Psychology and Psychiatry Review*, **5**, 148–56.

Hutchings, J., Appleton, P., Smith, M., Lane, E. and Nash, S. (2002). Evaluation of two treatments for children with severe behaviour problems: child behaviour and maternal mental health outcomes. *Behavioural and Cognitive Psychotherapy*, **30**, 279–95.

Johnson, C. R. and Babbitt, R. L. (1993). Antecedent manipulation in the treatment of primary solid food refusal. *Behaviour Modification*, **17**, 510–21.

King, N. J. and Ollendick, T. H. (1997). Annotation: treatment of childhood phobias. *Journal of Child Psychology and Psychiatry*, **38**, 389–400.

Linscheid, T. R., Budd, K. S. and Rasnake, L. K. (1995). Pediatric feeding disorders. In M. C. Roberts (ed.), *Handbook of Pediatric Psychology*, 2nd edn., New York: Guilford Press, pp. 501–16.

Mathisen, B., Skuse, D., Wolke, D. and Reilly, S. (1989). Oral motor dysfunction and failure to thrive among inner city infants. *Developmental Medicine and Child Neurology*, **31**, 293–302.

Minde, K., Faucon, A. and Falkner, S. (1994). Sleep problems in toddlers: effects of treatment on their daytime behaviors. *Journal of the Academy of Child and Adolescent Psychiatry*, **33**, 1114–21.

Minde, K., Popiel, K., Leos, N., Falkner, S., Parker, K. and Handley-Derry, M. (1993). The evaluation and treatment of sleep disturbances in young children. *Journal of Child Psychology and Psychiatry*, **34**, 521–33.

Pugiliese, M. T., Weyman-Daum, M., Moses, N. and Lifshitz, F. M. (1987). Parental health beliefs as a cause of non-organic failure to thrive. *Pediatrics*, **80**, 175–81.

Rapee, R. M. (1997). Potential role of child rearing practices in the development of anxiety and depression. *Clinical Psychology Review*, **17**, 47–67.

  (2001). The development of generalized anxiety. In M. W. Vasey and M. R. Dadds (eds.), *The Developmental Psychopathology of Anxiety*. New York, Oxford University Press.

Roth, J. H. and Dadds. M. R. (1999). Prevention and early intervention strategies for anxiety disorders. *Current Opinion in Psychiatry*, **12**, 169–74.

Schauster, H. and Dwyer, J. (1996). Transition from tube feedings to feedings by mouth in children: preventing eating dysfunction. *Journal of the American Dietetic Association*, **96**, 277–81.

Stallard, P. (2002). Cognitive behaviour therapy with children and young people: a selective review of key issues. *Behavioural and Cognitive Psychotherapy*, **30**, 297–309.

Wolf, L. S. and Glass, R. (1992). *Feeding and Swallowing Disorders in Infancy: Assessment and Management*. Tucson, AZ: Therapy Skill Builders.

Wolfson, A. R. (1998). Working with parents on developing efficacious sleep/wake habits for infants and young children. In J. H. Briesmeister and C. E. Schaefer (eds.), *Handbook of Parent Training: Parents as Co-therapists for Children's Behaviours*, 2nd edn. New York: John Wiley and Sons, pp. 347–84.

Wolfson, A., Lacks, P. and Futterman, A. (1992). Effect of parent training on infant sleeping patterns, parents' stress and perceived parental control. *Journal of Consulting and Clinical Psychology*, **60**, 41–8.

13

Conduct disorders in young children

Veira Bailey

Maudsley Hospital, London, UK

Conduct disorder (CD) is a term used to describe behaviour which includes: excessive levels of fighting or bullying; cruelty to animals or other people; severe destructiveness to property; fire-setting, stealing and repeated lying; frequent and severe temper tantrums; defiant provocative behaviour and persistent severe disobedience; and truanting from school and running away from home. As a child grows, not only do problems escalate but the response to treatment is reduced (Olweus, 1979; Patterson, 1982). Longitudinal studies indicate that CD is relatively stable over time and predicts antisocial behaviour in adult life: there are increased rates of delinquency and antisocial personality disorders (Farrington, 1995). Follow-up studies suggest high rates not only for alcoholism, substance abuse, physical illness, suicide and accidental death but also for widespread social dysfunction, with poor work records and difficulties in all relationships, including marital relationships (Robins and Rutter, 1990).

The prediction of antisocial behaviour is stronger for men than for women. For girls, CD in childhood predicts depression and anxiety disorders more strongly than antisocial behaviour and substance abuse (Robins and Price, 1991).

In addition to antisocial behaviours, there may be coexisting attention deficit and hyperactivity, frequently including cognitive deficits and academic failure (Moffitt, 1990a,b; Moffitt and Henry, 1991; Farrington, 1995). This is associated with particularly poor outcome (Sturge, 1982; Taylor et al., 1996).

Younger children are more likely to show the signs of oppositional defiant disorder (ODD) which is classified as a subtype of CD in ICD-10 (World Health Organization, 1996), characterized by markedly defiant, disobedient and disruptive behaviour that does not include delinquent acts or the more extreme forms of aggressive or antisocial behaviour. In Diagnostic and Statistical Manual of Mental Disorders-IV (DSM-IV) (American Psychiatric Association, 1994), ODD

Cognitive Behaviour Therapy for Children and Families, ed. Philip J. Graham.
Published by Cambridge University Press. © Cambridge University Press 2004.

is classified as a separate condition which may be a developmental precursor of CD.

Antisocial behaviour in younger children is usually present by the age of 3 years, and frequently continues through life. It is associated with hyperactivity, behavioural impulsiveness, irritability, lower IQ and has a high degree of heritability. This is designated 'early onset – lifetime persistent' type antisocial behaviour and is differentiated from an 'adolescence-limited' type where the antisocial behaviour generally occurs in the company of deviant peers and does not persist into adulthood (Moffitt, 1993).

Disruptive and antisocial children are often unpopular with other children and are extruded from groups of normally functioning children, associating only with other antisocial children and becoming part of a deviant subculture (Kupersmidt et al., 1990). They, therefore, lack pro-social models and do not learn how to negotiate and fit in with the pro-social mainstream cultural group. Anti-authority attitudes and an inability to settle in class lead to a lack of satisfaction with the school and increasing alienation, disaffection and disruptive behaviour.

Parents of children with CD engage in incompetent child management practices associated with the inadvertent development and maintenance of aggressive and antisocial child behaviours (Patterson, 1982). Escalating cycles of coercive behaviour occur when the parent and the child use negative reinforcement to maintain the behaviour e.g. giving in when the child has a tantrum or complying only when threatened with being hit (Patterson, 1980). Parents of antisocial children are identified as being deficient in their child-rearing skills by: failing to tell their children how to behave; failing to monitor the behaviour of their children to ensure it is desirable; and failing to enforce rules promptly and clearly with positive and negative consequences (Patterson, 1982). Webster-Stratton and Spitzer (1991) found the management style of parents to involve more violence and criticism, to be more permissive, erratic and inconsistent, and to fail in monitoring their child's behaviour, thus reinforcing inappropriate behaviours. Pro-social behaviour was characteristically ignored or punished.

Such parental behaviour is often elicited by the temperamental characteristics of the children involved. Children with attention deficit hyperactivity disorder (ADHD) are difficult to rear. They may elicit more negative, controlling and coercive management from their parents and are vulnerable to develop comorbid CD. Younger children with ADHD whose parents are less critical have been found to develop fewer conduct problems by age 17 than those whose parents are highly critical (Taylor et al., 1996).

Other factors associated with the development of CD include deficits in reading, lower IQ, generally poor academic performance, association with deviant peers, parental disharmony, neighbourhood cultural factors and child abuse. Of the multiple influences on CD, parenting stands out as a key point of influence on children's behaviour (Burke *et al.*, 2002).

13.1 Rationale for using cognitive behaviour therapy

Children with CD have been shown to have a range of cognitive deficits and distortions (Crick and Dodge, 1994). They recall high rates of hostile cues in social situations, attend to few cues when interpreting the meaning of others' behaviour and attribute the behaviour of others in ambiguous situations to hostile intentions (Dodge and Newman, 1981; Dodge, 1986; Dodge *et al.*, 1990). When in conflict with others, children with CD underestimate their own level of aggression and responsibility in the early stages of a disagreement (Lochman, 1987). When problem-solving, children with CD generate fewer verbal assertive solutions and many more action-orientated and aggressive solutions to interpersonal problems (Dodge and Newman, 1981).

When upset, or in situations that might cause upset feelings, such children show an unusual pattern of affect labelling; they anticipate fewer feelings of fear or sadness. When highly aroused, the feeling is interpreted as anger and increasingly action-orientated responses result. However, when aggressive children are encouraged to use deliberate rather than quick automatic responses, their rates of competent and assertive solutions can increase (Lochman *et al.*, 1991). Children with CD/ODD, with ADHD only and with both disorders show deficient problem-solving, encoding fewer social cues and generating fewer responses. Those with CD/ODD only and with both disorders also select aggressive responses more often than those with ADHD alone (Matthys *et al.*, 1999).

A positive view of aggression and its use to solve social problems appears to be incorporated into the belief system of children with CD; they expect their aggressive actions to reduce negative consequences, they think aggressive behaviour enhances their self-esteem and they value social goals of dominance and revenge more than affiliation (Slaby and Guerra, 1988).

Cognitive deficits in children with CD can be addressed through emotional education, self-reinforcement, social perspective-taking and social problem-solving. These are components of most problem-solving skills training (PSST) and aim to teach children how to approach interpersonal problem-solving adopting a step-by-step approach (Kazdin *et al.*, 1987).

Distorted cognitions may be dealt with in parallel with problem-solving skills training by continued reference to concepts of fairness, safety and what the other person feels. In this chapter, a cognitive behavioural approach to CD in 6–11-year-old children is described. Management of such problems in adolescents is discussed by Lochman *et al.* in Chapter 25.

13.2   Assessment for treatment

Assessment should be broadly based and needs not only to include the diagnosis of disorder in the child but also an assessment of parenting competence. The possibility of child abuse, treatable mental illness in the parent and the presence or absence of support systems for parents in the community should all be considered. An assessment needs to be made of the child's social functioning at school with adults and with peers and of the nature and extent of academic difficulties. A psychometric assessment should be made to detect any cognitive deficit.

It is important to detect comorbid hyperkinetic disorder. The presence of severe antisocial symptoms with undoubted poor parenting and possibly abuse can dominate the picture. This may lead to a classic diagnostic pitfall, as hyperkinetic disorder, if untreated, is associated with a high risk of persisting antisocial behaviour (Moffitt, 1990a, b). Cognitive behavioural approaches to hyperkinetic disorder are described in Chapter 14.

Another diagnostic difficulty may be presented by the child who is well engaged with an experienced clinician and symptom free at interview but impulsive and distractible in other situations. The use of standardized questionnaires (Conners, 1969; Behar and Springfield, 1974; Routh, 1978; Barkley, 1990; Goodman, 1997; Goodman *et al.*, 1998) may help in diagnosis. A different problem occurs when the diagnosis of hyperkinetic disorder – manifest by inattention, overactivity and impulsiveness – is made correctly but because a broad-based assessment has not been carried out, CD may be missed.

The presence of depression or anxiety should be considered. The cocky anti-authority presentation of many children with CD may mask coexisting emotional problems. This also occurs with children of below average IQ whose lack of cooperation when tested may be attributed to CD and whose cognitive deficits only become apparent when they are found to have severe difficulties in problem-solving. Lack of social skills may be related not only to poor parenting but also to constitutional deficits in the ability to empathize.

A social assessment may be necessary in some cases, not only to provide a child protection risk assessment but also to assess the need for respite provision and advice on housing and finances.

13.3   Interventions: general considerations

With the range of risk factors identified as influencing the development of CD, successful treatment is most likely when multiple risk domains are targeted in treatment.

A multimodal treatment approach will need careful orchestration of the various elements involved and should include regular networking and consultation with other agencies, such as education and social services, in order to avoid conflict and confusion. Occasionally, children may need admission to local authority care or to an inpatient unit. Satisfactory controlled studies of inpatient versus community care are limited. One comparison, though somewhat flawed, showed that community placement produced at least as favourable a result as inpatient treatment (Wimsberg *et al.*, 1980).

There is substantial evidence for multisystemic treatment being effective in older adolescents. However, the effectiveness of the intervention in 6–12-year-old children is largely untested (Farmer *et al.*, 2002). In these younger children, parent management training is essential to change the powerful modelling and reinforcement of antisocial behaviour which is otherwise likely to persist. This may need to involve a cognitive component to help parents whose maladaptive cognitions or negative automatic thoughts, such as 'I can't let him have the last word' or 'spare the rod . . .', interfere with their ability to carry out effective positive parenting.

13.4   Parent management training

The theoretical and practical basis for this work was developed by Patterson, Reid and colleagues at the Oregon Social Learning Center (OSLC). They describe an escalating cycle of coercive interactions between parent and child – the *coercive hypothesis*. This postulates that children learn to escape or avoid parental criticism by escalating their negative behaviours (such as temper tantrums and defiance), which leads to increasingly negative parental behaviour (such as telling the child off, yelling or hitting the child). Over time, the 'coercive training' in the family continues with an increasing rate and intensity of parent and child aggressive behaviour. Thus, both parents and child are caught in the 'negative reinforcement trap' which effectively trains children to develop CD (Patterson, 1982).

In addition to the negative reinforcement, the child also experiences effective modelling of antisocial behaviours from observation of parental aggression. Parents may also positively reinforce the child's misbehaviour – e.g. by paying attention to the child only when he or she is shouting or behaving badly and ignoring the child when playing quietly.

Five family management practices form the core components of the OSLC programme:

(1) Parents are taught how to pinpoint the problem behaviours and track them at home – e.g. recording compliance versus non-compliance.

(2) Parents are taught reinforcement techniques such as praise, points systems, treats and rewards.

(3) When parents see their children behaving inappropriately, they learn to apply a mild consequence or a short-term deprivation of privileges – e.g. 1 hour loss of television time or bike use.

(4) Parents are taught to 'monitor' (or supervise) the children at all times, even when they are away from home. This involves parents knowing where their children are at all times, what they are doing and when they will be returning home.

(5) Finally, the parents are taught problem-solving and negotiating strategies. They also become increasingly responsible for designing their own programmes.

This programme typically requires 20 hours of direct contact with individual families and includes home visits in order to improve the generalization of parenting strategies.

Another individual parent-training programme (Helping the Non-Compliant Child) designed to treat non-compliance in young children aged 3–8 was developed by Forehand and McMahon (1981). This incorporated the idea of *alpha* and *beta* commands based on the observation that parents with reasonably obedient children give more so-called alpha commands and parents with children with CD give more negative beta comments. Alpha commands are characterized by being clear, specific and direct, being given one at a time and being followed by a waiting of 5 seconds for compliance. Beta commands are streams of ineffectual nagging, vaguely phrased chains of instruction and comment, often delivered as a question and frequently followed by rationalization. An example of a beta command is: 'How many times have I told you, if you don't come away from there, Tony . . . I don't know how I'm going to keep my hands off you . . . Tony, what have I told you . . . you know I've had a bad day, what with that letter from the welfare people and now the TV's on the blink!' As an alternative, parents are taught to give alpha commands using clear, specific and direct instructions and waiting 5 seconds for compliance. The child is also named and eye contact is achieved. Parents are encouraged to use a firm but not a cold voice and are encouraged to refrain from telling their children what to stop doing.

Parent–Child Interaction Training (PCIT) uses two phases of training: child-directed interaction in which the parents are trained in non-directive play skills to alter the quality of the relationship and parent-directed interaction which focuses on improving parenting skills by teaching parents to give clear instructions, praise for compliance and time out for non-compliance. Treatment is carried out in a clinic playroom, equipped with a one-way mirror, and includes the coaching of parents in the use of appropriate parenting behaviour by means of an 'ear bug'. This is frequently called the *Parent–Child Game*. As it involves naturalistic play settings, it is most useful for younger children.

Scott (2002) summarizes the characteristics of effective parent-training programmes which are effective when used for individual families or for groups.

Content

- Structured sequence of topics, introduced in set order over 8–12 weeks. Subjects include play, praise, incentives, setting limits and discipline, emphasis on promoting sociable self-reliant child behaviour and calm parenting.
- Constant reference to parents' own experience and predicament.
- Theoretical basis informed by extensive empirical research and made explicit.
- Detailed manual available to enable replicability.

Delivery

- Collaborative approach acknowledging parents' feelings and beliefs.
- Difficulties normalized and humour and fun encouraged.
- Parents supported to practise new approaches during sessions and through homework.
- Parent and child seen together in individual family work – just parents in some group programmes.
- Crèche, good quality refreshments and transport provided if necessary.
- Therapists supervised regularly to ensure adherence and to develop skills.

13.5 Group discussion videotape modelling for parents

The Group Discussion Videotape Modelling Programme (GDVM) was developed by Webster-Stratton as a parent-training programme for young children with CD. It includes components of the Forehand, McMahon and Patterson programmes as well as problem-solving and communication skills (D'Zurilla and Nezu, 1982; Webster-Stratton, 1982).

The basic parent-training programme consists of a series of ten videotape programmes, modelling parenting skills. There are 250 vignettes, each of which lasts approximately 1–2 minutes. These are shown by a therapist to groups of 8–12 parents per group. After each vignette, the therapist leads the group discussion of the relevant interactions and encourages parents' ideas and problem-solving as well as role play and rehearsal. Parents are given homework exercises to practise a range of skills at home, but the children do not attend. Great efforts are made to use models of different sexes, ages, cultures, socioeconomic backgrounds and temperament in order to enhance the power of the modelling by enabling parents to identify with the models.

The programme has also been used by parents of children with CD as a self-administered intervention, viewing the video vignettes and completing the homework assignment without therapist feedback or group support. A recent development has been a further six videotape programmes called ADVANCE, which focus on family issues other than parenting skills, including anger management, coping with depression, marital communication skills, problem-solving strategies and how to teach children to problem-solve and manage their anger more effectively (Webster-Stratton, 1994). Enhancing parent management training by including work on parental concerns such as job stress, family disputes and personal worries has enabled behavioural gains for children to be maintained (Dadds *et al.*, 1987) and has reduced attrition (Prinz and Miller, 1994). For mild behavioural problems, the provision of a brochure alone is often sufficient to produce behavioural change (Clark *et al.*, 1976; McMahon and Forehand, 1978).

The major advantages of effective group parent-training programmes are the lower drop-out rates compared with those found in individual practice (10–20% versus 30%) and the lower cost (approximately one-quarter) compared with individual interventions with which they are equally effective.

Recent findings of the effectiveness of the replication of the Webster-Stratton Programme in ordinary clinical settings using regular clinic staff are particularly encouraging as they included interventions in socially deprived communities (Scott *et al.*, 2001b).

13.6   Working with individual families

Family therapy techniques have emphasized general principles rather than the contingency management of antecedents and consequences of specific target behaviours. The emphasis has been on altering maladaptive patterns of interaction and communication through broad principles of child management, the strengthening of generational boundaries, the interpersonal interactions of family members and marital relationships and improving the self-esteem of carers.

Individual behavioural programmes for children with CD using parents as co-therapists have been shown to be most successful when attention is paid both to the antecedents and to the consequences of the targeted behaviour. This makes use of the ABC model, a helpful mnemonic for parents as well as therapists (Herbert, 1987):

A. stands for **A**ntecedents events – what happens immediately before the targeted behaviour.

B. stands for targeted **B**ehaviour.

C. stands for the **C**onsequences – what happens after the targeted behaviour. Paying attention to the antecedents and consequences of targeted behaviours leads to intervention programmes which aim to increase pro-social behaviours by giving clearer instructions and positive reinforcement ('catch the child doing something good') for desirable behaviours.

Antisocial behaviour can be decreased by a range of techniques such as extinction, overcorrection, time out from positive reinforcement and, most importantly, teaching and reinforcing pro-social behaviour that is incompatible with the antisocial behaviour.

13.7   Behavioural and cognitive techniques used in working directly with the child

Social skills training approaches (see Chapter 23) have been increasingly used with young children with CD. Initially, *operant techniques* were developed, rewarding pro-social behaviour and discouraging antisocial behaviours. *Modelling strategies* were also used, teaching by allowing children to observe appropriate social behaviour modelled by adult or child models. *Coping modelling* with a therapist or other model talking through the task, including how to deal with setbacks and frustration, has been found to be more effective than a mastery model demonstrating ideal or perfect behaviour (Meichenbaum and Goodman, 1971). *Coaching* was used in which principles of competent social behaviour were taught, often using role play of problem situations such as what to do when hit by another child or punished unfairly by a teacher.

An approach used by the Hahnemann Programmes (Spivack *et al.*, 1976) emphasizes deficits in *alternative thinking*, the ability to generate multiple solutions to interpersonal problems; *consequential thinking*, the ability to foresee the immediate and long-term consequences of the solution; and *means-end thinking*, the ability to plan a series of actions to attain the goal, devising ways around obstacles within a realistic timeframe. They use simple word concepts as a foundation for problem-solving – e.g. *or* and *different* to help generate alternatives: 'I can hit him *or* I can tell him I am upset' – 'hitting is *different* from telling'.

Interpersonal cognitive problem-solving training (ICPS) emphasizes the paramount importance of interpersonal communications and negotiating skills, seeing the other person's point of view and achieving compromise within the social situation. The training develops thinking processes: *how* to think rather than *what* to think.

The aim of therapy for children with CD is to remedy the deficits and distortions in behaviour and cognitions. Several programmes and models have been developed for PSST and most have several elements in common. *Emotional education* enables the child to identify and label different emotions and the situations in which they occur. The therapist may model expression of feelings and empathizing with others in addition to using pictures and games to increase the repertoire. *Self-monitoring* of behaviour and of feelings whose intensity can be rated enables children to be empowered and to manage their own behaviour and feelings. *Self-instruction* may use a 'Stop! Think! What can I do?' approach to inhibit or slow automatic responses, while *self-reinforcement techniques* teach children to use *positive self-talk* – e.g. 'Well done, I didn't answer back' – to enhance the development of pro-social skills. *Social perspective taking* uses vignettes, modelling, role play and feedback in order to help children become aware of the intentions of others in social situations.

The core elements of *problem-solving* are: defining the problem; generating alternative solutions; assessing the pros and cons of each solution; deciding on a plan to tackle the problem; and carrying out the plan and monitoring it. These core elements can be adapted for different age groups. In very young children, the generation of alternatives before moving on to assess the advantages and disadvantages of each may be too difficult and cause confusion. For children of junior school age, the 'Think Aloud Programme' (Camp and Bash, 1985) uses a cartoon of Ralph the Bear to teach a self-instructional approach to problem-solving: 'What is the problem? What can I do about it? Is it working? How did I do?' In generating alternative solutions, an element of fun can be used to loosen rigid thinking by asking, for example, what the little green man from Mars might suggest. It is also important to remember that 'no change' has to be included as one of the alternatives in the evaluation.

In a group setting, the generation of alternatives and the evaluation of solutions can be highly productive, as (hopefully pro-social) peer modelling and ideas of other children will broaden the repertoire of group members (Bailey and Vickers, 2003). Children with CD often need help to identify their problems appropriately as they are particularly liable to attribute their problems to the hostile intentions of others. They are also likely to need encouragement to consider assertive and non-aggressive alternative solutions to interpersonal difficulties.

Children can be taught self-control procedures such as the Turtle Technique where the child retires into an imaginary shell to consider the problem. Cognitive strategies to control impulsivity are provided in the *Stop and Think Workbook* (Kendall, 1989).

Cognitive restructuring can be introduced in parallel to problem-solving by including consideration of concepts of fairness, safety and what the other person would feel, the aim being to change basic beliefs and attitudes. Therapists can model expression of feelings and appropriate empathizing with others.

The central aspects of cognitive restructuring include: thought identification and monitoring; linking thoughts, feelings and behaviours; challenging and changing distorted and dysfunctional thoughts; and learning alternative ways of coping with difficult situations. For young children, thought bubbles and cartoons can be used as a way of eliciting thoughts and images while older children can manage a simple thought diary or log. It is important, at all ages, that the child should understand that it is only their thought that is being challenged. They should not see themselves as being told they are 'wrong' or that they are being told off.

In order to encourage the generalization of pro-social behaviours learned in therapy at home and at school, goal setting and operant techniques should be used. Goals should always be specific and attainable and must be carefully monitored. The contingent use of social reinforcement (e.g. praise, particularly the approval of a valued person), activity reinforcements (treats) and tangible reinforcements (rewards) can be tailored to a particular child's need. Pairing social reinforcement by parents, teachers or therapists with other reinforcements is particularly important for children with CD as they often have poor relationships with authority figures and are minimally motivated by adults' reinforcement. Other techniques may focus particularly on anxiety (Garrison and Stolberg, 1983) or anger management (Lochman *et al.*, 1987) and may use group feedback with whiteboards, flipcharts, video feedback, role play and group discussion. Interventions which explicitly target anger-coping skills, especially recognizing the triggers (anger cue recognition), and which rehearse specific coping strategies appear to produce more positive outcomes, whether with CD or ADHD (Hinshaw *et al.*, 1984; Lochman and Curry, 1986).

13.8   Group work with children

The techniques described above can easily be adapted for use in a group setting. They should be incorporated into a matrix of enjoyable activities in order for therapy itself to be enjoyable for the child. When working with groups, the therapist must pay attention to group composition and be able to manage and control the behaviour of the group using behavioural methods such as positive reinforcement for participation so that disruptive behaviour is contained and therapy can proceed.

There should be some caution in assembling a homogeneous group of children with disruptive behaviour disorders. Not only will this be a difficult group for therapists to manage but, in older children, iatrogenic effects have been described which may make behaviours worse (Mulvey *et al.*, 1993; Dishion *et al.*, 1999).

The Dinosaur Child Training Curriculum for young children aged 4–8 who have early-onset conduct problems has been developed, making use of video-tape scenes depicting children coping with stressful situations in a variety of ways (Webster-Stratton *et al.*, 2001). They may be seen controlling their anger with the 'Turtle Technique'; problem-solving at home and at school; making friends; coping with rejection and teasing; paying attention to teachers; finding alternatives to bothering a child sitting next to them in the classroom; and cooperating with family members, teachers and class-mates. At the 'Dinosaur School', children were taught how to handle themselves in time out and what self-talk to use while they were there – e.g. 'I can cope with this and calm down', 'I can go back and be successful' and 'I'm OK, I just made a mistake'. The interactive video modelling was based on a coping model where children were encouraged to discuss the use of positive social skills in different situations and to find new solutions for typical problems such as being told off by a teacher. Children were encouraged to identify the feelings of the children on the videotapes and to discuss the possible reasons for their feelings in order to increase their ability to empathize.

13.9   Liaison with schools

Teacher liaison is necessary in order to aid generalization by reinforcing the development of pro-social behaviours and to change inappropriate beliefs or behaviours by the teacher. Teachers may also be helped by advice on management and structuring of the classroom (Wheldall and Lam, 1987), in training in positive teaching methods (Wheldall and Merrett, 1991) and in teaching problem-solving (Kendall and Bartel, 1990). It may also be necessary to integrate specific educational remediation for a child whose educational attainments are retarded. School approaches to bullying (Olweus, 1994) are useful in reducing a school culture of antisocial behaviour.

A very promising approach is the SPOKES Intervention Programme for children at risk of social exclusion (S. Scott, personal communication). This is a community-based intervention with two aspects. It delivers both a general parenting programme based on Webster-Stratton Group Discussion Videotape Modelling techniques and a parent-led literacy programme for children. This programme combines two evidence-based interventions (Sylva and Hurry, 1995; Scott *et al.*, 2001b) and has been found to be effective in substantially improving children's social behaviour and reading. Held in a local primary school, the programme was felt to be non-stigmatizing, had a good take up and reasonable attendance and provided a very high level of parent satisfaction.

13.10   Outcome

Parent management training (PMT) strategies are well established as being among the most effective in the treatment of disruptive behaviour disorders, with clinically significant and sustained improvements for at least two-thirds of children treated (Brestan and Eyberg, 1998). However, improvements at home are not necessarily accompanied by improvements at school. Furthermore, some parents are unwilling to participate in PMT and others have difficulty in implementing or sustaining the skills learned. Children with CD have more negative and hostile attributions, deficits in their social skills, deficient problem-solving ability and reduced self-control which contribute to their difficulties in relationships including poor peer relationships (Webster-Stratton and Hammond, 1997).

In direct interventions with children, randomized controlled trials have shown that, particularly when used together with PMT, interventions focusing on social skills, problem-solving and conflict management strategies effectively reduce conduct problems (Kazdin *et al.*, 1992; Kazdin, 1996, 1997; Webster-Stratton and Hammond, 1997) and promote better peer relationships (Webster-Stratton and Hammond, 1997). Effects were maintained in both interventions 1 year later.

Unfortunately, the characteristics of parents which lead to parenting difficulties are those which are also associated with poorer outcomes (Webster-Stratton, 1989a; Patterson, 1991). These factors include multiple social problems, marital problems, single parents of low socioeconomic status and a strong punishment ideology in the parents. Components can, therefore, be added to address these difficulties as in the 'advanced' Webster-Stratton programme. Close liaison with social services will be helpful where there are multiple social problems, perhaps using family aides support or respite care to reduce stress, while couple therapy to address problems in the parents' relationship may reduce marital difficulties interfering with their parenting.

Other components successfully added to PMT have been cognitive behaviour therapy for depressed mothers (Sanders and McFarland, 2000) and partner communication and support (Dadds *et al.*, 1987).

The underlying behaviour principles of parent management training have a face validity which parents appreciate and which may increase their compliance. Programmes generally have high parental ratings of acceptability and consumer satisfaction (Webster-Stratton, 1989b). However, while teaching parenting skills empowers parents, it also makes demands on them, with consequent difficulties in engaging in therapy and high drop-out rates (Kazdin *et al.*, 1992).

Although programmes treating children with CD are steadily developing and the therapeutic elements are being evaluated in randomized controlled trials, the central problems of working with families who are difficult to engage remain. Despite being highly effective and well received by parents, parent training is not routinely available in any country in the world (Hoagwood, 2001; Scott, 2002). A survey of current practice at clinics in the UK found that 24% offered no parent training either in a group or individually and, of those offering programmes, staff training in evidence-based effective programmes was variable (Richardson and Joughin, 2002). Furthermore, it appears helpful to recognize that CD is a chronic condition and that 'booster sessions' may be necessary.

When compared with children in the general population (up to the age of 27 years), the cost of using public services (including foster and residential care and remedial education services) is ten times greater for children with CD (Scott *et al.*, 2001a).

While public anxiety about delinquency and violence is high, it is important to emphasize the cost–benefit and potential health gain of early intervention with children with CD (Offord, 1989; Light and Bailey, 1993), as well as the opportunities afforded to therapists for creative therapeutic interventions.

13.11   REFERENCES

American Psychiatric Association (1994). *Diagnostic and Statistical Manual of Mental Disorders*, 4th edn. Washington, DC: American Psychiatric Association.

Bailey, V. and Vickers, B. (2003). Cognitive behavioural group work with children. In E. Garralda and C. Hyde (eds.), *Managing Children with Psychiatric Problems*. London: BMJ Books, pp. 79–95.

Barkley, R. A. (1990). *Attention-Deficit Hyperactivity Disorder. A Handbook for Diagnosis and Treatment*, 2nd edition. New York: Guilford Press.

Behar, L. B. and Springfield, S. (1974). A behaviour rating scale for the preschool child. *Developmental Psychology*, **10**, 601–10.

Brestan, E. V. and Eyberg, E. M. (1998). Effective psychosocial treatments of children with CD and adolescents: 29 years, 82 studies and 5272 kids. *Journal of Clinical Child Psychology*, **27**, 180–9.

Burke, J. D., Loeber, R. and Birnaher, B. (2002). Oppositional defiant disorder and conduct disorder: a review of the past ten years. Part II. *Journal of the American Academy of Child and Adolescent Psychiatry*, **41**, 1275–93.

Camp, B. W. and Bash, M. A. S. (1985). *Think Aloud: Increasing Social and Cognitive Skills – A Problem-Solving Programme for Children*. Champaign, IL: Research Press.

Clark, H. B., Risley, T. R. and Cataldo, M. F. (1976). Behavioral technology for the normal middle-class family. In E. J. Mash., L. A. Hamerlynk and L. C. Hardy (eds.), *Behavior Modification and Families*. New York: Brunner/Mazel.

Conners, C. C. (1969). A teacher rating scale for use in drug studies with children. *American Journal of Psychiatry*, **126**, 884–6.

Crick, N. R. and Dodge, K. A. (1994). A review and reformulation of social information processing mechanisms in childrens' social adjustment. *Psychological Bulletin*, **115**, 74–101.

Dadds, M. R., Schwartz, S. and Sanders, M. R. (1987). Marital discord and treatment outcome in behavioral treatment of child conduct disorders. *Journal of Consulting and Clinical Psychology*, **55**, 396–403.

Dishion, T. J., McCord, J. and Paulin, E. (1999). When interventions harm: peer groups and problem behaviour. *American Psychologist*, **54**, 755–64.

Dodge, K. A. (1986). Attributional bias in aggressive children. In P. C. Kendall (ed.), *Advances in Cognitive-Behavioral Research and Therapy*. San Diego: Academic Press, pp. 71–100.

Dodge, K. A. and Newman, J. P. (1981). Biased decision-making processes in aggressive boys. *Journal of Abnormal Psychology*, **90**, 375–9.

Dodge, K. A., Price, J. M., Bachorowski, J. and Newman, J. P. (1990). Hostile attributional biases in severely aggressive adolescents. *Journal of Abnormal Psychology*, **99**, 385–92.

D'Zurilla, T. J. and Nezu, A. (1982). Social problem-solving in adults. In P. C. Kendall (ed.), *Advances in Cognitive Behavioral Research and Therapy*, Volume 1. New York: Academic Press.

Farmer, E. M. Z., Compton, S. N., Burus, J. B. and Robertson, E. (2002). Review of the evidence base for treatment of childhood psycopathology: externalizing disorders. *Journal of Consulting and Clinical Psychology*, **70**, 1267–302.

Farrington, D. P. (1995). The development of offending and anti-social behaviours from childhood: key findings from the Cambridge Study in Delinquent Development. *Journal of Child Psychology and Psychiatry*, **36**, 929–64.

Forehand, R. L. and McMahon, R. J. (1981). *Helping the Non-Compliant Child: A Clinician's Guide to Parent Training*. New York: Guilford Press.

Garrison, S. T. and Stolberg, A. G. (1983). Modification of anxiety in children by affective imagery training. *Child Psychology*, **11**, 115–30.

Goodman, R. (1997). The strengths and difficulties questionnaire: a research note. *Journal of Child Psychology and Psychiatry*, **38**, 581–6.

Goodman, R., Meltzer, H. and Bailey, V. (1998). Strengths and difficulties questionnaire: a pilot study on the validity of the self-report measure. *European Child and Adolescent Psychiatry*, **7**, 125–30.

Herbert, M. (1987). *Behavioural Treatment of Children with Problems: A Practice Manual*. London: Academic Press/Harcourt Brace Jovanovich.

Hinshaw, S. P., Henker, B. and Whalen, C. K. (1984). Cognitive behavioral and pharmacological interventions for hyperactive boys: comparative and combined effects. *Journal of Consulting and Clinical Psychology*, **52**, 739–49.

Hoagwood, K. (2001). Evidence-based practice in children's mental health services: what do we know? Why aren't we putting it to use? *Report on Emotional and Behavioral Disorders in Youth*, I, 84–7.

Kazdin, A. E. (1996). Combined and multimodal treatments in child and adolescent psychotherapy: issues, challenges and research directions. *Clinical Psychology: Science and Practice*, **3**, 69–100.

(1997). Practitioner review: psychosocial treatments for conduct disorder in children. *Journal of Child Psychology and Psychiatry*, **38**, 161–78.

Kazdin, A. E., Esveldt-Dawson, K., French, A. E. and Unis, A. S. (1987). Problem-solving skills training and relationship therapy in the treatment of antisocial child behavior. *Journal of Consulting and Clinical Psychology*, **55**, 76–85.

Kazdin, A. E., Siegel, T. and Bass, D. (1992). Cognitive problem-solving skills and parent management training in the treatment of antisocial behaviors in children. *Journal of Consulting and Clinical Psychology*, **60**, 733–47.

Kendall, P. C. (1989). *Stop and Think Workbook*. Merrion Station, PA: Workbooks.

Kendall, P. C. and Bartel, N. R. (1990). *Teaching Problem-Solving for Students with Learning and Behavior Problems: A Manual for Teachers*. Merrion Station, PA: Workbooks.

Kupersmidt, J. G., Core, J. D. and Dodge, K. A. (1990). The role of peer relationships in the development of disorders. In G. R. Asher and J. D. Coie (eds.), *Peer Rejection in Childhood*. Cambridge: Cambridge University Press, pp. 274–308.

Light, D. and Bailey, V. (1993). Pound foolish. *Health Service Journal*, **11**, 16–18.

Lochman, J. E. (1987). Self and peer perceptions and attributional biases of aggressive and non-aggressive boys in dyadic interactions. *Journal of Consulting and Clinical Psychology*, **55**, 404–10.

Lochman, J. E. and Curry, J. F. (1986). Effects of social problem-solving training and self-instruction with aggressive boys. *Journal of Consulting and Clinical Psychology*, **15**, 159–64.

Lochman, J. E., Lampron, L. B., Gemmer, T. C., Harris, R. and Wyckoff, G. M. (1987). Anger coping intervention with aggressive children: a guide to implementation in school settings. In P. A. Keller and S. R. Heyman (eds.), *Innovations in Clinical Practice: A Source Book*. Professional Resource Exchange, pp. 339–56.

Lochman, J. E., White, K. J. and Wayland, K. K. (1991). Cognitive behavioral assessment and treatment with aggressive children. In P. C. Kendall (ed.), *Child and Adolescent Therapy: Cognitive Behavioral Procedures*. New York: Guilford Press, pp. 25–65.

Matthys, W., Cuperus, J. M. and Van Engeland, H. (1999). Deficient social problem-solving in boys with ODD/CD with ADHD and with both disorders. *American Academy of Child and Adolescent Psychiatry*, **38**, 311–21.

McMahon, R. J. and Forehand, R. (1978). Non-prescriptive behavior therapy: effectiveness of a brochure in teaching mothers to correct their child's inappropriate mealtime behaviours. *Behaviour Therapy*, **9**, 814–20.

Meichenbaum, D. and Goodman, J. (1971). Training impulsive children to talk to themselves: a means of developing self-control. *Journal of Abnormal Psychology*, **77**, 115–26.

Moffitt, T. E. (1990a). The neuropsychology of delinquency: a critical review of theory and research. In N. Morris and M. Tonry (eds.), *Crime and Justice: An Annual Review of Research*, Vol. 12. Chicago: University of Chicago Press, pp. 99–169.

(1990b). Juvenile delinquency and attention deficit disorder: boys' developmental trajectories from age 3 to age 15. *Child Development*, **61**, 893–910.

(1993). Adolescence-limited and life-course-persistent antisocial behaviors: a developmental taxonomy. *Psychological Review*, **100**, 674–701.

Moffitt, T. E. and Henry, B. (1991). Neuropsychological studies of juvenile delinquency and juvenile violence. In J. S. Milner (ed.), *Neuropsychology of Aggression*. Boston: Kluwer Academic Publishers, pp. 67–91.

Mulvey, E., Ashton, M., Reppucci, N. (1993). The prevention and treatment of juvenile delinquency. *Clinical Psychology Review*, **13**, 133–67.

Offord, D. R. (1989). Conduct disorders: risk factors and prevention. In D. Shaffer, I. Philips, N. B. Enzer and M. M. Silverman (eds.), *Prevention of Mental Disorders, Alcohol and Other Drug Use in Children and Adolescents*. Rockville, MD: US Department of Health and Human Services, pp. 273–307.

Olweus, D. (1979). Stability of aggressive behavior patterns in males: a review. *Psychological Bulletin*, **86**, 852–75.

(1994). Bullying at school: basic facts and effects of a school based intervention programme. *Journal of Child Psychology and Psychiatry*, **35**, 1171–90.

Patterson, G. R. (1980). Mothers: the unacknowledged victims. *Monographs for the Society for Research in Child Development*, **45**, 1–64.

(1982). *Coercive Family Process*. Eugene, OR: Castalia.

(1991). Performance models for antisocial boys. *American Psychologist*, **41**, 432–44.

Prinz, R. J. and Miller, G. E. (1994). Family based treatment for childhood antisocial behavior: experimental influence on dropout and engagement. *Journal of Consulting and Clinical Psychology*, **62**, 645–50.

Richardson, J. and Joughin, C. (2002). *Parent Training Programmes for the Management of Young Children with CDs: Findings from Research*. London: Royal College of Psychiatrists.

Robins, L. N. and Price, R. K. (1991). Adult disorders predicted by childhood conduct problems: results from the NMH Epidemiologic Catchment Area Project. *Psychiatry*, **54**, 116–32.

Robins, L. N. and Rutter, M. (eds.) (1990). *Straight and Devious Pathways from Childhood to Adulthood*. Oxford: Oxford University Press.

Routh, D. K. (1978). Hyperactivity. In P. Magrab (ed.), *Psychological Management of Pediatric Problems*, 2. Baltimore: University Park Press.

Sanders, M. R. and McFarland, M. T. (2000). Treatment of depressed mothers with disruptive children: a controlled study of cognitive behavioral family intervention. *Behavior Therapy*, **31**, 89–112.

Scott, S. (2002). Parent training programmes. In M. Rutter and E. Taylor (eds.), *Child and Adolescent Psychiatry*. Oxford: Blackwell Publishing, pp. 949–67.

Scott, S., Knapp, M., Henderson, J. and Maughan, B. (2001a). Financial cost of social exclusion: follow-up study of antisocial children into adulthood. *British Medical Journal*, **323**, 194–7.

Scott, S., Spender, Q., Doolan, M., Jacobs, B. and Aspland, H. (2001b). Multicentre controlled trial of parenting groups for child antisocial behaviour in clinical practice. *British Medical Journal*, **323**, 194–7.

Slaby, R. G. and Guerra, N. G. (1988). Cognitive mediators of aggression in adolescent offenders: 1. Assessment. *Developmental Psychology*, **24**, 4, 580–8.

Spivack, G., Platt, J. J. and Shure, M. B. (1976). *The Problem-Solving Approach to Adjustment*. San Francisco: Jossey-Bass.

Sturge, C. (1982). Reading retardation and antisocial behaviours. *Journal of Child Psychology and Psychiatry*, **23**, 21–31.

Sylva, K. and Hurry, J. (1995). *Early Intervention in Children with Reading Difficulties*. Research Monograph Series. London: School Curriculum Assessment Authority.

Taylor, E., Chadwick, O., Heptinstall, E. and Danckaerts, M. (1996). Hyperactivity and conduct problems as risk factors for adolescent development. *Journal of the American Academy of Child and Adolescent Psychiatry*, **35**, 1213–26.

Webster-Stratton, C. (1982). Teaching mothers through video tape modelling to change their children's behaviors. *Journal of Paediatric Psychology*, **1**, 279–94.

   (1989a). Predictors of treatment outcome in parent training for children with CD. *Behaviour Therapy*, **16**, 223–43.

   (1989b). Systematic comparison of consumer satisfaction of three cost-effective parent training programmes for conduct problem children. *Behaviour Therapy*, **20**, 103–15.

   (1994). Advancing videotape parent training: a comparison study. *Journal of Consulting and Clinical Psychology*, **62**, 583–93.

Webster-Stratton, C. and Hammond, M. (1997). Treating children with early-onset conduct problems: a comparison of child and parent training interventions. *Journal of Consulting and Clinical Psychology*, **65**, 93–109.

Webster-Stratton, C. and Spitzer, A. (1991). Development, reliability and validity of a parent's daily telephone discipline interview: DDI. *Behavioural Assessment*, **13**, 221–39.

Webster-Stratton, C., Reid, J. and Hammond, M. (2001). Social skills and problem-solving training for children with early onset conduct problems: who benefits? *Journal of Child Psychology and Psychiatry*, **42**, 943–52.

Wheldall, K. and Lam, Y. Y. (1987). Rows versus tables. II. The effects of two classroom seating arrangements on classroom disruption rate, on-task behaviour and teacher behaviours in three special school classes. *Educational Psychology*, **7**, 303–12.

Wheldall, K. and Merrett, F. (1991). Effective classroom behaviour management: positive teaching. In K. Wheldall (ed.), *Discipline in Schools: Psychological Perspectives on the Elton Report*. London: Routledge, pp. 46–65.

Wimsberg, B. G., Bialer, I., Jupietz, S., Botti, E. and Balka, E. (1980). Home versus hospital care of children with behavior disorders. *Archives of General Psychiatry*, **37**, 413–18.

World Health Organization (1996). *Multiaxial Classification of Childhood and Adolescent Psychiatric Disorders: The ICD-10 Classification of Mental and Behavioural Disorders in Children and Adolescents*. Cambridge: Cambridge University Press.

14

Attention deficit hyperactivity disorder

William E. Pelham Jr. and Kathryn S. Walker

State University of New York, Buffalo, New York, USA

Restlessness, inattention and impulsiveness are common problems in children of school age and indeed in those of preschool years. When these problems are shown in extreme form, impairing the social and educational functioning of children involved, they can be considered to be signs of a psychiatric or psychological disorder. There are currently two major categorizations of such disorder. The first is that defined as Hyperkinetic Disorder in the International Classification of Diseases (ICD) (World Health Organization, 1994); this is the classification used in most European countries. Using this definition, approximately 1–2% of children of school age are affected (Danckaerts and Taylor, 1995). The second is that defined in the Diagnostic and Statistical Manual (DSM) of the American Psychiatric Association as Attention Deficit Hyperactivity Disorder (ADHD). There are less stringent criteria for the diagnosis of ADHD, and the prevalence rate is 3–5% of boys and 1–2% of girls. Nevertheless, ADHD is a chronic and impairing childhood mental health disorder (American Psychiatric Association, 1994). In this chapter, discussion of assessment and management will be based around the concept of ADHD.

Children with ADHD by definition present with abnormally high levels of inattention, impulsivity and hyperactivity, and these children often suffer substantial impairment in their daily life functioning in home, school and recreational settings. The behaviour of children with ADHD is often characterized as developmentally inappropriate and is now known to follow a developmental trajectory persisting into adolescence and adulthood. ADHD, once considered an acute disorder, has been broadly reconceptualized as a chronic, life-spanning disorder (American Academy of Pediatrics, 2001). Each of the three core symptoms of ADHD can present quite dangerous and expensive consequences for these children, their families and peers, as well as society at large, as children

Cognitive Behaviour Therapy for Children and Families, ed. Philip J. Graham.
Published by Cambridge University Press. © Cambridge University Press 2004.

with the condition develop into affected adolescents and adults. For these reasons and others, effective treatment for childhood ADHD has long been a major concern for parents, teachers, doctors and mental health professionals.

Children with ADHD are typically identified and referred to treatment by parents or through schools. Teachers may be the first people to recognize the behaviour problems of children with ADHD, perhaps because they are better able than parents to compare the child's behaviour with that of unaffected children, or because the demands for attention and impulse control are greater in school than at home (e.g. sitting in a desk for the day, completing tasks that require sustained attention). Once identified by the school, the most common referral is to primary health care professionals and thence to mental health professionals for diagnosis and treatment.

A strong case conceptualization for treatment of ADHD, no different from other disorders presented in other chapters in this volume, involves a well-integrated, *seamless* approach to assessment, treatment and case follow-up. By this we mean: (1) careful selection of assessment measures and tools that can double as goal attainment and follow-up measures; and (2) thorough functional analysis during the assessment phase that leads to a treatment plan that focuses on treating the child in the settings and domains where they show functional impairments. In an age where practitioners are constrained to keep session numbers to a minimum, the importance of streamlining the entire therapeutic process cannot be understated. Our approach minimizes the initial process of diagnosis and instead emphasizes the treatment side of the therapeutic endeavour. In this view, assessment is best conducted by clinicians who have an eye on subsequent treatment plans and who can craft individualized, evidence-based treatments that are tailored to the presenting problems of the referred child.

14.1 Assessment

Proper assessment of ADHD begins with diagnosis, but it does not end there. As any well-versed practitioner or clinician can attest, children with the same parent- and teacher-endorsed symptoms of inattention, impulsivity and hyperactivity may present in a clinic completely differently. In part, this is due to the subjective nature of parent and teacher ratings, as well as the fact that only a subset of the symptom list is required for diagnosis. This variability is also in part due to the differing functional impairments with which the children present, as well as the settings in which they are most salient. Indeed, it is not typically the DSM-IV symptoms of disorders, including ADHD, that motivate parents or teachers to seek treatment (Angold *et al.*, 1999); more often, it is the functional impairment that they experience in the social and academic domains. With this in mind, it is crucial that professionals explore the spectrum of impairment that each child experiences.

Diagnosis of childhood ADHD should be based on parent and teacher endorsement of DSM-IV criteria (American Psychiatric Association, 1994). There are three subtypes based on symptom clusters: predominantly inattentive, predominantly hyperactive–impulsive or combined subtypes. To meet diagnostic criteria, children must experience these symptoms at an early age (i.e. onset before age 7) and for at least 6 months. The child must show demonstrable impairment in at least two settings (e.g. home, school or recreational settings), or be endorsed by at least two adults not in the same setting (usually teacher and parent).

The American Academy of Pediatrics (2000) provides guidelines for a thorough approach to the assessment of ADHD. Assessment or rating scale information should be gathered from adults well acquainted with the child in their natural environment and should ascertain both symptom endorsements *and* the degree to which symptoms cause impairments for children in their daily life functioning in home, school and recreational environments. Structured interviews with mothers are commonly used for diagnosis; parent and teacher rating scales that incorporate DSM symptoms of ADHD are cost-efficient tools for this purpose. Unfortunately, impairment has not been well measured by the rating scales traditionally utilized for childhood mental health assessment. However, a brief, simple parent and teacher rating scale that measures impairment in several domains important to ADHD children (adult and peer relationships, family and classroom functioning and academic achievement) has been developed and validated (G. A. Fabiano and colleagues, unpublished data).

The American Academy of Pediatrics' guidelines for diagnosis emphasize that no medical (e.g. neuropsychological examinations) or psychological (e.g. neuropsychological battery) tests or tasks are diagnostic, although they may help in the diagnosis or exclusion of comorbid disorders (such as learning disabilities and seizure disorder). The guidelines also note that if an ADHD child behaves well and fails to exhibit symptoms during a visit to a clinic, that information cannot be used to rule out ADHD; however, if a child readily exhibits impairments and symptoms during an office visit, these observations may serve to confirm reports by parents, teachers and others in the child's natural environment. Because ADHD children tend to be poor/inaccurate raters of their externalizing behaviour problems, interviewing the child has little utility for diagnosing ADHD. Children with ADHD often have inaccurate self-perceptions, systematically inflating their self-worth and demonstrating a lack of insight into their difficulties (Hoza *et al.*, 2002). These difficulties may result in the limited effects that cognitive therapies have had on these children, which will be discussed further below. Talking to a child with ADHD may, however, shed light on comorbid internalizing disorders or thought disturbance, and may be useful for those purposes. Although talking with and listening to children may have little value in the diagnosis of ADHD, most clinicians would regard it as helpful to take the opportunity of direct observation of the child in a clinic setting, hoping to gain further insight into the nature and severity of the child's problems and to observe the interaction between parent(s) and child.

As mentioned above, although historically most researchers and clinicians in the psychiatric community have strongly emphasized the importance of making an accurate DSM diagnosis for ADHD and using DSM symptoms of ADHD as targets in treatment and measures of treatment outcome, there has been a recent shift towards the belief that appropriate targets for treatment centre on the child's impairment in daily life functioning and not on symptoms (Scotti *et al.*, 1996). The central role that impairment plays in assessment and treatment of ADHD can be borne out by the fact that: (1) impairment – that is, problems in daily life functioning that result from symptoms – rather than symptoms themselves is why children are referred to treatment (Angold *et al.*, 1999); and that (2) impairment in key domains of functioning (e.g. peer relationships, parenting skills, academic achievement) – not symptoms themselves – mediate long-term outcome for children with disruptive behaviour disorders (Hinshaw, 1992; Chamberlain and Patterson, 1995; Coie and Dodge, 1998). Thus, assessment of impairment in daily life functioning becomes the most important element of initial evaluation, and plants the seed for effective treatment planning. The major reasons for referral can be turned into effective, socially relevant individualized targets or objectives of treatment.

Similarly, impairment rather than symptoms should be the focus of treatment, and ongoing assessment of the presenting problems in daily life functioning is necessary to evaluate whether it is necessary to calibrate and/or modify treatment. Treatment development and adjustment may only be achieved through a comprehensive functional analysis. A functional analytic approach includes an A-B-C analysis – an analysis that describes the functional relationship between the antecedents of the behaviour (A; i.e. settings, people, time of day), the behaviour itself (B) and the consequences of the behaviour (C; i.e. what the child obtains from the behaviour – attention, removal of demands) (see Mash and Terdal 1997, for an expanded discussion of how to conduct a functional analysis in the initial stages of treatment planning). It is important to note that assessment and treatment conceptualization is an ongoing process as the child's presenting problems change over time and require ongoing monitoring and modification.

14.2   Behavioural treatment

In a book giving comprehensive coverage of cognitive behavioural therapies (CBT), this chapter may differ significantly from others. Specifically, although CBT has been shown to be effective or evidence based for many other disorders, it has not been shown to be an effective treatment for ADHD. Although the core symptoms of ADHD (inattention, impulsivity and hyperactivity) would seem to make this disorder a good candidate for CBT, 15 years of cognitive behavioural interventions utilized on inattentive and impulsive children show that they are quite refractory to these types of interventions. Many different types of CBTs have been applied to children with ADHD, including verbal self-instructions, problem-solving strategies, cognitive modelling, self-monitoring, self-evaluation, self-reinforcement and others. Reviews of these studies have consistently documented the lack of efficacy of cognitive mediational approaches in ADHD children (Abikoff, 1987; Hinshaw, 2000; Pelham, 2002). Thus, recent clinical trials for ADHD have involved primarily non-cognitive, behavioural interventions (e.g. MTA Cooperative Group, 1999).

Because cognitively mediated treatment approaches have not been considered to be empirically supported (Pelham *et al.*, 1998), the treatments summarized here will be largely behavioural as opposed to cognitive behavioural. However, cognitively mediated approaches will be discussed when contradictory examples occur. Although it has not yet been well validated, there is evidence that CBTs can be relatively successful *adjuncts* to operant behavioural interventions, and they will be described in the context of child-directed and multi-component treatments for ADHD summarized below. Indeed, it is noteworthy that cognitive interventions were originally developed in the 1970s to enhance *generalization* of well-established behavioural treatments with children – particularly those with problems in impulsivity.

14.3   Comprehensive treatment of ADHD

Several recent reviews have now established the effectiveness of behaviour modification in both school and home settings for the treatment of ADHD (Pelham *et al.*, 1998; DuPaul and Eckert, 1997; G. A. Fabiano and W. E. Pelham, unpublished data). Behaviour therapy and stimulant medication are the only two

Table 14.1 Components of effective, intensive behaviour modification treatment for ADHD

Parent training

Behavioural approach; therapist teaches parents contingency management techniques to use with the child and the parent implements the treatment

Focus on specific target behaviours that reflect impairment in multiple domains of functioning (e.g. peer and adult relationships, sibling relationships, homework, classroom and family functioning)

Typical model is group-based, weekly sessions with therapist initially, then contact faded

Adherence to treatment components regularly checked, and treatment goals are continually added, deleted or modified based on an ongoing functional analysis of behaviour

Continued support and contact as long as necessary (e.g. years versus weeks or months)

Programme for maintenance and relapse prevention (e.g. develop plans for dealing with backsliding – e.g. booster sessions – or concurrent cyclic parental problems – e.g. adjunctive sessions for coping with stress)

Re-establish contact for major developmental transitions (e.g. adolescence)

School intervention

Behavioural approach; therapist teaches contingency management techniques to teacher and the teacher implements the treatment with the child

Focus on specific target behaviours that reflect impairment in multiple domains of functioning (e.g. peer and adult relationships, academic progress, classroom functioning)

Consultant works with teacher – initial weekly face-to-face or phone sessions, then contact faded

Adherence to treatment components regularly checked, and treatment goals are continually added, deleted or modified based on an ongoing functional analysis of behaviour

Continued support and contact for multiple school years after initial consultation (as long as necessary)

Programme for maintenance and relapse prevention (e.g. school-wide programmes, in-service training all school staff, including administrators; train parent to work with the teacher and monitor/modify classroom programmes)

Re-establish contact for major developmental transitions (e.g. move from primary (elementary) school to secondary (middle) school)

Child intervention

Behavioural and developmental approach – involving direct work in natural or analogue settings, *not* clinic settings

Focus on specific target behaviours that reflect impairment in multiple domains of functioning (e.g. friendships, peer interactions, adult relationships, academic skills, classroom and family functioning)

Paraprofessional implemented

If available, intensive treatments such as summer treatment programmes (9 hours daily for 8 weeks), and/or school-year, after-school and Saturday (6-hour) sessions

Table 14.1 (*cont.*)

Adherence to treatment components regularly checked, and treatment goals are continually
added, deleted or modified based on a current functional analysis of behaviour

Provided as long as necessary (e.g. years versus weeks or months)

Programme for generalization and relapse prevention (e.g. integrate with school and parent
treatments, booster sessions, buddy systems)

Re-establish contact for major developmental transitions (e.g. move from primary (elementary)
to secondary (middle) school)

Adjunctive stimulant medication

Only used as a first-line treatment with pervasive, moderately or severely impairing disorders

Need determined following initiation of behavioural treatments, timing depends on child's
severity and responsiveness to behavioural treatments, parental preferences and parent/
school resources

Individualized, randomized, school-based medication trial should be conducted to determine
need and minimal dose to complement the behavioural intervention

Need for frequency and duration of medication determined during ongoing assessment based
on child's impairment across settings, with repeated monitoring of main and side effects to
adjust dosages and justify need

evidence-based treatments for ADHD (American Academy of Pediatrics, 2001).
In general, behavioural interventions examined in these studies consistently
reveal considerable improvement relative to control conditions. Our belief is
that four building blocks make up a comprehensive treatment for ADHD: Parent
Training, Teacher Consultation, Child Intervention and Concurrent Medication
with a central nervous system stimulant (see Table 14.1). The first three comprise
behaviour modification and are necessary components of a comprehensive treatment. We believe that psychosocial treatments for ADHD should always be a
first-line treatment, and that, *although others may differ*, medication should be
added as an adjunctive treatment to behavioural interventions when they have
proven to be insufficient. When comprehensive behavioural treatments are utilized, only a minority of ADHD children (25%) will need adjunctive medication
(MTA Cooperative Group, 1999). *These are likely to be the children with moderate
and severely impairing disorders, pervasive across settings.*

As mentioned above, the targets of behavioural treatment should be the
most socially relevant and face-valid problems in daily life functioning that the
child exhibits. These are those that if changed would probably lead to improved
long-term outcomes for the child with ADHD: difficulties in peer relationships,
academic functioning and family relationships. Presenting problems should be

targeted for every domain of impairment the child experiences, starting with those in which the most problematic behaviour occurs, and, where possible, bridging across settings (e.g. home, school, after-school activities).

It is important that clinicians do not begin a behavioural intervention with a child until there has been clear indication from the parents and school that they are dedicated and committed to the implementation of behavioural interventions. Sometimes parents expect that they are taking the child to a psychologist who will see their child in individual therapy and return a cured child to the parents. Parents need first to be disabused of that notion and motivated to work with the therapist on their child's difficulties from a social learning approach. It may be useful for clinicians to utilize some of the techniques from the motivational interviewing literature to create readiness for treatment in parents who do not have it as a preliminary step in behavioural interventions (see Chapter 5). It is also important that parents come to terms with the fact that ADHD is a chronic and pervasive disorder that lasts into adolescence and adulthood, although the presentation of impairment and symptoms will vary. As such, parents must buy into the fact that psychosocial treatment will need to be long term and intensive and used across the child's environment as long as is necessary. When done well, clinicians who interface weekly with both the school and home for 10–12 weeks can cause clinically significant change in most children with ADHD. These changes will be maintained with appropriate procedures in place to foster maintenance of treatment gains.

14.4   Behavioural interventions in the home

Behavioural parent-training programmes make up the first of two classes of well-established treatments for ADHD (Pelham *et al.*, 1998). Parent-training packages that are manualized and widely utilized for children with ADHD include those developed by Barkley (1998), Webster-Stratton (2003), Hembree and McNeil (1995), Sanders *et al.* (1998) and Cunningham *et al.* (1993). All of these programmes, as well as others, have a solid evidence base behind them. They are discussed elsewhere in this book in more detail (see Chapter 13).

Table 14.2 illustrates a typical sample sequence of parent-training sessions, taken from the COPE (Community Parent Education) programme (Cunningham *et al.*, 1993). Typical parent-training programmes are run for 8–16 weeks, either individually or in groups, with possible additions of maintenance sessions afterwards. In all of these programmes, parents are first educated about the nature and prognosis over the long term for children with ADHD. They are told that medication, even if indicated, as will be the case in only a

Table 14.2   Sample 10-week COPE parent-training curriculum

Session	Content
1	Introductory Night and Introduction to ADHD
2	Attending, Rewards, Balanced Attending Among Siblings
3	Planned Ignoring
4	Point Systems 1
5	Transitional Warnings and When-Then
6	Planning Ahead
7	Point Systems II (Response Cost)
8	Time Out from Positive Reinforcement 1
9	Time Out from Positive Reinforcement II
10	Problem Solving and Closing

minority of affected children with ADHD, will require supplementation with behavioural approaches, because only behavioural changes caused by lifestyle and parenting changes on the parent's part will have long-term impact on the child's prognosis. Techniques are then taught that focus on behavioural shaping of their child's behaviour: rewarding and praising, punishing and modelling appropriate behaviour themselves. Parents are given readings and weekly homework assignments where they track their children's behaviours and implement the newly learned parenting strategies.

Techniques taught sequentially in parent training range from simple notions such as increasing contingent praise and teaching better commands to more complex techniques that include time out and point systems. A simplified version of what is typically a complex component of a home programme – a token or point system – can be downloaded without charge from http://wings. buffalo.edu/adhd. It is a simple, 20-page, self-instructional programme for establishing a point system at home. The point system is called a Home Daily Report Card, and it is integrated with the School Daily Report Card described below.

Although most programmes focus on behavioural contingencies parents can utilize with their children, adjunctive work is increasingly being incorporated in parent-training programmes to address such additional domains as child-rearing disagreements among parents, parental stress and depression and parental ADHD (A. M. Chronis et al., unpublished data). Parent training is easily supplemented with other treatments, such as those targeting parental psychopathology or stress management, and dealing with these cyclic and debilitating parental problems may be necessary to maximize the impact of behavioural parent training.

Although traditional parent-training programmes have been didactic and run in clinic settings, constraints of time and financial resources have contributed to the increasing utilization of group parent-training programmes (see Chapter 13). Thus, contemporary parent training is typically run in groups, with the addition of supplementary individual sessions where needed. Given a chronic disease model and the developmental changes that occur in ADHD (i.e. puberty, changes in school, parent–child relationships), it will often be helpful for clinicians to re-establish contact with the family at times of major developmental transitions – e.g. adolescence, when the problems of children with ADHD often worsen at the same time as they become *most* reluctant to take medication. This speaks to the need for consistent and monitored oversight and contact on the part of the treating professional with these families.

Most of the parent-training programmes noted above employ similar didactic formats. One that is different is the COPE programme (Cunningham *et al.*, 1993) that the authors use in their clinic. The COPE programme differs from a typical parent training approach in several ways. First, it is done in large groups of 15–30 parents in each group, making it very cost-effective. Secondly, rather than being a didactic approach, COPE Parent Training Leaders utilize brief videotaped vignettes and Socratic questioning to engage the group and allow group members to do most of the talking, thereby increasing group activity and group cohesion. Parents themselves end up helping each other develop the plans that they adopt to use with their children. It has been our observation that parents who are able to generate and evaluate parenting skill options as a group instead of having a professional tell them what to do are better able to problem solve on their own and therefore apply the skills they have learned to their unique environment.

14.5   Behavioural interventions in the school

As the vast majority of children with ADHD are referred for school problems in North America, and, in Europe, all children with the condition are affected in their school behaviour, treatment in the school context is central to the treatment of ADHD. Many training programmes, manuals, handbooks and texts have been developed over the years for classroom management, including for students who have ADHD, and are designed to run in both regular education classes and special education classes (Walker and Walker, 1991; Pfiffner, 1996; DuPaul and Stoner, 2003). Many of the materials that are useful for teachers implementing instructional modifications for a student with ADHD can be created ahead of time by the clinician and brought to the teacher. Table 14.3

Table 14.3 Sample teacher consultation sequence

Session	Content
1	Introduction to ADHD, rationale for and overview of treatment; obtain teacher/school commitment, introduction to behavioural principles
2	Establish and post operationalized classroom rules
3	Home–School Daily Report Card (essential)
4	Structural/instructional modifications for an individual child
5	Attending, praising, rewarding skills
6	Giving effective commands and reprimands, enforcing rules and when-then contingencies
7	Classwide interventions
8	Group contingencies
9	Response cost/reward point or token system for the target child
10	Time out (classroom, office, systematic exclusion)
11	Discussion of special services or special class placement

illustrates a sample 11-week sequence that clinicians can use as a guide for teacher consultation.

As with parents, the first step for most classroom interventions is to provide information about ADHD and collaborate with the teacher to implement behaviour management strategies. Techniques, of which teachers are often well aware, include simple interventions that can be incorporated into the classroom as a whole – e.g. developing and implementing a good set of classroom rules. The classroom rules that the authors have developed for their Summer Treatment Program (STP) classroom are: 'be respectful of others', 'obey adults', 'work quietly', 'stay in assigned seat/area', 'use materials and possessions appropriately', 'raise hand to speak or ask for help' and 'stay on task/complete assignments' (Pelham *et al.*, 1997). These rules have been compiled after many years of working in the schools and amalgamating the most common rules that teachers use. Children with ADHD need to be informed immediately of rule violations and need to have systematic consequences for following and violating class rules.

Teachers may also need encouragement to use consistent praise of appropriate behaviours while ignoring a child's inappropriate behaviours and trying to ensure they are not reinforced by peer attention. Studies on classroom management from the 1970s have shown that teachers issue three times as many negative comments to children as positive comments. Teachers can be encouraged to reverse that ratio, with praise outnumbering reprimands/commands by at least a 3:1 ratio. Teachers can also be encouraged to use the same techniques as are parents for giving commands that maximize the likelihood of compliance (Walker and Walker, 1991).

The most important component of school intervention for a child with ADHD is an individualized Daily Report Card (DRC). A DRC is a daily school–home communication tool that: (1) lets the child know what his/her daily goals are at school and how he or she has done at achieving them; and (2) provides for school–home communication through which the teacher can inform parents how a child has performed. A DRC can be a separate document or can be inserted in the child's homework folder. Teachers choose behavioural targets for the child to meet and provide regular feedback, and rewards are provided daily both in school and at home for goal attainment. Such a system allows parents and teachers to be on the same page in their dealings with the child. A 10-page instructional template for establishing a school DRC can be downloaded at no charge from http://wings.buffalo.edu/adhd. It can be easily integrated with the home DRC noted above.

School rules, learning good commands, contingent praising and DRCs are necessary components of school-based interventions for ADHD, but they are often not sufficient to deal with the behaviour in school settings. When the DRC is helpful but there is still room for improvement with the child, there are more complex behavioural interventions that can be used in the classroom, including point/token systems, time out, classwide and group contingencies. These are more potent interventions than DRCs but they are also more complex and difficult for a teacher to do unaided. If a DRC is insufficient, the choice for a parent and teacher is often whether to step up to more intensive behavioural interventions or whether to add a low dose of medication to a DRC regimen. Parent and teacher preferences and resources/limitations are key factors in such a decision (see discussion below).

14.6   Child-focused interventions

Child-focused interventions for ADHD are useful as adjuncts to the parent-training and classroom management strategies that rely on parents and teachers to manipulate environmental antecedents, consequences and contingencies (Pelham and Fabiano, 2000). However, as noted above, child-focused interventions for ADHD typically do not involve cognitive behavioural interventions and traditional therapy, both of which rely on some insight into the fact that the child has difficulties. Instead, child-focused interventions for ADHD are particularly important for working directly on poor peer interactional skills displayed by many children with ADHD (Pelham and Hoza, 1996; also see Chapter 23) and for teaching competencies and skills to improve self-efficacy with the child. In the context of a comprehensive or multi-component treatment package, some examples of adjunctive child-directed treatment components include: (1) social skills or social problem-solving training programmes (which often make use of cognitive behavioural or self-mediated strategies); (2) playground interventions; (3) academic interventions; (4) anger management training; or (5) sports skills training.

As Table 14.2 reflects, professionals who incorporate child interventions into their treatment plan should take a behavioural as well as a developmental approach, and should focus on target behaviours that reflect impairment in the multiple domains of functioning (e.g. friendships, peer interactions, academic skills) that are relevant for treatment directed towards skill development in the child. These targets are best treated in direct work in the child's natural setting. They cannot be adequately dealt with in a clinic-based setting. Often, child-focused interventions are implemented in the context of larger treatment packages, including school-based or, if available, Saturday, after-school or summer treatment programmes, in which they are integrated with parent-training and school interventions.

Therapeutic summer camps (STP) (Pelham and Hoza, 1996; Pelham et al., 1997) that incorporate numerous evidence-based behavioural treatments in the context of recreational and classroom settings (e.g. point system with reward and response–cost components, social reinforcement, time out, social skills and problem-solving training, and peer tutoring) combine potent behavioural techniques with skills training in academic subjects and common children's sports. They have been widely studied and have a substantial evidence base (Pelham et al., in press). A comprehensive behavioural treatment package that included the STP, behavioural parent training and behavioural teacher consultation – all as outlined in Table 14.1 – was utilized in the Multimodal Treatment Study for ADHD (MTA Cooperative Group, 1999; Pelham et al., 2000). Results showed that the comprehensive behavioural treatment package was very effective, with results that reflected major changes in multiple domains of impairment. These changes were maintained 1 year after treatment such that 68% of the children who received the behavioural treatment were functioning so well that their parents had discontinued their medication (MTA Cooperative Group, in press). Information about how to conduct an STP can be obtained at http://www.summertreatmentprogram.com.

The STP is an example of child-focused treatments for ADHD that focus on peer relationships. It has a major impact on ADHD children's functioning, but it cannot be easily implemented in a contemporary mental health setting. Clinicians who would like to utilize some of the components of the STP can incorporate aspects of it into social skills training groups that they conduct on a weekly basis integrated with behavioural parent training. Although such interventions are far less intensive than the STP, there is some evidence that they may be useful adjuncts to parent training for the domain of peer relationships (Pfiffner and McBurnett, 1997).

14.7 Medication

Many studies in the area of ADHD treatment have shown that medication alone is an effective short-term treatment for ADHD and that combined behavioural and pharmacological treatments show incremental benefits over behavioural treatments on their own (Swanson *et al.*, 1995; Pelham and Waschbusch, 1999). Why then do we suggest medication only as a second-line treatment option? The foremost reason is the maxim 'do no harm'. Behavioural treatments have no known adverse effects, while medication with a central nervous system stimulant has several potentially serious side effects. If a less dangerous and less invasive treatment is available, that should always be tried before a more invasive one. Secondly, as noted above, recent studies have shown that nearly two-thirds of ADHD children treated with comprehensive behavioural treatment will do so well that medication is not necessary (MTA Cooperative Group, in press). The only way for parents to know whether their children can be treated effectively without medication is to give an adequate trial of behaviour modification first. It should be added that a number of clinicians believe that there are occasions when it is justifiable to use medication as a first-line treatment, especially if the condition is pervasive and severe. This view is controversial, and these authors do not agree with it.

Medication as a stand-alone treatment has several limitations, of which clinicians and parents should be aware. Even when helpful, stimulant medication often fails to 'normalize' children with this condition. In one recent study, only one-quarter to one-half of children with ADHD were normalized with medication alone (Swanson *et al.*, 2001). Further, no studies yet have demonstrated that there are long-term beneficial effects of pharmacological treatments on important outcomes for ADHD individuals. Even after a decade of treatment, medication does not positively affect any of the domains of worsening impairments for which such children are at risk as they move into adolescence and adulthood (Swanson *et al.*, 1995). Secondly, medication works only as long as it is in the system, which for the majority of medicated children is during the school day. This would allow for improvement in the teacher–child relationship and in the peer domain but leaves the family environment for the most part untouched. Even for children who receive long-acting or *frequent* dosing, medications are not active at bedtime and early in the morning. Any clinician who has worked with families of children with ADHD can concur that morning routines (getting ready for school) and evening routines (getting ready for bed) are very often problematic, and sole reliance on medication would leave a gap in treatment for these time periods. Some areas of impairment will not be affected by medication even when it is active, including problem-solving strategies, parent–child relationships, parenting skills, children's knowledge of and proficiency in sports, academic achievement and social skills. Psychosocial treatments are necessary to effect change in these domains.

Another limitation of stimulants is that we now know that the majority of adolescents with ADHD discontinue their medication, giving it questionable effectiveness with that population. Medication may have the deleterious effect of discouraging parents from learning and consistently implementing good parenting practices, if they rely on medication to control their children's behaviour. In contrast, teaching parents and teachers fundamental behavioural management skills yields long-term changes in the child and also enables generalization to the other children in parents' and teachers' lives. Finally, medication may have potentially serious long-term side effects that are not currently well understood. For example, recent data suggest that growth suppression is a larger problem than previously thought (MTA Cooperative Group, in press).

For these reasons and others, our belief is that medication should be brought in as an adjunct to behaviour therapy only after behavioural strategies have been tried and adjusted and the child's problems continue to be refractory. For more severe cases of ADHD – perhaps one-third of the cases – adjunctive pharmacological treatment can substantially improve functioning. Psychostimulants are the most commonly prescribed medications for ADHD, including methylphenidate (Ritalin) and amphetamine compounds (Dexedrine, Adderall). Long-acting forms of these are now gaining popularity and include Adderall XR, Concerta, Ritalin LA and Metadate. Second-line treatment agents, none of which have been approved by the Federal Drug Administration, include antidepressants (tricyclics, selective serotonin reuptake inhibitors, Wellbutrin), clonidine, major tranquillizers, lithium and others (e.g. anti-anxiety agents). These second-line agents sometimes are combined with stimulants, but there is little evidence that they are effective treatments for ADHD and little evidence on their safety. Thorough discussions of risk–benefit analyses of using second-line agents at all should be conducted with parents before physicians prescribe them.

A final issue regarding medication is how often children should be medicated and how much medication they should take. Some experts recommend that all children be treated three times a day, 7 days a week, 52 weeks per year. The authors disagree with this approach. Just as with any other treatment, stimulants are used to reduce impairment and improve functioning in target domains. Therefore, medication regimens should be based firmly on impairment. A child should be medicated only in settings and during times when impairment is experienced and when other treatments do not alleviate it. For some children, this may mean school time only, while for others it may mean medicating for coverage at home in the evenings and on weekends. Regarding medication dosage, recent guidelines call for doses to be optimized or maximized – increasing until there is no further room for improvement (American Academy of Pediatrics, 2001). Such a strategy ignores the fact that there are diminishing returns as stimulant dose is increased beyond a moderate dose level (e.g. 0.3 mg/kg or 10 mg methylphenidate equivalent per dose); side effects are increased and incremental gains in beneficial effects are small. All things considered, minimizing a child's lifetime dose of medication is an important goal. By medicating for impairment rather than across the board regardless of need, and by using the lowest rather than the highest effective dose, this goal can be accomplished.

If medication is employed, it is obviously important that its use should only be carried out in consultation with psychologists who are involved in implementing behavioural programmes as well as with teachers. Decisions regarding frequency of medication and dosage cannot be made effectively without feedback from such professionals.

14.8   Discussion

The treatment of ADHD requires a comprehensive, individualized approach to treatment. Treatment needs to be truly comprehensive if it is to alleviate impairment associated with ADHD. Assessment, ideally with an Impairment Rating Scale, needs to be continual and ongoing, with DRC targets constantly monitored and adjusted both at home and at school. Parent training, teacher training with regular report back, child intervention for peer difficulties and, on occasions, medication are likely to be the cornerstones of successful treatment.

All of these intervention components are evidence based. Because we know that ADHD is a chronic disorder, comprehensive and sustained treatment should be the rule rather than the exception. For most children with ADHD, this will mean years, rather than weeks or months, of treatment.

14.9 REFERENCES

Abikoff, H. (1987). An evaluation of cognitive behavior therapy for hyperactive children. In B. B. Lahey and A. E. Kazdin (eds.), *Advances in Clinical Child Psychology*. New York: Plenum Press, pp. 171–216.

American Academy of Pediatrics (2000). Clinical practice guideline: diagnosis and evaluation of the child with attention-deficit/hyperactivity disorder. *Pediatrics*, **105**, 1158–70.

(2001). Clinical practice guideline: treatment of the school-aged child with attention-deficit/hyperactivity disorder. *Pediatrics*, **108**, 1033–44.

American Psychiatric Association (1994). *Diagnostic and Statistical Manual of Mental Disorders*, 4th edn. Washington, DC: American Psychiatric Association.

Angold, A., Costello, E. J., Farmer, E. M. Z., Burns, B. J. and Erkanli, A. (1999). Impaired but undiagnosed. *Journal of the American Academy of Child and Adolescent Psychiatry*, **38**, 129–37.

Barkley, R. A. (1998). *Attention-Deficit Hyperactivity Disorder: A Handbook for Diagnosis and Treatment*. New York: The Guilford Press.

Chamberlain, P. and Patterson, G. R. (1995). Discipline and child compliance in parenting. In M. Bornstein (ed.), *Handbook of Parenting, Volume 4. Applied and Practical Parenting*. Mahwah, NJ: Lawrence Erlbaum Associates, pp. 205–25.

Coie, J. D. and Dodge, K. A. (1998). Aggression and antisocial behavior. In W. Damon (Series ed.) and N. Eisenberg (Vol. ed.), *Handbook of Child Psychology, Volume 3. Social, Emotional, and Personality Development*, 5th edn., New York: John Wiley and Sons, Inc, pp. 779–862.

Cunningham, C. E., Bremner, R. and Secord-Gilbert, M. (1993). *The Community Parent Education Program: A School Based Family Systems Oriented Workshop for Parents of Children with Disruptive Behavior Disorders*. Available from www.summertreatmentprogram.com

Danckaerts, M. and Taylor, E. (1995). The epidemiology of childhood hyperactivity. In F. Verhulst and H. Koot (eds.), *The Epidemiology of Child and Adolescent Psychopathology*. Oxford: Oxford University Press, pp. 178–209.

DuPaul, G. J. and Eckert, T. L. (1997). The effects of school-based interventions for attention deficit hyperactivity disorder: a meta-analysis. *School Psychology Review*, **26**, 5–27.

DuPaul, G. J. and Stoner, G. (2003). *ADHD in the Schools: Assessment and Intervention Strategies*. New York: The Guilford Press.

Hembree, T. L. and McNeil, C. B. (1995). *Parent-Child Interaction Therapy*. New York: Plenum Press.

Hinshaw, S. P. (1992). Academic underachievement, attention deficits, and aggression: comorbidity and implications for intervention. *Journal of Consulting and Clinical Psychology*, **60**, 893–903.

(2000). Attention-deficit/hyperactivity disorder: the search for viable treatments. In P. C. Kendall (ed.), *Child and Adolescent Therapy, Cognitive Behavioral Procedures*. New York: The Guilford Press, pp. 88–128.

Hoza, B., Pelham, W. E., Dobbs, J. and Owens, J. (2002). Do boys with attention-deficit/hyperactivity disorder have positive illusory self-concepts? *Journal of Abnormal Psychology*, **111**, 268–78.

Mash, E. J. and Terdal, L. G. (1997). Assessment of child and family disturbance: a behavioral-systems approach. In E. J. Mash and L. G. Terdal (eds.), *Assessment of Childhood Disorders*, 3rd edn. New York: The Guilford Press, pp. 3–68.

MTA Cooperative Group (1999). 14-month randomized clinical trial of treatment strategies for attention deficit hyperactivity disorder. *Archives of General Psychiatry*, **56**, 1073–86.

MTA Cooperative Group (in press). The NIMH MTA follow-up: 24-month outcomes of treatment strategies for attention-deficit/hyperactivity disorder (ADHD). *Pediatrics*.

Pelham, W. E. (2002). Psychosocial interventions for ADHD. In P. S. Jenson and J. R. Cooper (eds.), *Attention Deficit Hyperactivity Disorder: State of the Science – Best Practices*. Kingston, NJ: Civic Research Institute, pp. 1–36.

Pelham, W. E. and Fabiano, G. A. (2000). Behavior modification. *Child and Adolescent Psychiatric Clinics of North America*, **9**, 671–88.

Pelham, W. E. and Hoza, B. (1996). Intensive treatment: a summer treatment program for children with ADHD. In E. Hibbs and P. Jensen (eds.), *Psychosocial Treatments for Child and Adolescent Disorders: Empirically Based Strategies for Clinical Practice*. New York: APA Press.

Pelham, W. E. and Waschbusch, D. A. (1999). Behavioral intervention in attention deficit/hyperactivity disorder. In H. C. Quay and A. E. Hogan (eds.), *Handbook of Disruptive Behavior Disorders*. New York: Kluwer Academic/Plenum Publishers, pp. 255–78.

Pelham, W. E., Fabiano, G. A., Gnagy, E. M., Greiner, A. R. and Hoza, B. (in press). The role of summer treatment programs in the context of comprehensive treatment for ADHD. In E. Hibbs and P. Jensen (eds.). *Psychosocial Treatments for Child and Adolescent Disorders: Empirically Based Strategies for Clinical Practice*. New York: APA Press.

Pelham, W. E., Gnagy, E. M. Greiner, A. R. *et al.* (2000). Behavioral vs. behavioral and pharmacological treatment in ADHD children attending a summer treatment program. *Journal of Abnormal Child Psychology*, *28*, 507–26.

Pelham, W. E., Greiner, A. R. and Gnagy, E. M. (1997). *Summer Treatment Program Manual*. Buffalo, NY: Comprehensive Treatment for Attention Deficit Disorders, Inc.

Pelham, W. E., Wheeler, T. and Chronis, A. (1998). Empirically supported psychosocial treatments for attention deficit hyperactivity disorder. *Journal of Clinical Child Psychology*, *27*, 190–205.

Pfiffner, L. J. (1996). *All About ADHD: The Complete Practical Guide for Classroom Teachers*. New York: Scholastic Professional Books.

Pfiffner, L. J. and McBurnett, K. (1997). Social skills training with parent generalization: treatment effects for children with attention deficit disorder. *Journal of Consulting and Clinical Psychology*, **65**, 749–57.

Sanders, M. R., Markie-Dadds, C. and Turner, K. M. T. (1998). *Facilitator's Kit for Enhanced Triple P*. Brisbane: Families International.

Scotti, J. R., Morris, T. L., McNeil, C. B. and Hawkins, R. P. (1996). DSM-IV and disorders of childhood and adolescence: can structural criteria be functional? *Journal of Consulting and Clinical Psychology*, **64**, 1177–91.

Swanson, J. M., Kraemer, H. C., Hinshaw, S. P. *et al.* (2001). Clinical relevance of the primary findings of the MTA: success rates based on severity of ADHD and ODD symptoms at the end of treatment. *Journal of the American Academy of Child and Adolescent Psychiatry*, **40**, 168–79.

Swanson, J. M., McBurnett, K., Christian, D. L. and Wigal, T. (1995). Stimulant medication and treatment of children with ADHD. In T. H. Ollendick and R. J. Prinz (eds.), *Advances in Clinical Child Psychology*, Volume 17. New York: Plenum, pp. 265–322.

Walker, H. M. and Walker, J. E. (1991). *Coping with Noncompliance in the Classroom: A Positive Approach for Teachers.* Austin, TX: Pro-Ed.

Webster-Stratton, C. (2003). *The Incredible Years.* http://www.incredibleyears.com

World Health Organization (1994). *ICD-10: Classification of Mental and Behavioural Disorders.* Geneva: World Health Organization.

15

Children with developmental disabilities and their parents

Jeremy Turk

St. George's Hospital Medical School, London, UK

The term 'developmental disabilities' as used in this chapter refers to inborn, early-onset developmental delays leading to substantial impairments in mental functioning; in the case of 'intellectual disability' (also known widely throughout the UK as 'learning disability'), these are consistent with performance on a test of intellectual functioning which would give an intelligence quotient (IQ) of below 70. The term is synonymous with the older terms 'mental handicap', 'mental subnormality' and 'mental retardation'. It must be distinguished from the North American use of the term 'learning disability' which corresponds to what is usually described as 'specific developmental delays' such as dyslexia or dyscalculia. Having a marked and generalized learning difficulty is associated with an increased risk of emotional and behavioural disturbance for a variety of reasons (see Turk, 1996a for review). Having a child with severe learning difficulties also causes great problems for parents (Gath, 1977; Dupont, 1986; Romans-Clarkson et al., 1986) and siblings (Gath and Gumley, 1987; Gath, 1989). The major determinants of familial adjustment are the associated behavioural disturbances rather than the level of intellectual impairment. However, there is good evidence that the likelihood of having a psychiatric disorder, and of its being severe, are associated with the degree of learning difficulty and the related central nervous system dysfunction (Rutter et al., 1970; Bernal and Hollins, 1995).

In the case of 'autistic spectrum disorders' or 'pervasive developmental disorders', the disabilities take the form of multiple, qualitative impairments in the domains of social interactional skills, language and communication, ritualistic/obsessional tendencies and imagination deficits (Wing, 1996). These can manifest in a number of different ways. Individuals may be 'aloof', neither initiating nor responding to social overtures. They may be 'passive', responding when approached socially by others, but tending not to initiate social interactions

Cognitive Behaviour Therapy for Children and Families, ed. Philip J. Graham.
Published by Cambridge University Press. © Cambridge University Press 2004.

themselves. Many present as 'active and odd', making frequent social approaches and interactions but in a highly chaotic, inappropriate, naive, bizarre and one-sided fashion. Autistic spectrum disorders can occur in conjunction with any level of intellectual functioning. However, there is an association between autistic features and diminished intellectual ability. As many as two-thirds of individuals with autistic spectrum disorders have an IQ below 70, while the rate of autistic features increases with diminishing level of intellectual ability. Thus, as many as 50% of individuals with moderate to profound intellectual disability (consistent with an IQ score below 50) are diagnosable as having typical or atypical autism.

For a family with a developmentally disabled child, cognitive behavioural therapy (CBT) may be focused on the child personally. More often, other family members will be employed as co-therapists, or indeed may be the focus of therapy themselves. Work with developmentally disabled individuals and their carers has confirmed just how intellectually or socially impaired a person may be yet still have the potential to benefit from cognitively based approaches (Kushlick, 1989). The important issue is whether the individual can entertain alternative hypotheses and appreciate that these can be evaluated practically. Earlier suspicions that such sophisticated thinking develops late during childhood have been superseded by an awareness of just how young, or developmentally delayed, a person can be yet still benefit from cognitive techniques.

This chapter commences with a definition of cognitive behavioural psychotherapy as applied to families who have a child with developmental difficulties. Important components of CBT relating to this are then reviewed. This is followed by a discussion of the relevance of distinguishing between cognitive deficiencies and cognitive distortions. The importance of a functional analysis of behaviour and cognitions is described, along with examples of common logical errors and useful cognitive techniques applicable to these client groups. The chapter concludes with descriptions of areas of theory particularly relevant to this area: attributional style (Alloy et al., 1984) and chronic sorrow (Wikler et al., 1981).

15.1 Definition

Cognitive behavioural psychotherapy as applied to families who have a child with developmental difficulties can be defined as:

any psychotherapeutic process addressing behaviour and/or thoughts directly, whether with the individual or with carers, as a means of producing change in the functioning of the young person with developmental difficulties, parents or siblings either individually or together.

This definition emphasizes that a wide range of techniques is available and applicable to this field of work. Furthermore, the focus of psychotherapy, and desired outcomes, will vary with family, presenting problem and psychotherapist. Certain fundamental principles of cognitive approaches are particularly applicable. These are based on the tenet that in CBT the therapist does not act to persuade the client or family that their views are illogical or inconsistent with reality. The skill of the psychotherapist is to assist the client and family in discovering this for themselves.

15.2   Important components of cognitive behavioural psychotherapy

Cognitive behavioural psychotherapy deals with the present ('the here and now'). This is particularly useful because of the frequently limited capacity for individuals with developmental difficulties to reflect extensively and deeply on innermost feelings in a verbally articulate way. Also, sense of time elapsing can be markedly impaired in individuals with intellectual disability or autistic spectrum disorders. In particular, the social and communicative impairments which characterize the autistic spectrum disorders dictate that psychotherapies reliant exclusively on talking and introspection will prove to be most difficult. Often, such talking therapies rely on the very aspects of mental life which are impaired in autism. These include perspective taking, introspection, use of metaphor, symbolism and hidden meanings within language and communication. Psychodynamically oriented approaches (Sinason, 1992) are extremely labour intensive and often continue over protracted time periods. Furthermore, the evidence base for their efficacy relies very much on individual case reports by the small number of enthusiasts in this field of endeavour. In contrast, cognitive behavioural approaches are brief, problem-focused, collaborative interventions involving partnership between therapist, client and family ('collaborative empiricism'). The priority given to clarifying and defining specific problems to be worked on and the use of ratings of outcome are highly beneficial not only in terms of confirming the nature and extent of change for therapist and family but also in justifying such approaches clinically and financially. As a means to this end, clear definitions are paramount, as are practical homework tasks whereby the 'theory' shared during psychotherapy sessions is applied back in the real world and the results analysed in subsequent meetings. A main therapeutic role is to coax and encourage the child and family to consider and test out alternative hypotheses in a practical fashion. The important components of cognitive behavioural psychotherapy:

- deal with the present ('here and now');
- are problem orientated;

- are objective;
- have clear definitions;
- are collaborative;
- include practical homework tasks; and
- provide encouragement to consider and test out alternative hypotheses in a practical fashion.

The therapeutic approach also lends itself to skill acquisition through structured, repeated and appropriately reinforced behaviour rehearsal sessions. These are the foundation of a number of currently popular approaches to facilitating development in young people with autistic spectrum disorders, such as the Treatment and Education of Autistic and Communication Handicapped Children (TEACCH) programme (Panerai *et al.*, 2002) and Lovaas approach.

Kendall and Lochman (1994) usefully describe the 'mental attitude' of the cognitive behavioural therapist working with young people as one which combines the qualities of *consultant* (collaborating in the evaluation of ideas), *diagnostician* (integrating and decoding information) and *educator* (teaching through experience with involvement). These same attributes are relevant to the therapist when working with families and familial subunits where there is a child with developmental difficulties. They complement the well-established 'non-specific' therapeutic variables of unconditional positive regard, empathy, warmth and genuineness.

15.3   Cognitive deficiencies versus cognitive distortions

Traditionally, cognitive psychotherapy focuses on cognitive distortions which mar the ability to appraise situations in a realistic and productive fashion. However, individuals with developmental difficulties have more generalized and pervasive developmental delays. This means that useful cognitive processes are more often underdeveloped or inadequate (see Figure 15.1).

In addition, there may be *specific* areas of cognitive deficiency such as the absence of a theory of mind (Baron-Cohen, 1989), inability to understand and label emotions (Hobson, 1986) and central coherence weaknesses (Happé, 1994) in many individuals who have autism. Cognitive deficiencies or distortions may lead to inappropriate and/or detrimental states of mind, behavioural patterns and emotions. However, the cause of such pathological mental states remains important because intervention will vary as a result. Cognitive deficiencies can be helped by psychoeducational strategies as well as tutored exercises in developing the ability to consider different perspectives (e.g. 'Well, maybe somebody else might see things differently. If you were somebody else seeing what you

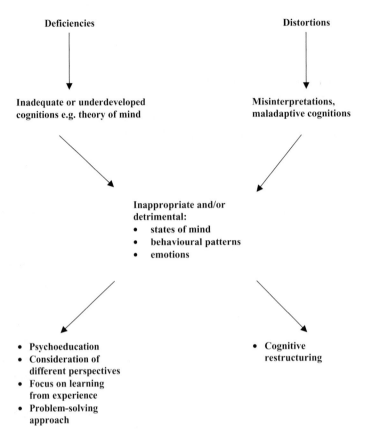

Figure 15.1   Cognitive deficiencies versus cognitive distortions.

were doing and how you were thinking and feeling, what might *they* think? What would *they* do?'). Such an approach is far from easy with individuals who have an autistic spectrum disorder. Never underestimate the impairment in perspective taking and understanding of another person's thoughts and feelings, which can be associated with even well-above average intelligence in an individual with autism. In this respect, it often becomes frankly misleading to refer to individuals with Asperger syndrome (Wing, 1996) as having 'high-functioning autism' simply because their IQ is within the average or above-average range. A more appropriate definition of Asperger syndrome is: 'a severe form of autistic spectrum disorder, complicated by the frequent association with at least average intelligence and often tortuous insight into one's developmental disabilities'.

Cognitive *deficiencies* can be remedied partially by focusing on learning from experience and the development of a problem-solving approach. The problem-solving approach includes the following:

(1) identify specific problems to be worked on;
(2) decide in which order to tackle problems;
(3) negotiate realistic goals;
(4) clarify steps needed to achieve goal(s);
(5) generate as many solutions as possible;
(6) weigh up advantages and disadvantages of each solution;
(7) decide on task required to tackle first step of chosen solution;
(8) undertake exercise;
(9) review with evaluation of success and, if necessary, reappraisal of how it could have gone better; and
(10) decide on next step and proceed.

In contrast, cognitive *distortions* are often better tackled by more traditional techniques of cognitive restructuring. Attwood (2003) illustrates these issues by highlighting the importance of evaluating and acknowledging the individual's developmental stage in terms of social and friendship skills, when developing a framework for cognitive behavioural intervention. He explains that the complexity lies in the frequent *combination* of *delay* and *distortion* in acquisition of social and communicatory abilities in those with autistic spectrum disorders. Thus, modifications to therapeutic approach are needed to accommodate the client's profile of cognitive skills – social and communicatory as well as intellectual. Nonetheless, Attwood (2003) illustrates the usefulness of a wide range of cognitive behavioural approaches for individuals with autistic spectrum difficulties who are experiencing the frequently witnessed secondary mood disorders of depression and anxiety. These include practical ways of managing anxiety, depression and anger; education about mood states; cognitive restructuring; stress management; self-reflection; and practise. The same author has also published an excellent and understandable practical guide to Asperger syndrome and its management which has become something of a best seller (Attwood, 1997).

Similar approaches are described by Bauminger (2002) in the report of a project which attempted to facilitate social–emotional understanding and social interaction in children with autism and good intellectual abilities. The 7-month programme focused on teaching interpersonal problem-solving, affective knowledge and social interaction. Initially, rates of positive social interactions improved. This was evidenced by improved frequency and quality of eye contact, ability to share experiences with peers and improved interest in peers. However, the intensity and duration of such interventions required to bring about change were clearly substantial; they also need to be maintained in the long term. Thus, such programmes should be developed within day-to-day settings such as school and home with a goal of carers maintaining input long term while therapeutic support from professionals is faded out.

15.4   The cognitive triad

Maladaptive beliefs in families who have a child with developmental difficulties can be grouped into three areas, just as they can with other client groups, referred to as the so-called 'cognitive triad' (Beck, 1976). This cognitive triad consists of core beliefs relating to oneself, the future and one's surroundings. It is construed as underlying most other assumptions and attributions ('core role constructs'). Thus, low self-esteem in an individual with developmental difficulties, as well as other family members, is a common occurrence as evidenced by such statements as: 'I'm a failure, I'm dim and stupid and ugly. I'm no good at making friends. Every time I try to do something it goes wrong'. A negative view of the future is also frequently witnessed in statements such as: 'It's going to go from bad to worse, I know it. You can't pull the wool over our eyes, doctor'. Negative views of people and happenings around one are shown in many ways. An example might be: 'People are well meaning but they really don't understand what we're going through and they really can't help'. Some psychological perspectives may be entirely appropriate and indeed may be the goal of psychotherapy. For example, full awareness and understanding of the nature and extent of the child's developmental limitations and their implications may be necessary to prevent potentially maladaptive and detrimental action and interventions by carers. These can arise from familial depressive tendencies resultant from having a family member with a disability, as well as from grief and chronic sorrow issues (see below). There are also often highly practical considerations such as the family's continuing search for the cause of the child's disability in the absence of any identifiable aetiology. In this respect, the therapist must guard against detrimental instructions to cease this search (which is usually seen as patronizing and unhelpful by the family anyway, and may even intensify the family's maladaptive behaviours). It is more appropriate in such circumstances to engage the family in discussion of what investigations have been undertaken, what results were obtained and with what meaning, and what value there may be in further similar pursuits. For example, there may be good psychological reasons for undertaking genetic and neuroimaging investigations if this will satisfy the family that all possible avenues of enquiry have been exhausted. There is, of course, the further issue that such investigations have undergone substantial recent refinement and will sometimes uncover aetiologically important data of use not only in facilitating resolution of the family's grief reaction and orientating them towards the future but also in terms of possible genetic counselling implications and more appropriate multidisciplinary interventions (see Turk and Sales, 1996 for full discussion of the importance of diagnosis). For most individuals with autism, a specific cause cannot be found, although it is well known that there is a strong genetic basis. However, in a significant minority, a specific aetiology can be identified – e.g. fragile X syndrome (Turk and Graham, 1997), tuberous sclerosis (Harrison and Bolton, 1997), Smith–Magenis syndrome (Vostanis *et al.*, 1994) and untreated phenylketonuria (Hackney *et al.*, 1968).

Given the developmental nature of intellectual, social and communicatory difficulties, and the frequently entrenched family perspectives which accompany these, the combination of behavioural with cognitive approaches becomes particularly useful. For a depressed and physically and psychologically inert family, behavioural strategies such as graded task assignments are applicable and useful. For example, a socially isolated and introspective family can be encouraged to undertake outings and other enjoyable activities even if this may be against their nature and inclination and at odds with the prevailing mood ('It doesn't matter if you don't feel up to it. Just do it. Do what you would do if you were happier – or what you used to do when you were happy'). Reassurances against common beliefs of personal selfishness are also of value ('You need to look after number one and ensure your own welfare and psychological health if you are going to be able to do your best for your child with disabilities'). So too are prompts to reflect on and explore the psychological impact on other family members ('How are his brothers and sisters getting on? Do you think they have been affected by his disabilities and challenging behaviours?'). As problems lighten, cognitive approaches can be instituted, thereby shifting the emphasis from activity-based interventions to tackling thoughts and assumptions. It seems that, while activity schedules are efficient at producing change, the re-evaluation of long-held thoughts, attributions and assumptions is important in ensuring enduring benefit for all family members and avoiding relapse. The critical issue is that behavioural and cognitive approaches are complementary and are usually used simultaneously (the proportion of each varying) whatever the severity of the problem and whatever the child's nature, severity and profile of developmental difficulties.

The applicability of both behavioural and cognitive approaches when working directly with individuals with intellectual disability has also been shown scientifically. For example, Bramston and Spence (1985) compared behavioural and cognitive approaches with social skills training for institutionalized individuals with moderate intellectual disability. The authors found that the *behavioural* package produced significant improvement in basic social skill performance. However, the *cognitive* intervention package was associated with significant increases in the generation of alternative solutions. Hence, both approaches have a role in terms of different aspects of improvement. Sadly, but perhaps predictably, the authors also found that training approaches did not produce lasting benefits and that skill improvements were not associated with changes in global ratings of social competence made by staff.

15.5   The functional analysis

Much of the time spent with families who have a child with developmental difficulties is focused on undertaking a functional analysis of the presenting challenging behaviours. Such behaviours are far from being a necessary accompaniment to having learning disabilities. They can and should be treated and ameliorated, even if the total extinction of such behaviours remains unlikely. Challenging behaviours are a common reason for clinical referral. They are serious, disruptive and destructive. Frequent presentations include severe self-injury, aggression, chaotic and disorganized hyperactive behaviour and social inappropriateness. Diary keeping of the nature, frequency and severity of targeted behaviours in vivid detail must be complemented by information on antecedents (where, when, with whom, what was happening?). There must also be data on the consequences of the behaviour (Did she get more attention as a result? Was he allowed to get away with what he was doing? Did she manage to secure solitude and freedom from pressure to interact socially? Did the behaviour seem to serve some self-stimulatory function?). This approach comprises the celebrated ABC chart technique for identifying possible behavioural reinforcers which may be triggering and perpetuating the inappropriate behaviours to the exclusion of more adaptive tendencies (see Oliver, 1995 for a detailed discussion of the role of functional analyses in evaluating self-injurious tendencies in children with learning difficulties).

The cognitive equivalent of ABC charting is of equal use. In this situation, an Activating event triggers a Belief based on past experience and attributional tendencies which results in Consequential behaviour and feelings. The sequence may begin extremely early in the development of the family with a disabled member. For example, the birth of a child with an obvious learning disability syndrome may create a belief that all family activities will be negative, distressing and unfulfilling, and lead to depressive feelings and withdrawal from social and other enjoyable pursuits. The onset of maladaptive cognitions may be later, for example, when a younger child overtakes the child with developmental difficulties academically, creating parental beliefs that there will be little, if any, further intellectual development. This can lead to similarly depressive feelings with associated behaviours which may further reinforce family beliefs that all life must revolve around the child with learning difficulties.

Documentation of multiple examples of behavioural and cognitive functional analyses, both in the therapy session and as part of homework exercises, helps in gaining understanding of how particular behaviours and beliefs are triggered and reinforced, and how these behaviours and beliefs can in turn encourage either useful or maladaptive mood states and behaviours.

15.6   Logical errors

Human ingenuity would seem to know no bounds in reconstruing events to coincide with developing views of self, surroundings and future. However, there are a number of recognized logical errors which recur in the assessments made by cognitive psychotherapists. By being alert to these, the therapist can intervene strategically to force discussion of often deeply held belief systems within the family or individual and to seize the moment in an attempt to produce cognitive, and hence emotional and behavioural, change.

Arbitrary inference describes the tendency to draw a negative conclusion on the basis of subjective impressions even in the absence of concrete evidence to support these views. For example: 'Families are only ever happy with an academically and socially successful child. We will never be happy.'

Selective abstraction is repeatedly judging a situation on the basis of a fragment of information available, focusing only on certain negative aspects and ignoring contradictory factors. For example: 'You say we need to take a long-term view of his development, steering clear of untested fad therapies. Well, he made no progress for 2 years, but now thanks to the alternative approach we commenced 2 months ago he is starting to walk and talk after all this time.'

Magnification or *catastrophizing* is exaggerating the intensity, stress or significance of events, and embellishing situations with surplus meaning that is not supported by objective evidence. For example: 'She would not settle to sleep last night. There's no hope for us.'

Personalization or *self-reference* is the tendency to relate external events to oneself. For example: 'His autistic features became noticeable when I started back at work part-time. I am responsible for his decline'.

Dichotomous or *all-or-nothing thinking* is thinking in extreme, absolute 'black and white' terms. For example: 'Either you are bright or dim, successful or unsuccessful, a happy fulfilled family or a sad unfulfilled one. There are no in-betweens, there is no middle road.'

Superstitious thinking is the belief in cause–effect relationships between non-contingent events. For example: 'If only we could find a way for her to communicate then everything would be all right'.

15.7 Cognitive techniques

The varieties of cognitive techniques available have in common the aim of encouraging more rational appraisal of the evidence for and against holding certain beliefs. Studies confirm that they can be used successfully with learning disabled individuals with depression (Lindsay *et al.*, 1993), recurrent stereotypic nightmares (Bradshaw, 1991) and even sex offending (Lindsay *et al.*, 2000). In addition, the cognitive behavioural techniques of contingency management, deceleration procedures, verbal instruction, self-management programmes and visual instruction and imagery have been described as being of particular benefit (Whitman, 1994).

Thought catching describes the active therapist intervention of interrupting the family's or individual's flow of conversation to focus on a particular thought or attribution as a means of evaluating its validity – e.g. 'Hold it right there . . . hang on . . . you just said that one thing that depresses you most is your son's problems expressing his feelings. Why is that? Did your partner/son/other children know of this? Does this depress him/them? Is this actually true all the time? This can link effectively with *psychoeducational strategies*. Knowledge imparted at strategic points in therapy can be particularly effective in orientating the child and family towards reality. Also, awareness of newly learnt facts may have a direct impact on emotional state and, consequently, on behaviour. For example, acknowledgement of the behavioural deterioration in adolescents with autism (normal adolescent changes, hormonal fluctuations, changes in routine, increasing awareness of personal limitations and dependency, growing familial anxieties regarding the future) can help alleviate feelings of guilt and reorientate family members towards greater mutual support and more appropriate management and survival strategies.

Hypothesis testing and the generation of alternatives lie at the heart of cognitive problem-solving approaches. They emphasize the shared, interactional and collaborative nature of cognitive behavioural psychotherapies and the importance of developing valid tests for particular points of view.

Cognitive restructuring is facilitated by a cognitive functional analysis (see above). It can be helped along by the therapist encouraging the rephrasing of sentences to *cut out absolutes* ('never say never') – e.g. 'He must attend a mainstream school. We can't cope with the idea of special education'. Parents can be encouraged to reframe such phrases in terms such as: 'We would really prefer him to attend mainstream school. The prospect of special education is one we are having particular problems coming to terms with'. Such shifts are, of course, not easy but the appreciation that situations can be viewed in a different light, and with greater flexibility, can be highly beneficial.

Self-monitoring follows on from such approaches. Once the child and family are aware of the importance of cognitive processes and how they can be analysed and adapted, they should be encouraged to develop an automatic tendency to monitor their own thoughts and to become their own cognitive therapists, thereby helping to limit the duration of therapy and to minimize therapist dependency. *Depersonalizing* techniques help counteract the tendency to believe that everything revolves around oneself (egocentricity). It is very common for families with a disabled member to hold double standards whereby they judge themselves far more harshly than others ('We should be able to cope, we only have ourselves to blame for not coping. There are other families who are far worse off than us'). Exhortations to the family to explain the logic underlying such statements can trigger therapeutic and constructive discourse. *Reattribution* can be of relevance to professionals as well as families. A speaker at a scientific meeting, addressing the needs of a family with a learning disabled member, referred to 'the learning disabled family'. He did, of course, mean a family with a learning disabled member. However, there was some important truth in the speaker's perception of how the family perceived themselves as a result of having a child with learning difficulties, which again opened up areas for cognitive work.

15.8   Attributional style

Just as behaviours usually have a situational basis determined by time, location and company, so too do cognitions. It has been appreciated, however, that there is wide individual variability in the extent to which people are influenced by happenings ('It is not things themselves which disturb us but the view we take of them'). There are three dimensions to attributional style which Seligman *et al.* (1984) have identified as contributing to what they term 'the word in your heart'. The *internal–external* dimension is akin to the older notion of locus of control. Some individuals will feel responsible for events happening to them while others tend to feel themselves the victims of circumstances. Conversely, when things go well, some individuals attribute this to their own actions while others feel them to be the result of lucky coincidence. The more in control of events you believe yourself to be, the more you will feel able to modify things positively.

Similarly, the less you habitually feel responsible for negative happenings, the greater your self-esteem. Thus, many individuals seem able from early on to appreciate that 'change has to come from within' and that their own appraisal of happenings and adaptation to them is crucial. Others will feel adrift in a sea of unpredictable currents wafting them randomly in varying directions. This latter perspective is a common one in adolescents with developmental difficulties and their families, confronted with the apparently insoluble struggle of continuing dependency versus the apparent impossibility of true autonomy (Kymissis and Leven, 1994). Individual work can be undertaken to challenge the all-or-nothing aspect of this appraisal and to work on areas of life where personal control and influence over events can be usefully developed.

The *global-specific* dimension addresses the situationality of one's mental state. Feeling depressed or helpless may be linked with particular circumstances or situations (which by inference could then be worked on) or may be perceived as a pervasive tendency unrelated to specific events. The view at one extreme could be of one's entire life being blighted and unrewarding in contrast to a perspective that certain situations or events will produce or rekindle profound feelings of grief and loss while others may promote a sense of reasonable well-being, even if happiness still proves to be elusive. The *stable–unstable* dimension describes the time corollary of the above. Are events always destined to be negative or are they so just at a particular time (or for particular reasons)? On the basis of these three dimensions, Seligman *et al.* (1984) has derived an optimism scale. Seligman and colleagues speculate that those who score highest on this scale tend to: be more successful, be healthier, improve under pressure, endure stress better and, even, live longer. Such optimistic claims are extreme but there is a strong face validity to the notion that the prevailing attributional style on the three dimensions is a useful phenomenon to consider, as well as having some predictive value as to how events will be construed and hence what the prevailing behaviours and emotions are likely to be.

More recent research has confirmed the importance of peoples' habitual patterns of subjective beliefs about the cause of events ('Things going wrong are always the result of her learning difficulties') (Seligman *et al.*, 1990). It does seem that this *explanatory style* can predict not only prevailing mental state but also physical accomplishment – e.g. in athletic pursuits. Seligman *et al.* (1990) have usefully applied the analogy of a habit or addiction to such habitual attribution patterns about causality with families with a learning disabled child. Most people can appreciate the deeply ingrained nature of ways of thinking and the often painful withdrawal process with intermittent cravings for earlier pathological modes of thinking. It is unclear why this urge to readopt unhelpful cognitive attribution patterns should occur but it may be linked to the small but compelling literature suggesting a genetic basis to ways of thinking (Schulman *et al.*, 1993).

15.9   Bereavement and chronic sorrow

An essential component of psychotherapy skills when working with families who have a child with developmental difficulties is an understanding of the bereavement and grieving process. Families experiencing the arrival of a child with disability will tend to go through a series of psychological stages reflecting their grief at the loss of the anticipated idealized child and the arrival of the child with disabilities (Bicknell, 1983). Denial of reality is common and varies from a momentary inability to understand or acknowledge the news ('shock') to long-term refutation of the child's disabilities and needs. Subsequent protest and anger is often directed to the breaker of bad news but may also be directed to oneself as guilt and depression with irrational self-blame for events seen as having contributed to the problem. Searching behaviour can be of oneself ('soul-searching') or seen in more concrete terms – e.g. 'shopping around' for multiple professional opinions or trying out many fad therapies of dubious potential benefit. Usually, these phases are replaced by the slow gaining of a new individual and family identity ('adaptation').

As well as bereavement, a phenomenon of 'chronic sorrow' has been recognized. Here, repeated reminders of the disabled family member's problems and differences from others rekindle grief feelings and some of the above processes (Wikler *et al.*, 1981). Such events usually coincide with times which emphasize the child's differences from others – e.g. falling behind a younger sibling developmentally, needing a statement of special educational need, not being able to play sport or socialize like other children or returning to a dependent life at home after schooling. Wikler and colleagues (1981) found that only 25% of parents had experienced time-bound grief. Most parents were enduring a succession of ups and downs with no general upwards course. It also seemed that professionals overestimated how upsetting early experiences were, yet underestimated how upsetting later experiences were. Chronic sorrow rather than time-bound adjustment seemed to characterize the experiences of parents of children with learning disabilities. This sorrow was periodic rather than continuous. The important cognitive message for therapists and families is that chronic sorrow is not an abnormal response. It is a normal reaction to an abnormal situation. Many of the above described techniques will be useful in addressing this crucial change of perspective. While chronic sorrow is a normal response, cognitive techniques can facilitate its progress through understanding and the development of useful coping strategies.

15.10   Specific evaluations and evidence of effectiveness

The potential for individuals with even quite severe learning difficulties to benefit from cognitive approaches has been confirmed (Kushlick, 1989). Studies have also demonstrated the efficacy of cognitive techniques in helping people with learning difficulties who have depression (Lindsay *et al.*, 1993) and recurrent nightmares (Bradshaw, 1991). Work suggesting benefits from specific cognitive behavioural techniques has been reviewed above (Whitman, 1994).

From a family perspective, early parental understanding of the nature and implications of their child's disorder is crucial to parental acceptance and the early institution of appropriate remedial and preventative interventions. There is evidence that parental acceptance and reality orientation depend on how and when this delicate information is conveyed. How this information is shared is as important as who does it. Parents want to be told the truth, however painful, and earlier rather than later. Time and multiple meetings are required in order to combat inevitable shock and denial associated with this breaking of bad news (Cunningham *et al.*, 1984). Counselling by a well-informed person is essential. Both over- and underoptimism by the informant can be extremely upsetting (Carr, 1985). Dissatisfaction with disclosure of diagnosis and impairments is not inevitable, but can have profound long-term adverse effects.

Tunali and Power (1993) have emphasized that, rather than trying to determine whether families of handicapped children adjust or not, one should identify variables that are associated with family adaptation. In reviewing the literature, they identify several predictors of successful adjustment including marital satisfaction, harmony and quality of parenting, presence of both parents at home and acceptance and understanding of the handicapping condition. Active problem-solving approaches are positively associated with adjustment, whereas approaches such as avoidance and wishful thinking are related to higher levels of distress. However, Tunali and Power (1993) make the point that it is often difficult to tell whether such 'predictors' are indeed predictors or whether they are consequences of successful coping. They proceed to outline a model of adaptation to inescapable situations where a need is under threat, based on 'redefinition'. The example is given of forced behavioural change in the family (e.g. less time available for leisure pursuits) being associated with additional cognitive changes that parallel the changes in the situation (e.g. devaluation of leisure activities).

Such inputs can be viewed as tertiary prevention strategies – aimed at reducing the complications and disability associated with established disorders, particularly those which have become chronic (Turk, 1996b). Thus, tertiary prevention includes not only active intervention aimed at the presenting condition itself but also rehabilitation to reduce potential secondary problems, minimize disability and prevent handicaps despite the persistence of impairment.

15.11   Future research

There is a need for further structured evaluations of cognitive behavioural approaches for young people with developmental difficulties and their families. Techniques need to be clearly defined – e.g. problem-solving approaches, psychoeducation and hypothesis testing. So too do the presenting difficulties – e.g. morbid familial grief, chronic sorrow and depression. A good example of the degree of detail required in these respects is provided by Willner *et al.* (2002) in their randomized controlled trial of the efficacy of a cognitive behavioural anger management group for clients with learning disabilities. Treatment consisted of nine 2-hour group sessions. Techniques employed comprised brainstorming, role play and homework. Topics addressed included triggers evoking anger, physiological and behavioural components of anger, behavioural and cognitive strategies to avoid build-up of anger and acceptable ways of displaying anger. Evaluation comprised two inventories of anger-provoking situations, completed by clients and their carers before and after the intervention. A 3-month follow-up showed maintained improvements over time.

Long-term follow-up is required to determine how durable the psychological and behavioural gains are. This will require further refinement of rating scales for emotional and behavioural disturbance in young people with learning difficulties. However, there is already good evidence for the benefits of time-limited, problem-focused, cognitive approaches with this client group. The applicability of particular approaches to specific problems, and the nature and intensity of therapist training required, still needs clarification.

15.12   REFERENCES

Alloy, L. B., Peterson, C., Abramson, L. Y. and Seligman, M. E. (1984). Attributional style and the generality of learned helplessness. *Journal of Personality and Social Psychology*, **46**, 681–7.

Attwood, T. (1997). *Asperger's Syndrome: A Guide for Parents and Professionals*. London: Jessica Kingsley.

(2003). Framework for behavioral interventions. *Child and Adolescent Psychiatric Clinics of North America*, **12**, 65–86.

Baron-Cohen, S. (1989). The autistic child's theory of mind: a case of specific developmental delay. *Journal of Child Psychology and Psychiatry*, **30**, 285–97.

Bauminger, N. (2002). The facilitation of social-emotional understanding and social interaction in high-functioning children with autism: intervention outcomes. *Journal of Autism and Developmental Disorders*, **32**, 283–98.

Beck, A. T. (1976). *Cognitive Therapy and the Emotional Disorders*. New York: International Universities Press.

Bernal, J. and Hollins, S. (1995). Psychiatric illness and learning disability: a dual diagnosis. *Advances in Psychiatric Treatment*, **1**, 138–45.

Bicknell, J. (1983). The psychopathology of handicap. *British Journal of Medical Psychology*, **56**, 167–78.

Bradshaw, S. J. (1991). Successful cognitive manipulation of a stereotypic nightmare in a 40 year old male with Down's syndrome. *Behavioural Psychotherapy*, **19**, 281–3.

Bramston, P. and Spence, S. H. (1985). Behavioural versus cognitive social-skills training with intellectually handicapped adults. *Behaviour Research and Therapy*, **23**, 239–46.

Carr, J. (1985). The effect on the family of a severely mentally handicapped child. In A. M. Clarke, A. D. B. Clarke and J. M. Berg (eds.), *Mental Deficiency: The Changing Outlook*, 4th edn. London: Methuen, pp. 512–48.

Cunningham, C., Morgan, P. and McGrucken, R. B. (1984). Down syndrome: is dissatisfaction with disclosure of diagnosis inevitable? *Developmental Medicine and Child Neurology*, **26**, 33–9.

Dupont, A. (1986). Socio-psychiatric aspects of the young severely mentally retarded and the family. *British Journal of Psychiatry*, **148**, 227–34.

Gath, A. (1977). The impact of an abnormal child upon the parents. *British Journal of Psychiatry*, **13**, 405–10.

(1989). Living with a mentally handicapped brother or sister. *Archives of Disease in Childhood*, **64**, 513–16.

Gath, A. and Gumley, D. (1987). Retarded children and their siblings. *Journal of Child Psychology and Psychiatry*, **28**, 715–30.

Hackney, I. M., Hanley, W. B., Davidson, W. and Lindsao, L. (1968). Phenylketonuria: mental development, behavior and termination of the low phenylalanine diet. *Journal of Pediatrics*, **72**, 646–55.

Happé, F. (1994). *Autism: An Introduction To Psychological Theory*. London: UCL Press.

Harrison, J. E. and Bolton, P. F. (1997). Annotation: tuberous sclerosis. *Journal of Child Psychology and Psychiatry*, **38**, 603–14.

Hobson, R. P. (1986). The autistic child's appraisal of expressions of emotion. *Journal of Child Psychology and Psychiatry*, **27**, 321–42.

Kendall, P. C. and Lochman, J. (1994). Cognitive-behavioural Therapies. In M. Rutter, E. Taylor and L. Hersov (eds.), *Child and Adolescent Psychiatry: Modern Approaches*. Oxford: Blackwell Scientific, pp. 844–57.

Kushlick, A. (1989). *Helping Caring Adults to Enjoy Working Directly with People with Learning Difficulties who Also Have Severely Challenging Behaviours*. Oxford: World Congress of Cognitive Therapy, Abstracts.

Kymissis, P. and Leven, L. (1994). Adolescents with mental retardation and psychiatric disorders. In N. Bouras (ed.), *Mental Health and Mental Retardation – Recent Advances and Practices*. Cambridge: Cambridge University Press, pp. 102–7.

Lindsay, W. R., Howells, L. and Pitcaithly, D. (1993). Cognitive therapy for depression with individuals with intellectual disabilities. *British Journal of Medical Psychology*, **66**, 135–41.

Lindsay, W. R., Olley, S., Baillie, N. and Smith, A. H. W. (2000). Treatment of adolescent sex offenders with intellectual disabilities. *Mental Retardation*, **37**, 201–11.

Oliver, C. (1995). Annotation: self-injurious behaviour in children with learning disabilities. Recent advances in assessment and intervention. *Journal of Child Psychology and Psychiatry*, **30**, 909–27.

Panerai, S., Fewante, L. and Zingale, M. (2002). Benefits of the Treatment and Education of Autistic and Communication Handicapped Children (TEACCH) programme as compared with a non-specific approach. *Journal of Intellectual Disability Research*, **46**, 318–27.

Romans-Clarkson, S. E., Clarkson, J. E., Dittmer, I. D. *et al.* (1986). Impact of a handicapped child on mental health of parents. *British Medical Journal*, **293**, 1395–7.

Rutter, M., Graham, P. and Yule, W. (1970). *A Neuropsychiatric Study in Childhood*. Clinics in Developmental Medicine, No. 35/36. London: Heinemann/Spastics International Medical Publications.

Schulman, P., Keith, D. and Seligman, M. E. (1993). Is optimism heritable? A study of twins. *Behaviour Research and Therapy*, **31**, 569–74.

Seligman, M. E., Abramson, L. Y., Semmel, A. and von Baeyer, C. (1984). Depressive attributional style. *Southern Psychologist*, **21**, 18–22.

Seligman, M. E., Nolen-Hoeksema, S., Thornton, N. and Thornton, K. M. (1990). Explanatory style as a mechanism of disappointing athletic performance. *Psychological Science*, **1**, 143–6.

Sinason, V. (1992). *Mental Handicap and the Human Condition: New Approaches from the Tavistock*. London: Free Association Books.

Tunali, B. and Power, T. G. (1993). Creating satisfaction: a psychological perspective on stress and coping in families of handicapped children. *Journal of Child Psychology and Psychiatry*, **34**, 945–57.

Turk, J. (1996a). Working with parents of children who have severe learning disabilities. *Clinical Child Psychology and Psychiatry*, **1**, 583–98.

(1996b). Tertiary Prevention of Childhood Mental Health Problems. In T. Kendrick, A. Tylee and P. Feeling (eds.), *The Prevention of Mental Illness in Primary Care*. Cambridge: Cambridge University Press, pp. 265–80.

Turk, J. and Graham, P. (1997). Fragile X syndrome, autism and autistic features. *Autism*, **1**, 175–97.

Turk, J. and Sales, J. (1996). Behavioural phenotypes and their relevance to child mental health professionals. *Child Psychology and Psychiatry Review*, **1**, 4–11.

Vostanis, P., Harrington, R., Prendergast, M. and Farndon, P. (1994). Case reports of autism with interstitial deletion of chromosome 17 (p11.2–p11.2) and monosomy of chromosome 5 (5pter–5p15.3). *Psychiatric Genetics*, **4**, 109–11.

Whitman, T. L. (1994). Mental retardation. In L. W. Craighead, W. E. Craighead, A. E. Kazdin and M. J. Mahoney (eds.), *Cognitive and Behavioral Interventions: An Empirical Approach to Mental Health Problems*. Boston: Allyn and Bacon.

Wikler, L., Wasow, M. and Hatfield, E. (1981). Chronic sorrow revisited: parent vs. professional depiction of the adjustment of parents of mentally retarded children. *American Journal of Orthopsychiatry*, **51**, 63–70.

Willner, P., Jones, J., Tams, R. and Green, G. (2002). A randomized controlled trial of the efficacy of a cognitive-behavioural anger management group for clients with learning disabilities. *Journal of Applied Research in Intellectual Disabilities*, **15**, 224–35.

Wing, L. (1996). *The Autistic Spectrum*. London: Constable.

16

Depressive disorders

Richard Harrington

Royal Manchester Children's Hospital, Manchester, UK

There is no longer a debate about the existence of major depressive disorder in late childhood and adolescence. Reported prevalence in adolescence ranges from 1% to 6% of the general population, with a recent British study finding that approximately 2% of adolescents had had a recent episode of major depression (Meltzer *et al.*, 2000). Rates in children are much less, probably in the order of one per 1000. There is a great deal of comorbidity with other emotional disorders and also with conduct disorder. Follow-up studies have demonstrated that young people with depression have a greater risk of subsequent episodes than non-depressed psychiatric cases. There is also an increased risk of both attempted and completed suicide.

A variety of treatments are now available for major depression in young people. For example, recent findings suggest that the serotonin-specific reuptake inhibitors (SSRIs) can be effective (Emslie *et al.*, 1997; Keller *et al.*, 2001; Emslie *et al.*, 2002). However, in many cases, psychological treatments are currently the preferred first line of treatment. Several different psychological treatments have been evaluated for depressed children and adolescents. Probably the best evaluated are the cognitive behavioural therapies (CBTs).

This chapter provides a practical account of CBT for depression in late childhood and adolescence. The chapter begins with a brief overview of the theory behind CBT and some general principles of treatment. The core CBT techniques are then described. The chapter concludes with a brief overview of the evidence base for CBT.

Cognitive Behaviour Therapy for Children and Families, ed. Philip J. Graham.
Published by Cambridge University Press. © Cambridge University Press 2004.

16.1   Theoretical basis

16.1.1   The cognitive model of depression

CBT for depression includes techniques based on a variety of different theoretical models of depression which, essentially, focus on different aspects of symptomatology as primary.

The cognitive model of depression and the work of Aaron Beck (Beck, 1967, 1983) are familiar to most mental health professionals. In the cognitive model of depression, thoughts are the primary experience of depression; affective and behavioural components are secondary. Beck described characteristic cognitions of depressed individuals, which involve distortion of reality with feelings of low self-worth, self-blame, a sense of overwhelming responsibilities and a desire to escape (see Figure 16.1). Typical cognitive processes in depression include irrational thinking such as overgeneralization and exaggerating negative features of experience. The major cognitive patterns are a negative view of the self, of one's past and present experiences and of the future. Thus, depressed individuals systematically distort their experience in keeping with their beliefs and increasingly avoid activity because they anticipate a negative outcome. Cognitive therapy, therefore, progresses from focusing on symptoms and behaviours to working on situation-specific thoughts and, finally, focusing on the central beliefs and philosophy of the individual, which are known as schemata (see Figure 16.1). The therapy relies on identifying the negative thoughts that are associated with feelings of depression. In addition, from a behavioural perspective, there is an emphasis on engaging in more activities that are positive and rewarding.

16.1.2   Cognitive models of depression in young people

Depressive disorder is much less common in children than in adolescents (Angold et al., 1998) and the question therefore arises as to how old children must be before they can experience the full range of cognitive symptoms found in adult depressive disorder. Children are capable of recognizing their own emotional states from as young as 2 years and, during the preschool years, they start to differentiate the basic emotions and to understand their meaning (Kovacs, 1986). However, even if they experience repeated failure, preschool children are not easily discouraged and they only rarely show evidence of learned helplessness (Rholes et al., 1980). With the onset of concrete operational thinking (age range 7–11 years), the child begins to discover what is consistent in the course of any change or transformation (Piaget, 1970). Egocentrism declines and the child starts to develop self-consciousness and to evaluate his own competence by

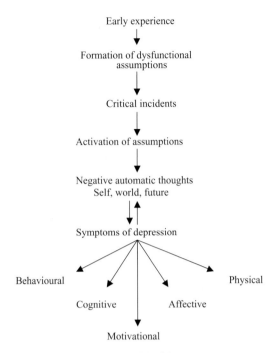

Figure 16.1   Cognitive model of depression.

comparison with others (Dweck and Elliot, 1983). Self is perceived more in psychological than physical terms and concepts such as guilt and shame become prominent. Enduring and relatively stable negative attributions about the self therefore become possible. In addition, children begin to understand the implications of certain kinds of adverse events. It is at around this age, for example, that most children can understand that death is permanent (Lansdown, 1992). At the same time, the child's emotional vocabulary expands, and children start to make fine grain distinctions between emotions such as sadness and anger. In other words, by around the age of 8–11 years, most children can both experience and report many of the cognitions that are found in adult depression.

Depressed children show a set of cognitive deficits and distortions that are similar to those found in depressed adults. They often have low self-esteem and cognitive distortions such as selectively attending to the negative features of an event (Kendall *et al.*, 1990). In addition, depressed are more likely than non-depressed children to develop negative attributions (Kaslow *et al.*, 1988). For example, Curry and Craighead (1990) found that adolescents with greater depression attributed the cause of positive events to unstable external causes.

16.1.3   Adaptations of CBT with young people

Beck's work with adults has been very influential in work with older children and adolescents. Wilkes and colleagues (Wilkes and Rush, 1988; Wilkes *et al.*, 1994) have described how Beck's method can be applied in work with depressed adolescents. Stark and colleagues have developed an evaluated and comprehensive programme for depressed 9–12-year-old children and their parents in a series of studies (Stark *et al.*, 1987; Stark, 1990; Stark *et al.*, 1991). Based on the assumption that depression arises from cognitive dysfunction and skill deficits, children and parents engage in a psychoeducational process aimed at acquiring more adaptive skills and cognitive problem-solving techniques. In Stark's studies, a group format is used.

Applying an alternative cognitive behavioural model, Lewinsohn and colleagues developed the 'Coping with Depression Course' with adults based on a more behavioural approach to depression. This course has subsequently been applied successfully to older children and adolescents (Clarke *et al.*, 1990; Lewinsohn *et al.*, 1990; Clarke *et al.*, 1992; Clarke *et al.*, 1995; Lewinsohn *et al.*, 1996; Clarke *et al.*, 1999). A key focus is on learning affective skills and coping with aversive events, which may lead to depression and self-reinforcement. The programme is available in a group format, with a parent programme to run in parallel.

16.2   Therapist stance

A core feature of all forms of CBT for adolescent depression is a collaborative stance. This means that the therapist should avoid behaving as someone who knows best and who routinely prescribes solutions to problems. Rather, the therapist is best viewed as a teacher, as someone who helps the adolescent to find his or her own solutions to the problems. Collaboration should be evident in all stages of therapy, and in all parts of the therapy session. For instance, the beginning of the therapy session should be a joint exercise between the adolescent and the therapist. Therapists must remember, however, that adolescents are not used to being asked about their point of view and may find it hard to deal with questions such as 'what shall we do today?' Rather, it may be better to ask the adolescent about his or her current problems, and then to help the adolescent to choose one or two problems during that session. Collaboration should also be modelled in the way that homework is dealt with (see later).

Another core feature of the therapist stance is the encouragement of empiricism. The term empiricism refers to two aspects of CBT. The first is that CBT uses empirical observations of behaviours and cognitions that are the basis for depression. Depression is not viewed as something that 'comes out of the blue' or is the result of unconscious processes. Rather, it is a problem that can be understood in terms of adversity, thinking and behaviours. The second empirical aspect of CBT is the use of an 'experimental approach to therapy'. The therapist does not have all the answers and will often prescribe experiments that the adolescent can test out. For example, a phone call to a father to confirm arrangements for a visit could be prescribed as an experiment, just to see if it worked.

An important feature of CBT is a problem-solving approach. Many depressed adolescents lead stressful and difficult lives and it is easy to collude with the adolescent's belief that nothing can be changed. The therapist must, however, adopt an optimistic problem-solving approach. At the same time, the therapist should recognize that some depressed adolescents live in extremely difficult situations and that certain cognitions may be realistic. For example, it may really be the case that it is impossible for the adolescent to establish a stable and loving relationship with an alcoholic and abusive parent. This means that in all cases there must be attempts to involve the family or other caretakers in therapy. Family members play an important role in development of the adolescent's beliefs about the world. There may, therefore, be a need to involve family members in some sessions, although the therapist should always bear in mind that CBT is essentially an individual therapy (see below and also Chapter 7, for a further account of issues involved in working with parents).

16.3   Structure of a cognitive behavioural programme

16.3.1   Structure of the sessions

The structure of the sessions is a vital part of CBT. Structure is important because it deals with problems effectively in the time available. A typical format for a CBT session would be:

(1)   review of the young person's state, including any recent events;
(2)   set agenda to review homework and targets area for this session;
(3)   review homework;
(4)   define session targets – e.g. defining problems, problem-solving, identifying negative thoughts and so on;
(5)   setting homework; and
(6)   feedback on session.

16.3.2   A typical CBT programme

Following referral for CBT, further assessment often involves detailed clarification of symptom status, by interview and questionnaires, to establish a baseline for measuring change. Useful questionnaires for children include the Children's Depression Inventory (Kovacs, 1981) and, for adolescents, the Mood and Feelings

Questionnaire (Angold *et al.*, 1987). Measures of anxiety, social skills and self-esteem may also be useful.

The goals of therapy are then discussed; these should be as specific as possible. They are likely to include a goal to feel less depressed, but may include a range of associated problems identified by the child or young person. An explanation of the therapeutic process is given and the importance of homework tasks emphasized.

During the early sessions, work focuses on clarifying the child's daily activities and diary keeping. With the change in mood state, depressed young people have often considerably reduced their activities, and diaries can be helpful in identifying the extent of this reduction. Children and their parents may be encouraged to increase activity levels.

A check is made on the child's vocabulary for describing feelings (*affective education*) and links are then made between activities and feelings. At this stage, homework tasks may be agreed, which increase the range or number of activities from which the child obtains a sense of achievement or pleasure. The emphasis is on reinstating previously enjoyed activities, which have ceased, and on normal day-to-day routines rather than trips out or adult treats (*activity scheduling*).

These behavioural interventions can often lead to a significant improvement in mood. At this stage, it is usually clear whether or not the child or adolescent is able to work at a cognitive level and whether or not cognitive restructuring is suitable. For the less emotionally articulate, the introduction of problem-solving techniques at this stage may be useful – e.g. to work on peer group problems or issues at school.

The key aspect of cognitive therapy is identifying negative automatic thoughts. In children and young people, similarly to adults, this is approached by considering in detail the thoughts that are identified with specific situations. Explaining to children the technique can be likened to video replay; that is, playing back a situation as if in the mind's eye and describing the thoughts associated with it. If changes in affect are noticed during the therapy session, therapists may also ask about a specific thought while the child is talking about an experience. Diaries, creative writing or even statements from questionnaires can also be helpful in identifying maladaptive cognitions. The therapist asks if thoughts from these materials connect to everyday experience.

Processes of cognitive restructuring then involve working on irrational interpretations and identifying recurrent themes such as being unlovable. This may include examining in detail the evidence for particular thoughts and the advantages and disadvantages of each way of thinking. In practice, the techniques involve learning to recognize and challenge negative automatic thoughts, generating more realistic thoughts and increasing positive statements about the self.

It is important to bear in mind, however, that with children and adolescents cognitive restructuring is not always possible or appropriate. Much depends on the presenting problem and the developmental level of the young person.

16.4   Indications for CBT

Research and clinical experience suggest that those most likely to benefit from a cognitive behavioural approach will share a number of characteristics. First, the depressive disorder will be a prominent part of the presenting complaints. While little is known about the role of comorbidity in predicting outcome, clinical experience suggests that when the clinical picture is dominated by non-depressive problems (e.g. aggression and truancy) it is difficult to focus the young person and the family on the mood disorder. Secondly, the young person must acknowledge having a problem and want to do something about it for themselves. Thirdly, the family must also see that there is a problem, and be prepared to support the therapy. In addition, those who are successful with the cognitive behavioural approach will usually be able to participate in sessions. They will usually be prepared to do homework.

16.5   Contraindications to CBT

Although CBTs are widely used for child and adolescent depression, they are not a cure all. There are several relative contraindications to their use.

16.5.1   Developmental stage

Suppose Ben and Simon have just moved into another town and are going to their first party. As she drops him off at the party, Ben's mother says, 'try to remember the names of all the other children so you can tell me about them later'. Simon's father simply says, 'we will meet you here afterwards'. Which child will remember more names? If the children are younger than 7 or 8 years, they will recall roughly the same number of names. If they are aged 11 years or older, Ben will usually remember the names of more children than Simon. When children respond to instructions that they have been asked to remember, they are using *meta-cognition*. The term 'meta-cognition' refers to children's knowledge about their own cognitive processes. It is also used to describe *executive functions* such as planning, activating rules, monitoring learning and evaluating product.

Some of the techniques that are used in CBT require that the patient has knowledge about cognition, or is able to use executive processes or both. For example, many programmes require that the child completes homework assignments that may involve some degree of planning (e.g. phoning a friend to see if he is really cross). Young children are likely to find this difficult, as they are less likely to plan activities before carrying them out. Similarly, a key task in some cognitive programmes is to evaluate the evidence for and against a particular belief, such as that 'my friends don't want to know me'. However, the ability to hold mental representation of theory versus the evidence emerges only gradually during adolescence. Children less than 10 years tend to ignore evidence that goes against their beliefs. It is only by middle adolescence that most individuals develop the skill of separating theory from evidence (see also Chapters 2 and 8).

Adolescence, then, is a transitional period in cognitive development. Developmental stage is, therefore, an important determinant of the best technique for the child. As a general rule, older children and adolescents respond better to cognitive treatments than younger children. Different techniques may therefore be used with children at different ages.

16.5.2   Severity of disorder

There is evidence that severe cases respond less well to CBT than mild cases. For instance, Jayson and colleagues (Jayson *et al.*, 1998) reported that increased severity of social impairment was associated with reduced response to CBT in adolescents with major depression. As a general rule, adolescents who are so impaired by their depression that they cannot function in at least one social domain (e.g. not going to school at all) are much less likely to respond to CBT than those with mild or moderate impairment.

16.5.3   Social context

Depressive disorders in young people are deeply embedded in a social context. This has implications both for how the child's problems should best be managed and for the likely response to treatment. No treatment for the child is likely to succeed if basic needs such as adequate educational opportunities or security of family placement are not met. For instance, children who are moved frequently from one home to another are unlikely to be helped by CBT, or indeed by any other kind of psychological intervention.

16.6   Core techniques

16.6.1   Assessment, goal setting and initial formulation

The assessment aims to provide a detailed description of the presenting problem that is consistent with a cognitive behavioural formulation of the child's difficulties. The assessment should also provide information about the child's social context and about his or her strengths and weaknesses.

The initial interview begins with a thorough review of the presenting problems and any associated symptoms. In collaboration with the child and family, the therapist carries out a detailed analysis of what are often vaguely defined presenting complaints to generate more specific target problems. The aim is to generate a short list of problems that are most distressing to the child and carers and which are most amenable to treatment. Standardized measures of the child's behaviour or emotions may help in defining these problems and are often a good way of measuring change. The therapist then endeavours to identify the cognitive distortions or deficits that often accompany depression (see above). Finally, an assessment is made of the child's social context in respect of family, peer relationships, neighbourhood and education. There should be a particular emphasis on identifying strengths both within the child and within the child's family or wider social environment.

The cognitive behavioural formulation is based on information from the initial assessment. It should be a written explanation of the problem that highlights the key cognitive and behavioural factors that are thought to play a role in the onset or maintenance of the child's difficulties. It should also reflect the role of external factors, such as family difficulties or peer problems, on the young person's views of himself and his world. The formulation is likely, then, to be multilayered and to outline several priorities for treatment. The development of a formulation is an essential part of CBT with young people.

16.6.2   Education and engagement of the child and family

All forms of CBT should begin with an explanation of the diagnosis and the model of treatment for the child and family. The nature of this explanation depends on the child's level of cognitive development. Young people who have developed what Piaget (Piaget, 1970) called 'formal thinking skills' can usually understand the kind of explanation of CBT that would be given to adults. Such an explanation might, for instance, include the relationship between the way a person thinks about himself and his environment, and his behaviour or feelings. Many children and young adolescents find it difficult, however, to think about thinking and require explanations that are more appropriate for their developmental stage. For example, the therapist might present to the child a story about a social situation that could have several different interpretations (e.g. a stranger knocking at the door) and explore with the child the various different thoughts and feelings that could occur. How would the child feel, for example, if he or she thought the stranger looked like the murderer shown on the evening news? Children's stories such as the *The Emperor's New Clothes* can also be a useful way of getting over ideas such as the power of thought and belief in determining how we behave (Wilkes *et al.*, 1994).

Although the CBTs are usually viewed as individual or group treatments, there is a growing trend towards encouraging parents to have a role. Parental involvement is important for several reasons. First, parents or significant others can often be very helpful in implementing a therapeutic programme – e.g. they can help to reinforce homework assignments. Moreover, they can provide information about ongoing stresses in the child's life and about the continuation of certain symptoms that the child may be reluctant to talk about (e.g. peer relationship problems and antisocial behaviour). Secondly, there is the practical reason that it will often be the parents who bring the child for therapy. Thirdly, parental behaviours and attitudes may be important predisposing or maintaining factors for the child's problems.

16.6.3   Problem-solving

A basic ingredient of both cognitive and behavioural approaches to depression in children is problem-solving. Although the immediate antecedents of many depressive disorders can often be identified as specific cognitions or affects, these are usually provoked by some kind of external problem. These problems are commonly of an interpersonal nature, involving either the family or peers. Training children in problem-solving helps them to deal with these external problems and also provides a useful model for many cognitive behavioural procedures. Problem-solving in children involves much the same steps as in adults. The child is first encouraged to identify a solvable problem and then to generate as many potential solutions to it as possible. The best solution is chosen, the steps to carry it out are identified and the child tries it out. Finally, the whole process is evaluated.

16.7   Core cognitive techniques

In some children and adolescents, these techniques may be helpful, although, as noted above, less use is made of these techniques in children than in older adolescents or adults. At all ages, there is an emphasis on *self-monitoring* – that is, on charting thoughts and on recording the relationship between thoughts and other phenomena such as behaviours or recent experiences. In older adolescents, cognitions can be elicited using much the same techniques as in adults. In younger children, it is often necessary to use more developmentally appropriate methods. For instance, cartoon drawings such as the *Thought Detective* (Stark, 1990) can help to communicate the idea that the child is actively involved in the understanding of thinking and behaviour.

Cognitive restructuring forms an important part of many CBT programmes. The first step is to identify the thought. The thought itself should be noted down. Next, arguments and evidence to support the thought should be considered. Then, arguments and evidence that cast doubt on the thought should be identified. Finally, patients should reach a reasoned conclusion based on the available evidence, both for and against their thinking.

Problematic thoughts are often underpinned by characteristic attitudes and assumptions about the self or about the world. Typical examples include the view that in order to be happy the patient must be liked by everyone or that aggression is a legitimate way of dealing with interpersonal conflicts. These attitudes cannot usually be identified using the approach that is used to identify problem thoughts because they are not fully articulated in the patient's mind. Rather, they are implicit rules that often can only be inferred by the person's behaviour. In the later stages of therapy with older adolescents, it may be possible to encourage the patient to look for patterns in his or her reactions to situations that betray these *underlying assumptions*. These techniques may be particularly useful in preventing relapse.

16.8   Core behavioural techniques

In parallel with cognitive methods, the therapist also uses relevant behavioural techniques. *Exposure* techniques are used when the client is avoiding a feared situation, such as school. Many programmes include a system of *behavioural contingencies* in which a system of rewards is set up to reinforce desirable behaviours. Reward systems for children usually involve the parents, but in some programmes there is an emphasis on *self-reinforcement* in which the child rewards himself.

Most child psychiatric disorders are worsened by inactivity. *Activity scheduling* involves the scheduling of goal-directed and enjoyable activities into the child's day. The child, therapist and caretakers collaborate to plan the young person's activities for a day on an hour-by-hour basis. *Specific behavioural techniques* are also used to treat certain symptoms. For example, sleep disturbance may be reduced by sleep hygiene measures. *Relaxation training* may be useful for somatic anxiety symptoms.

16.9 Common technical problems

Randomized trials have indicated the promise of the CBTs in managing depressive disorders (see below). However, some patients fail to respond to the initial course of treatment, or drop out before treatment has been completed. There are several common problems that can occur during CBT with young people and which may partly explain lack of response.

16.9.1 Therapist factors

One of the most common mistakes made by trainees is taking on patients who are unsuitable for CBT. Most research studies of cognitive therapy have been based on selected cases. Clinical practice should generally be confined to the kinds of cases that have been included in these studies. Thus, for example, the effectiveness of therapy with depressed adolescents has been demonstrated almost entirely in samples without significant comorbidity (Harrington *et al.*, 1998b). It cannot be assumed that adolescents with, say, depression and severe conduct disorder will respond to treatment in the same way as those with 'pure' depression. Another common problem is the failure to construct an adequate cognitive behavioural formulation of the young person's difficulties. This can lead to the application of techniques in a 'cookbook' fashion, which is not tailored to the needs of the individual.

The attitudes of the therapist may lead to problems. For example, many children who are referred for therapy are in difficult life situations and believe that their predicament cannot be resolved. In such cases, the therapist may be drawn into the belief that 'anyone would feel like that' in the same situation. This view is generally incorrect. It is important that the therapist adopts an optimistic problem-solving approach and does not catastrophize the problem.

16.9.2 Patient factors

The patient's beliefs can also lead to difficulties during therapy. Some young people come to treatment with the belief that all of their problems will be cured by psychological therapy. It is important that they understand the limitations of cognitive therapy. Therapists must ensure that specific and realistic goals are set at the start of the course. Other youngsters denigrate the therapy in statements such as 'I've had five visits and nothing has changed at all'. In such cases, the therapist should explain that treatment often follows a variable course, with downs as well as ups.

Many technical problems can arise during CBT with young people. One of the most common is failure to complete homework assignments. In such cases, the therapist must first think back to the previous session to ensure that the homework tasks were adequately discussed. With younger patients, for example, it is important to get them to repeat the task back to ensure that they have understood it. Homework problems can often be prevented. Next, the therapist should rehearse the homework tasks during the session. The therapist must model persistence and not simply give up if homework has not been completed. Another common problem is the adolescent who does not talk in a session. In such cases, the therapist should try to take the pressure off the young person by, for example, saying that 'I will do the talking for a while'. Once the adolescent starts talking, the therapist can try to understand the source of the problem.

16.9.3   Parent factors

Parental attitudes can be a powerful determinant of the outcome of treatment. Some parents believe that their child is simply 'making it up' and does not really have a problem: e.g. 'He will grow out of it'. Some take the opposite view and believe that the child's problems are so severe and so much part of the personality that nothing can be achieved in therapy. Careful exploration of these beliefs by the therapist, followed by an appropriate explanation, can help to modify these attitudes.

16.10   Length of treatment and follow-up

Programmes for children with depression tend to be quite short, at around 12–16 sessions within 8 weeks (Clarke *et al.*, 1990). Versions of CBT as brief as eight sessions have been shown to be effective (Wood *et al.*, 1996).

Since depressive disorders tend to be relapsing and remitting, extended forms of CBT have also been developed. Two main varieties exist. The first involves continuation of treatment after the acute phase of symptoms has improved. At that point, the child enters into *maintenance therapy*, which typically involves CBT on a more intermittent basis than during the initial course of treatment. The development of continuation forms of CBT is at an early stage, but there is preliminary evidence that it may help to prevent relapse of depression (Kroll *et al.*, 1996). The second model involves periodic 'check-ups' in which the young person returns to the therapist from time to time (Kazdin, 1997). Any return of symptoms can be treated at an early stage.

16.11   The evidence base

CBT has been used in both school and clinical settings. There have been at least six randomized controlled studies of CBT in samples of children with depressive symptoms recruited through schools (Reynolds and Coats, 1986; Stark *et al.*, 1987; Kahn *et al.*, 1990; Liddle and Spence, 1990; Marcotte and Baron, 1993; Weisz *et al.*, 1997). The design has usually been to screen for depression with a questionnaire and then to invite those with a high score to a group CBT intervention. In three of the trials, CBT was significantly superior to no treatment. Although these results are promising, they may not necessarily apply to cases with depressive disorder. However, a meta-analysis (Harrington *et al.*, 1998a) of six randomized trials with clinically diagnosed cases of depressive disorder (Lewinsohn *et al.*, 1990; Reed, 1994; Vostanis *et al.*, 1996b; Wood *et al.*, 1996; Brent *et al.*, 1997; Clarke *et al.*, 1999) found that CBT was significantly superior to comparison conditions such as remaining on a waiting list or having relaxation training (pooled odds ratio of 2.2).

CBT is, therefore, a promising treatment for adolescent depression. Nonetheless, it has limitations. The first is that adolescents with severe depressive disorders respond less well than those with mild or moderately severe conditions (Clarke *et al.*, 1992; Brent *et al.*, 1998; Jayson *et al.*, 1998; Brent *et al.*, 1999). Secondly, although proponents of psychosocial treatments often claim long-term benefits for the adolescent's psychological development, this has yet to be conclusively demonstrated. Few trials have provided follow-up data for more than a few months, and those that do have not generally found long-term effects (Vostanis *et al.*, 1996a; Wood *et al.*, 1996; Birmaher *et al.*, 2000). Thirdly, it is unclear which psychological processes correlate with a better outcome. The therapeutic basis for change is therefore uncertain. Finally, although CBT has been described in detailed manuals (Clarke *et al.*, 1990), few centres offer training for therapists wishing to work with this age group.

16.12   Conclusions

All in all, this chapter has suggested that the CBTs are effective for mild and moderately severe depressive disorders. They are not, however, a 'cure all'. Future research will need to establish whether they are effective in severe forms of depressive disorder and how they are best combined with other treatments such as medication. Another key issue is how the results from research are disseminated into clinical practice.

16.13   Acknowledgements

Thanks are due to the National Coordinating Centre for Health Technology Assessment and to the PPP Foundation which support trials involving CBT in which the author is involved. The views and opinions expressed herein do not necessarily reflect those of either body.

16.14   REFERENCES

Angold, A., Costello, E. J., Pickles, A. and Winder, F. (1987). *The Development of a Questionnaire for Use in Epidemiological Studies of Depression in Children and Adolescents*. London: Institute of Psychiatry.

Angold, A., Costello, E. J. and Worthman, C. M. (1998). Puberty and depression: the roles of age, pubertal status and pubertal timing. *Psychological Medicine*, **28**, 51–61.

Beck, A. T. (1967). *Depression: Clinical, Experimental and Theoretical Aspects*. New York, Harper and Row.

(1983). Cognitive therapy of depression: new perspectives. In P. J. Clayton and J. E. Barrett (eds.), *Treatment of Depression: Old Controversies and New Approaches*. New York, Raven Press, pp. 265–84.

Birmaher, B., Brent, D., Kolko, D. *et al.* (2000). Clinical outcome after short-term psychotherapy for adolescents with major depressive disorder. *Archives of General Psychiatry*, **57**, 29–36.

Brent, D., Holder, D., Kolko, D. *et al.* (1997). A clinical psychotherapy trial for adolescent depression comparing cognitive, family, and supportive treatments. *Archives of General Psychiatry*, **54**, 877–85.

Brent, D. A., Kolko, D. J., Birmaher, B. *et al.* (1998). Predictors of treatment efficacy in a clinical trial of three psychosocial treatments for adolescent depression. *Journal of the American Academy of Child and Adolescent Psychiatry*, **37**, 906–14.

Brent, D. A., Kolko, D. J., Birmaher, B., Baugher, M. and Bridge, J. (1999). A clinical trial for adolescent depression: predictors of additional treatment in the acute and follow-up phases of the trial. *Journal of the American Academy of Child and Adolescent Psychiatry*, **38**, 263–70.

Clarke, G., Lewinsohn, P. and Hops, H. (1990). *Leaders' Manual for Adolescent Groups. Adolescent Coping with Depression Course*. Eugene, OR: Castalia Publishing Company.

Clarke, G. N., Hawkins, W., Murphy, M., Sheeber, L. B., Lewinsohn, P. M. and Seeley, J. R. (1995). Targeted prevention of unipolar depressive disorder in an at-risk sample of high school adolescents: a randomized trial of a group cognitive intervention. *Journal of the American Academy of Child and Adolescent Psychiatry*, **34**, 312–21.

Clarke, G. N., Hops, H., Lewinsohn, P. M., Andrews, J. A., Seeley, J. R. and Williams, J. A. (1992). Cognitive-behavioral group treatment of adolescent depression: prediction of outcome. *Behavior Therapy*, **23**, 341–54.

Clarke, G. N., Rohde, P., Lewinsohn, P. M., Hops, H. and Seeley, J. R. (1999). Cognitive-behavioural treatment of adolescent depression: efficacy of acute group treatment and booster sessions. *Journal of the American Academy of Child and Adolescent Psychiatry*, **38**, 272–9.

Curry, J. F. and Craighead, W. E. (1990). Attributional style in clinically depressed and conduct disordered adolescents. *Journal of Clinical and Consulting Psychology*, **58**, 109–16.

Dweck, C. and Elliot, E. (1983). Achievement motivation. In P. Mussen and M. Hetherington (eds.), *Handbook of Child Psychology, Volume 4. Social and Personality Development*. New York: Wiley, pp. 643–91.

Emslie, G., Rush, A., Weinberg, W. *et al.* (1997). A double-blind, randomized placebo-controlled trial of fluoxetine in depressed children and adolescents. *Archives of General Psychiatry*, **54**, 1031–7.

Emslie, G. J., Heiligenstein, J. H., Wagner, K. D. *et al.* (2002). Fluoxetine for acute treatment of depression in children and adolescents: a placebo-controlled randomized clinical trial. *Journal of the American Academy of Child and Adolescent Psychiatry*, **41**, 1205–15.

Harrington, R., Whittaker, J., Shoebridge, P. and Campbell, F. (1998a). Systematic review of efficacy of cognitive behaviour therapies in child and adolescent depressive disorder. *British Medical Journal*, **316**, 1559–63.

Harrington, R. C., Whittaker, J. and Shoebridge, P. (1998b). Psychological treatment of depression in children and adolescents: a review of treatment research. *British Journal of Psychiatry*, **173**, 291–8.

Jayson, D., Wood, A. J., Kroll, L., Fraser, J. and Harrington, R. C. (1998). Which depressed patients respond to cognitive-behavioral treatment? *Journal of the American Academy of Child and Adolescent Psychiatry*, **37**, 35–9.

Kahn, J. S., Kehle, T. J., Jenson, W. R. and Clark, E. (1990). Comparison of cognitive-behavioral, relaxation, and self-modeling interventions for depression among middle-school students. *School Psychology Review*, **2**, 196–211.

Kaslow, N. J., Rehm, L. P., Pollack, S. L. and Siegel, A. W. (1988). Attributional style and self-control behavior in depressed and nondepressed children and their parents. *Journal of Abnormal Child Psychology*, **16**, 163–75.

Kazdin, A. E. (1997). Practitioner review: psychosocial treatments for conduct disorder in children. *Journal of Child Psychology and Psychiatry*, **38**, 161–78.

Keller, M. B., Ryan, N. D., Strober, M. *et al.* (2001). Efficacy of paroxetine in the treatment of adolescent major depression: a randomized, controlled trial. *Journal of the American Academy of Child and Adolescent Psychiatry*, **40**, 762–72.

Kendall, P. C., Stark, K. D. and Adam, T. (1990). Cognitive deficit or cognitive distortion in childhood depression. *Journal of Abnormal Child Psychology*, **18**, 255–70.

Kovacs, M. (1981). Rating scales to assess depression in school aged children. *Acta Paedopsychiatrica*, **46**, 305–15.

(1986). A developmental perspective on methods and measures in the assessment of depressive disorders: the clinical interview. In M. Rutter, C. E. Izard and R. B. Read (eds.), *Depression in Young People: Developmental and Clinical Perspectives*. New York: Guilford Press, pp. 435–65.

Kroll, L., Harrington, R. C., Gowers, S., Frazer, J. and Jayson, D. (1996). Continuation of cognitive-behavioural treatment in adolescent patients who have remitted from major depression. Feasibility and comparison with historical controls. *Journal of the American Academy of Child and Adolescent Psychiatry*, **35**, 1156–61.

Lansdown, R. (1992). The child's concept of death. In C. Kaplan (ed.), *Bereaved Children*. London: Association of Child Psychology and Psychiatry, pp. 2–6.

Lewinsohn, P. M., Clarke, G. N., Hops, H. and Andrews, J. (1990). Cognitive-behavioural treatment for depressed adolescents. *Behavior Therapy*, **21**, 385–401.

Lewinsohn, P. M., Clarke, G. N., Rohde, P., Hops, H. and Seeley, J. R. (1996). A course in coping: a cognitive-behavioral approach to the treatment of adolescent depression. In E. Hibbs and P. S. Jensen (eds.), *Psychosocial Treatments for Child and Adolescent Disorders: Empirically Based Strategies for Clinical Practice*. Washington, DC: American Psychological Association, pp. 109–35.

Liddle, B. and Spence, S. H. (1990). Cognitive-behaviour therapy with depressed primary school children: a cautionary note. *Behavioural Psychotherapy*, **18**, 85–102.

Marcotte, D. and Baron, P. (1993). L'efficacite d'une strategie d'intervention emotivo-rationnelle aupres d'adolescents depressifs du milieu scolaire. *Canadian Journal of Counselling*, **27**, 77–92.

Meltzer, H., Gatward, R., Goodman, R. and Ford, T. (2000). *Mental Health of Children and Adolescents in Great Britain*. London: The Stationery Office.

Piaget, J. (1970). Piaget's theory. In P. H. Mussen (ed.), *Carmichael's Manual of Child Psychology*, Volume 1. New York: Wiley, pp. 703–32.

Reed, M. K. (1994). Social skills training to reduce depression in adolescents. *Adolescence*, **29**, 293–302.

Reynolds, W. M. and Coats, K. I. (1986). A comparison of cognitive-behavioural therapy and relaxation training for the treatment of depression in adolescents. *Journal of Consulting and Clinical Psychology*, **54**, 653–60.

Rholes, W., Blackwell, J., Jordan, C. and Walters, C. (1980). A developmental study of learned helplessness. *Developmental Psychology*, **16**, 616–24.

Stark, K. D. (1990). *Childhood Depression: School-Based Intervention*. New York, Guilford Press.

Stark, K. D., Reynolds, W. M. and Kaslow, N. (1987). A comparison of the relative efficacy of self-control therapy and a behavioral problem-solving therapy for depression in children. *Journal of Abnormal Child Psychology*, **15**, 91–113.

Stark, K. D., Rouse, L. W. and Livingston, R. (1991). Treatment of depression during childhood and adolescence: cognitive-behavioral procedures for the individual and the family. In P. C. Kendall (ed.), *Child and Adolescent Therapy: Cognitive-Behavioural Procedures*. New York, Guilford Press, pp. 165–206.

Vostanis, P., Feehan, C., Grattan, E. and Bickerton, W. (1996a). A randomized controlled out-patient trial of cognitive-behavioural treatment for children and adolescents with depression: 9-month follow-up. *Journal of Affective Disorders*, **40**, 105–16.

(1996b). Treatment for children and adolescents with depression: lessons from a controlled trial. *Clinical Child Psychology and Psychiatry*, **1**, 199–212.

Weisz, J. R., Thurber, C. A., Sweeney, L., Proffitt, V. D. and LeGagnoux, G. L. (1997). Brief treatment of mild-to-moderate child depression using primary and secondary control enhancement training. *Journal of Consulting and Clinical Psychology*, **65**, 703–7.

Wilkes, T. C. R. and Rush, A. J. (1988). Adaptations of cognitive therapy for depressed adolescents. *Journal of the American Academy of Child and Adolescent Psychiatry*, **27**, 381–6.

Wilkes, T. C. R., Belsher, G., Rush, A. J. and Frank, E. (eds.) (1994). *Cognitive Therapy for Depressed Adolescents*. New York: Guilford Press.

Wood, A. J., Harrington, R. C. and Moore, A. (1996). Controlled trial of a brief cognitive-behavioural intervention in adolescent patients with depressive disorders. *Journal of Child Psychology and Psychiatry*, **37**, 737–46.

17

Cognitive behavioural psychotherapy for obsessive compulsive disorders

John S. March

Duke University Medical Center, Durham, North Carolina, USA

Martin Franklin, Edna Foa

University of Pennsylvania School of Medicine, Philadelphia, Pennsylvania, USA

17.1 Introduction

At any given time, between 0.5% and 1% of children and adolescents suffer from clinically significant obsessive compulsive disorder (OCD) (Flament *et al.*, 1988). Among adults with OCD, one-third to one-half develop the disorder during childhood or adolescence (Rasmussen and Eisen, 1990). Although some children persevere in the face of OCD, the disorder typically disrupts academic, social and vocational functioning. Hence, besides reducing morbidity associated with paediatric OCD, improvements in treating the disorder early in life have the potential to reduce adult morbidity.

Over the past 15 years, cognitive behavioral therapy (CBT) has emerged as the initial treatment of choice for OCD across the lifespan (March *et al.*, 1997). Unlike other psychotherapies that have been applied, usually unsuccessfully, to OCD (March and Leonard, 1996), there is a logically consistent and compelling relationship between CBT, the disorder and the specified outcome (Foa and Kozak, 1991). Despite expert consensus that CBT is by far the best psychosocial treatment, clinicians routinely complain that patients will not comply with behavioural treatments and parents routinely complain that clinicians are poorly trained in CBT. Coupled with the lack of CBT-trained clinicians, the result is that many if not most children and adolescents are denied access to effective CBT. This unfortunate situation may be avoidable, given an increased understanding regarding the implementation of CBT in children and adolescents with OCD.

Cognitive Behaviour Therapy for Children and Families, ed. Philip J. Graham.
Published by Cambridge University Press. © Cambridge University Press 2004.

Following a discussion of the assessment of paediatric OCD, this chapter will move on to review the current status of CBT for OCD in children and adolescents. The principles that underlie the treatment will be reviewed. A brief review of our CBT protocol as used in both clinical and research settings will be provided (March and Mulle, 1998) and then empirical studies supporting the use of CBT and directions for future research will be discussed. We conclude with a set of clinical recommendations. The reader wishing to follow the protocol would be well advised to purchase and use the published version of the authors' treatment manual (March and Mulle, 1998).

17.2   Assessment

An adequate assessment of paediatric OCD should include a comprehensive evaluation of current and past OCD symptoms, current OCD symptom severity and associated functional impairment and a survey of comorbid psychopathology. In addition, the strengths of the child and family should be evaluated, as well as their knowledge of OCD and its treatment. There are many self-report and clinician-administered instruments that can be used to guide this type of assessment. The authors typically mail several relevant self-report questionnaires for the family to complete prior to the intake visit, and then review these materials prior to meeting with the child. If it is apparent from these materials that comorbid depression or other anxiety problems besides OCD are prominent, the focus will be on these symptoms as well in the intake. The Anxiety Disorders Interview Schedule for Children (ADIS-C) is a semi-structured interview that can be used to examine comorbid problems in greater detail; the authors use the ADIS in their current collaborative study examining the relative efficacy of CBT, sertraline, combined treatment and pill placebo (Franklin *et al.*, 2003). For surveying history of OCD symptoms and current symptom severity, we use the Children's Yale-Brown Obsessive Compulsive Scale (CY-BOCS) checklist and severity scale (Scahill *et al.*, 1997). Before administering this scale, it is important to determine whether the child should be interviewed with or without the parent present. In the authors' randomized controlled trial, a conjoint interview is conducted, directing questions to the child but soliciting parental feedback as well. In non-research settings, there is more flexibility, and the decision to interview the child alone or with a parent present can be made by discussing these choices with the parent in advance, observing the child's and family's behaviour in the waiting area and even during the interview if necessary. For example, if it becomes clear that a patient is reluctant to discuss certain symptoms with a parent present (e.g. sexual obsessions), the therapist can skip that item on the

CY-BOCS checklist and save some time at the end of the interview to revisit these potentially sensitive issues alone with the patient. Our mantra in the clinic is: 'get the information', meaning that if parental presence increases the validity of the assessment then do that – if not, interview the child alone.

Prior to administering the CY-BOCS, the therapist should explain the concepts of obsessions and compulsions, using examples if the child and/or parent have difficulty grasping the concepts. This opportunity can also be taken to tell children and adolescents about the prevalence, nature and treatment of OCD, which may increase their willingness to disclose their specific symptoms. Children may be particularly vulnerable to feeling as if they are the only ones on earth with obsessive fears of hurting a loved one, so prefacing the examples with 'I once met a kid who . . .' dispels this myth and minimizes the accompanying sense of isolation. During the intake, it is also important to observe the child's behaviour and enquire if certain behaviours (e.g. unusual movements and vocalizations) are compulsions designed to neutralize obsessions or to reduce distress. Tic disorders are commonly comorbid with OCD, and it is important to try to make a differential diagnosis as compulsions and tics would be targeted by different treatment procedures. Further, as mentioned above, some children who are aware of their obsessional content may be fearful of saying the fears aloud. Surveying common obsessions with a checklist instead of asking the child to disclose the fears tends to help with this problem, as does encouragement on the part of the therapist (e.g. 'lots of the kids I see have a hard time talking about these kinds of fears'). The authors have found that flexibility in the manner of disclosing the obsession is warranted. Thus, for example, the authors allow the child to write down the fears or nod their heads as the therapist describes examples of similar fears in order to help the child share their OCD problems. In this way, we can convey to the child and family that we recognize the difficulty associated with disclosure. The authors also use examples from children who have been evaluated in the past (e.g. 'I remember a few months ago when a kid about your age told me she would be scared to touch her dog for fear she might lose control and hurt him'), although they let the children and families know they are careful not to violate confidentiality when citing such examples. Below are brief descriptions of the core assessments.

17.2.1   CY-BOCS

The primary instrument for assessing OCD is the Y-BOCS, which assesses obsessions and compulsions separately on time consumed, distress, interference, degree of resistance and control. The authors use the paediatric version (Scahill et al., 1997) to record past and present OCD symptoms, initial severity, total OCD severity, relative preponderance of obsessions and compulsions and degree of insight. The CY-BOCS is a clinician-rated instrument merging data from clinical observation and parent and child report.

17.2.2   ADIS

The child and adolescent ADIS is a semi-structured interview for assessing Diagnostic and Statistical Manual IV (DSM-IV) (American Psychiatric Association, 1994) anxiety disorders in youth (Silverman and Albano, 1996). Relative to other available instruments, such as the Diagnostic Interview Schedule for Children (DISC), it has excellent psychometric properties for internalizing conditions. The ADIS utilizes an interviewer–observer format, thereby allowing the clinician to draw information from the interview and from clinical observations. Scores are derived regarding: (1) specific diagnoses and (2) level of diagnosis-related interference. Adequate psychometric properties have been demonstrated.

17.2.3   Children's OCD Impact Scale (COIS)

We also obtain child and parent versions of the OCD Impact Scale, which shows preliminary evidence favouring psychometric adequacy and sensitivity to change, for use in analyses of functional impairment from OCD (Piacentini et al., 2001). This instrument enables us to estimate whether the CY-BOCS improvements result in normalization as assessed by functional impairment. A new and shorter version of this scale has been developed recently, and the psychometric properties of this scale appear to be favourable (Piacentini et al., 2001).

17.2.4   Multidimensional Anxiety Scale for Children (MASC)

The MASC has four factors and six subfactors – physical anxiety (tense/restless, somatic/autonomic), harm avoidance (perfectionism, anxious coping), social anxiety (humiliation/rejection, performance anxiety) and separation anxiety – and is in use in a variety of National Institute of Mental Health (NIMH)-funded treatment outcome studies. The MASC shows high test–retest reliability in clinical (intraclass correlation coefficient (ICC)>0.92) and school samples (ICC>0.85); convergent/divergent validity is similarly superior (March, 1998b).

17.2.5   Children's Depression Inventory (CDI)

The CDI is a 27-item self-report scale that measures cognitive, affective, behavioural and interpersonal symptoms of depression (Kovacs, 1996). Each item consists of three statements, of which the child is asked to select the one statement that best describes his/her current functioning. Items are scored from

0 to 2; thus, scores on the CDI can range from 0 to 54. The CDI shows adequate reliability and validity. This scale is useful for assessment of symptoms of depression, which assists in tailoring the treatment plan.

17.2.6   Medical history

Paediatric OCD patients' medical histories should also be surveyed, with particular attention paid to the presence of recurrent streptococcal infection. Although children with streptococcal-precipitated OCD (Paediatric Autoimmune Neuropsychiatric Disorders Associated with Streptococcal Infection or PANDAS) may require somewhat different treatment(s), experts agree that the base rate of PANDAS developing OCD is currently unknown and that the diagnosis cannot be assigned retrospectively at this juncture (Swedo et al., 1998), although it is likely to be fairly common (Giulino et al., 2002). Current research diagnostic criteria for PANDAS require at least two prospectively documented episodes of exacerbations in OCD and tic symptoms associated with streptococcal infection. Unfortunately, an unambiguous retrospective diagnosis of PANDAS is next to impossible in a clinically referred population of youth with OCD (Giulino et al., 2002). Clinically, children who have unambiguous evidence of PANDAS should be referred for appropriate treatment of their group A β-haemolytic streptococcal (GABHS) infection. Once treated for the infection, the clinician should then also consider the CBT and / or selective serotonin reuptake inhibitor (SSRI) pharmacotherapy strategies described below.

In brief, the aforementioned scales, interviews and questionnaires may be useful in helping to generate relevant clinical information at pretreatment and in helping us to evaluate treatment gains once treatment has ended. In the authors' research-oriented settings, this is part of routine clinic practice. They hope the development of an efficient package for evaluating outcome may stimulate effectiveness research in real-world clinical settings. Until their measurements have been streamlined and boiled down to their essential components, however, financial, time and personnel constraints may limit the more general usefulness of their battery.

17.3   The application of CBT for paediatric OCD

17.3.1   Overview

A wide variety of dynamic, family and supportive psychotherapies have been and continue to be inconsistently and, in the light of current knowledge, inappropriately applied to children and adolescents with OCD. For the most part, insight-orientated psychotherapy, whether delivered individually or in the family setting, has proved to be disappointing in both youths and adults. Conversely, effective, flexible, empirically supported cognitive behavioural treatments are now available for many childhood mental illnesses, including OCD (March *et al.*, 2001).

In adults, the cognitive behavioural treatment of OCD generally involves a three-stage approach consisting of information gathering, therapist-assisted exposure and response prevention (EX/RP), including homework assignments, followed by generalization training and relapse prevention. Both graded exposure and flooding procedures have garnered strong empirical and clinical support (Franklin *et al.*, 2002). Component analyses suggest that both exposure and response prevention are active ingredients of treatment, with exposure reducing phobic anxiety and response prevention reducing rituals (Foa *et al.*, 1984). Relaxation has been shown to be an inert component of behavioural treatment for OCD and has been used as an active placebo in brief (4–6 weeks) studies in adults (Fals-Stewart *et al.*, 1993). Cognitive interventions, although found efficacious in some studies (e.g. van Oppen *et al.*, 1995), may be generally less potent than EX/RP in reducing OCD symptoms.

17.3.2   Tools

While CBT is routinely described as the psychotherapeutic treatment of choice for children and adolescents with OCD (King *et al.*, 1998), robust empirical support is only now emerging (March *et al.*, 2001). In practice, treatment components, especially EX/RP, generally similar to interventions in adults make up the typical CBT treatment package.

17.3.2.1   EX/RP

As applied to OCD, the exposure principle relies on the fact that anxiety usually attenuates after sufficient duration of contact with a feared stimulus. Thus, a child with a fear of germs must confront relevant feared but low-risk situations until his or her anxiety decreases. Repeated exposure is associated with decreased anxiety across exposure trials, with anxiety reduction largely specific to the domain of exposure, until the child no longer fears contact with specifically targeted phobic stimuli. Adequate exposure depends on blocking the negative reinforcement effect by rituals or avoidance behaviour, a process termed response or ritual prevention. For example, a child with germ worries must not only touch 'germy things', but must refrain from ritualized washing until his or her anxiety diminishes substantially. EX/RP is typically implemented in a gradual fashion (sometimes termed graded exposure), with exposure targets under the control of the patient or, less desirably, the therapist. Intensive approaches may be especially useful for treatment-resistant OCD or for patients who desire a very rapid response (Franklin *et al.*, 1998).

17.3.2.2   Cognitive therapy

A wide variety of cognitive interventions have been used to provide the child with a 'tool kit' to facilitate compliance with EX/RP (Soechting and March, 2002). The goals of cognitive therapy, which may be more or less useful or necessary depending on the child and nature of OCD, typically include increasing a sense of personal efficacy, predictability, controllability and self-attributed likelihood of a positive outcome within EX/RP tasks. Specific interventions include: (1) constructive self-talk; (2) cognitive restructuring; and (3) cultivating non-attachment or, stated differently, minimizing the obsessional aspects of thought suppression. Each must be individualized to match the specific OCD symptoms that afflict the child, and must mesh with the child's cognitive abilities, developmental stage and individual differences in preference among the three techniques. Such methods are often incorporated into EX/RP programmes, where the cognitive procedures are used to support and complement EX/RP rather than replace it.

17.3.2.3   Extinction

Because blocking rituals or avoidance behaviours remove the negative reinforcement effect of the rituals or avoidance, ritual prevention technically is an extinction procedure. By convention, however, extinction is usually defined as the elimination of OCD-related behaviours through removal of parental positive reinforcement for rituals. For example, with a child with reassurance-seeking rituals, the therapist may ask parents to refrain from gratifying the child's reassurance seeking. Extinction frequently produces rapid effects, but can be hard to implement when the child's behaviour is bizarre or very frequent. In addition, non-consensual extinction procedures often produce unmanageable distress on the part of the child, disrupt the therapeutic alliance, miss important EX/RP targets that are not amenable to extinction procedures and, most importantly, fail to help the child internalize a strategy for resisting OCD. Hence, as with EX/RP, placing the extinction programme under the child's control leads to increased compliance and improved outcomes.

17.3.2.4   Modelling and shaping

Modelling – whether overt (the child understands that the therapist is demonstrating more appropriate or adaptive coping behaviours) or covert (the therapist informally models a behaviour) – may help improve compliance with in-session EX/RP and generalization to between-session EX/RP homework. Intended to

increase motivation to comply with EX/RP, shaping involves positively reinforcing successive approximations to a desired target behaviour. Modelling and
shaping reduce anticipatory anxiety and provide an opportunity for practising
constructive self-talk before and during EX/RP. Since EX/RP has not proven
to be particularly helpful with obsessional slowness, modelling and shaping
procedures are currently the behavioural treatment of choice for children with
this OCD subtype. Unfortunately, relapse often occurs when therapist-assisted
shaping, limit setting and temporal speeding procedures are withdrawn.

17.3.2.5   Operant procedures

Clinically, positive reinforcement seems not to alter OCD symptoms directly, but
rather helps to encourage compliance with EX/RP and so produces a noticeable if indirect clinical benefit. In contrast, punishment (defined as imposition
of an aversive event) and response–cost (defined as removal of a positive event)
procedures have shown themselves to be unhelpful in the treatment of OCD.
Most CBT programmes use liberal positive reinforcement for EX/RP and pro-
scribe aversive contingency management procedures unless targeting disruptive
behaviour outside the domain of OCD. Since OCD itself is a powerful tonic
aversive stimulus, successful EX/RP breeds a willingness to engage in further
EX/RP via negative reinforcement (e.g. elimination of OCD symptoms boosts
compliance with EX/RP) as manifested by unscheduled generalization to new
EX/RP targets as treatment proceeds.

17.3.2.6   Individual versus family treatment

Family psychopathology is neither necessary nor sufficient for the onset of OCD;
nonetheless, families affect, and are affected by, the disorder (Amir *et al.*, 2000).
Hence, while empirical data are lacking, clinical observations suggest that a
combination of individual and family sessions is best for most patients.

17.3.3   A typical CBT protocol

The protocol used by March *et al.* in their NIMH study (discussed below), which
is fairly typical of a gradual exposure regimen (March and Mulle, 1998), consists of 14 visits over 12 weeks spread across five phases: (1) psychoeducation;
(2) cognitive training; (3) mapping OCD; (4) exposure and ritual prevention;
and (5) relapse prevention and generalization training. As shown in Table 17.1,
except for weeks 1 and 2, where patients come twice weekly, all visits are administered on a once per week basis, last 1 hour and include one between-visit,

Table 17.1 CBT treatment protocol

Visit number	Goals	Targets
Weeks 1 and 2	Psychoeducation	Neurobehavioural model
	Cognitive training	Labelling OCD as OCD
Week 2	Mapping OCD	Set up stimulus hierarchy
	Cognitive training	Cognitive restructuring
Weeks 3–12	Exposure and response prevention	Imaginal and *in vivo* EX/RP
Weeks 11–12	Relapse prevention	Targets, relapse and follow-up plans
Visits 1, 7 and 9	Parent sessions	Decrease reinforcement of OCD
		Enlist parents as co-therapists

10-minute telephone contact scheduled during weeks 3–12. Psychoeducation, defining OCD as the identified problem, cognitive training and development of a stimulus hierarchy (mapping OCD) take place during visits one to four, EX/RP takes up visits five to twelve, with the last two sessions incorporating generalization training and relapse prevention. Each session includes a statement of goals, review of the previous week, provision of new information, therapist-assisted practise, homework for the coming week and monitoring procedures.

Parents are centrally involved at sessions one, seven and 11, with the latter two sessions devoted to guiding the parents about their central role in assisting their child to accomplish the homework assignments. Session 13 and 14 also require significant parental input. Parents check in with the therapist at each session, and the therapist provides feedback describing the goals of each session and the child's progress in treatment. The therapist works with parents to assist them in refraining from insisting on inappropriate EX/RP tasks, which is a common problem in paediatric OCD treatment. The therapist also encourages parents to praise the child for resisting OCD, while at the same time refocusing their attention on positive elements in the child's life, an intervention technically termed differential reinforcement of other behaviour (DRO). In some cases, extensive family involvement in rituals and/or the developmental level of the child require that family members play a more central role in treatment. It is important to note that the CBT protocol provides sufficient flexibility to accommodate variations in family involvement dictated by the OCD symptom picture.

Crucial to the success of any CBT protocol is the ability to deliver protocol-driven treatments in a developmentally appropriate fashion (Clarke, 1995). In the authors' hands, CBT has been shown to be effective in children as young as

5 years. Developmental appropriateness is promoted by allowing flexibility in CBT within the constraints of fixed session goals. More specifically, the therapist adjusts the level of discourse to the cognitive functioning, social maturity and capacity for sustained attention of each patient. Younger patients require more redirection and activities in order to sustain attention and motivation. Adolescents are generally more sensitive to the effects of OCD on peer interactions, which in turn require more discussion. Cognitive interventions in particular require adjustment to the developmental level of the patient, so, for example, adolescents are less likely to appreciate giving OCD a 'nasty nickname' than younger children. Developmentally appropriate metaphors relevant to the child's areas of interest and knowledge are also used to promote active involvement in the treatment process. For instance, an adolescent male football player treated with CBT was better able to grasp treatment concepts by casting them in terms of offensive and defensive strategies employed during football games (e.g. 'picking up blitzes'). Patients whose OCD symptoms entangle family members will require more attention to family involvement in treatment planning and implementation than those without as much family involvement. However, although the CBT manual (March and Mulle, 1998) includes a section on developmental sensitivity that is specific for each treatment session, the general format and goals of the treatment sessions will be the same for all children.

17.3.3.1   Course of initial treatment

To illustrate a typical course of initial treatment, March and Mulle (1995) used a within-subject, multiple baseline design plus global ratings across treatment weeks to treat an 8-year-old girl with OCD with CBT alone. Eleven weeks of treatment produced complete resolution in OCD symptoms in this 8-year-old female with uncomplicated OCD; treatment gains were maintained at 6-month follow-up. Figure 17.1 illustrates the progress of treatment at each week for each symptom baseline. Each box represents a treatment week. The Y (vertical) axis represents fear thermometer scores for each symptom present at baseline on the symptom hierarchy; symptoms are depicted as bars on the X (horizontal) axis. Initially, symptom reduction within each baseline was specific to the exposure and/or response prevention targets for that baseline. As is often the case, however, once their patient 'got the idea', generalization across baselines appeared with some slowing down again as she reached the most difficult symptoms at the top of the symptom hierarchy. Improvement slows down at the high end of the

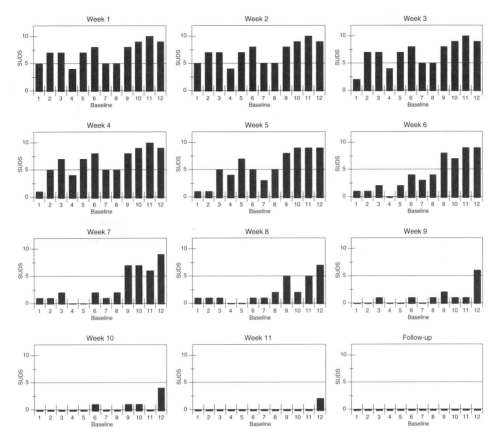

SUDS, subjective units of discomfort ascertained on a fear thermometer rated from 0 (no problem) to 10 (worst). Symptom key: 1, touching mouth; 2, snack after touching plants; 3, not washing for meals; 4, wearing turtlenecks again; 5, touching something sticky; 6, touching dish liquid; 7, use towel again; 8, touch cat; 9, use Ajax; 10, use windex; 11, toxic paint; 12, touching sick people.

Figure 17.1   Multiple baselines over time.

hierarchy, but progress continues until most, if not all, OCD symptoms remit and relapse and generalization training are appropriate.

17.4   Treatment outcome studies

17.4.1   Empirical studies

While the field still awaits the results of several currently running randomized controlled trials of CBT against control and active comparison treatments, existing literature is sufficiently robust to have resulted in widespread acceptance among experts of CBT as the initial treatment of choice for OCD in children and adolescents.

17.4.1.1   Efficacy

Uncontrolled evaluations published to date (Franklin *et al.*, 1998; March, 1998a; Franklin *et al.*, 2001; March *et al.*, 2001) have yielded remarkably similar findings: at post-treatment, the vast majority of patients were responders, with mean CY-BOCS reductions ranging from 50% to 67%. Although strong conclusions require a randomized controlled study, these reported CY-BOCS reductions associated with CBT are impressive. However, complicating interpretation of the findings is the fact that many, if not most, patients were on serotonin reuptake inhibitors prior to or during the course of CBT, and therefore the separate effects of CBT cannot be determined.

17.4.1.2   Dose and time response

Most of the published studies of CBT outcome in paediatric OCD have employed a weekly therapy regimen. In contrast, Wever and Rey (1997) used an intensive CBT protocol that included two information-gathering sessions followed by ten daily sessions of CBT over 2 weeks. Franklin *et al.* (1998) found no differences between 14 weekly sessions over 12 weeks or 18 sessions over 4 weeks, but interpretation of this finding is hampered by the lack of random assignment. Taken together, the available studies suggest that patients respond well to CBT delivered either weekly or intensively. Given the greater acceptability of weekly treatment for patients and providers, most providers will probably use the widely available 14-session, 12-week protocol (March and Mulle, 1998) that the authors evaluated in their collaborative NIMH study.

17.4.1.3   Durability

Epidemiological studies suggest that OCD is a chronic condition. However, clinical research in adults shows that long-term outcomes for patients successfully treated with CBT alone or CBT plus medication are generally favourable. Foa and Kozak (1996) concluded that gains achieved with behaviour therapy persist without continuing treatment, whereas those achieved with medication alone require continuing medication for maintenance. As in adults, OCD in children and adolescents is a chronic mental illness in many patients. For example, in the first NIMH follow-up study, 68% of patients had clinical OCD at follow-up (Flament *et al.*, 1990). In a subsequent more systematic 2–7-year follow-up study (Leonard *et al.*, 1993), 43% still met diagnostic criteria for OCD; only

11% were totally asymptomatic. Seventy per cent continued to take medication at the time of follow-up, plainly illustrating the limitations of the treatments received by these patients. The three paediatric OCD pilot studies that have included a follow-up evaluation (March *et al.*, 1994; Wever, 1994; Franklin *et al.*, 1998) support the durability of CBT, with therapeutic gains maintained up to 9 months post-treatment. Moreover, since relapse commonly follows medication discontinuation, the finding of March *et al.* (1994) that improvement persisted in six of nine responders following the withdrawal of medication provides limited support for the hypothesis that CBT inhibits relapse when medications are discontinued.

17.4.1.4   Direct comparison of CBT and pharmacotherapy

Results from a single small 'n' (number) randomized comparison of CBT and clomipramine indicated benefit for both CBT and clomipramine relative to baseline and superiority of CBT compared with clomipramine (de Haan *et al.*, 1998). In the study by Franklin and colleagues (Franklin *et al.*, 1998), which compared CBT outcomes in patients naturalistically provided medication or not, 12 of the 14 patients were at least 50% improved over pretreatment Y-BOCS severity, and the vast majority remained improved at follow-up; mean reduction in Y-BOCS was 67% at post-treatment and 62% at follow-up (mean time to follow-up of 9 months). No differences were apparent between those who received gradual versus intensive exposure or between those who received or did not receive medication. Thus, a definitive answer to the question of whether CBT and medication alone differ in outcome or whether the combination is equivalent or better than either monotherapy awaits the results of the Duke / Penn randomized controlled trial.

17.4.1.5   Availability, acceptability and tolerability

Experts have recommended CBT with a strong emphasis on EX / RP as a first-line treatment for OCD in children and adolescents (March *et al.*, 1997), yet several barriers may limit its widespread use. First, few therapists have extensive experience with CBT for paediatric OCD; thus, CBT typically, if available at all, is only obtainable in areas associated with major medical centres. Secondly, even when the treatment is available, some patients and families reject the treatment as 'too difficult'. Once involved in CBT, some patients find the initial distress when confronting feared thoughts and situations while simultaneously refraining from rituals so aversive they drop out of treatment. In the authors' protocol, hierarchy-driven EX / RP is used, actively involving the patient in choosing exposure exercises and including anxiety management techniques for the few who need them. As a result, the drop-out rates in the pilot studies and in the ongoing comparative treatment trial (unpublished data) are low, which in turn suggests that the vast majority of children and adolescents can tolerate and will benefit from CBT when delivered in a clinically informed and developmentally sensitive fashion.

17.4.2   Modifiers of treatment outcome

The question of paramount interest to clinicians and to researchers attempting to refine and improve treatment outcome is: 'which treatment for which child with what characteristics'.

Conventional wisdom holds that patients with OCD who benefit from CBT and medication differ in important if ill-understood ways. However, other than comorbid schizotypy (Baer *et al.*, 1992) and tic disorders (McDougle *et al.*, 1993), which may represent treatment impediments and possible indications for neuroleptic augmentation, the meagre empirical literature on moderators of treatment outcome in adults provides no clear support for any of the putative predictors proposed by Goodman *et al.* (1994) in their review of pharmacotherapy trials methodology in OCD. Conversely, predictors of a successful response to behaviour therapy include the presence of rituals, the desire to eliminate symptoms, ability to monitor and report symptoms, absence of complicating comorbidities, willingness to cooperate with treatment and psychophysiological indicators (Foa and Emmelkamp, 1983).

While many have suggested that the presence of comorbidity, especially with the tic disorders, lack of motivation or insight and the presence of family psychopathology might predict a poor outcome in children undergoing CBT, there is as yet little or no empirical basis on which to predict treatment outcome in children undergoing psychosocial treatment. In contrast, a rather extensive literature on the prediction of outcome for drug treatment has failed to identify any predictor variables. For example, in a recently published multicentre trial of sertraline and pill placebo in children and adolescents with OCD (March and Mulle, 1998), neither age, race, gender, body weight, baseline OCD score, baseline depression score, comorbidity, socioeconomic status nor plasma sertraline or desmethylsertraline level predicted the outcome of treatment.

Given that the research literature is as yet undecided on which treatments – CBT, pharmacotherapy with an SSRI or their combination – are best for which children with OCD, the candidate predictors summarized in Table 17.2 (which the authors will test as potential moderators of treatment outcome in their currently funded NIMH comparative treatment trial of CBT and medication alone and in combination) should be assessed when structuring treatment plans for children and adolescents with OCD.

Table 17.2 Sets of predictor variables

Set	Variables evaluated
Demographics	Age, sex, race; SES
Neurocognitive profile	Full-scale, verbal and performance IQ
Medical history	PANDAS, weight and height and obstetrical history
OCD specific factors	Symptom profile, initial severity, impact on functioning, insight and treatment history
Treatment expectancy	Treatment expectancy
Comorbidity	Internalizing and externalizing disorders and symptoms, tic disorders
Parental psychopathology	General symptoms, depression, anxiety and OCD
Family functioning	Parental stress, expressed emotion and marital distress

SES, socioeconomic status.

17.5 Future directions

17.5.1 Overview

Current research efforts are now (or shortly will be) focused on eight areas: (1) controlled trials comparing medications, CBT and combination treatment with controls to determine whether medications and CBT are synergistic or additive in their effects on symptom reduction; (2) follow-up studies to evaluate relapse rates, including examining the utility of booster CBT in reducing risk for relapse; (3) component analyses, such as a comparison of EX/RP, cognitive therapy and their combination, to evaluate the relative contributions of specific treatment components to symptom reduction and treatment acceptability; (4) comparisons of individual- and family-based treatments to determine which are more effective in which children; (5) development of innovative treatment for OCD subtypes such as obsessional slowness, primary obsessional OCD and tic-like OCD that do not respond well to EX/RP; (6) targeting treatment innovations to factors, such as family dysfunction, that constrain the application of CBT to patients with OCD; (7) exporting research treatments to divergent clinical settings and patient populations in order to judge the acceptability and effectiveness of CBT as a treatment for child and adolescent OCD in real-world settings; and (8) once past initial treatment, the management of partial response, treatment resistance and treatment maintenance and discontinuation.

17.5.2 Comparative treatment trial

Despite the by-now routine recommendation of CBT alone or the combination of CBT and an SSRI as the treatment of choice for OCD in the paediatric population (March *et al.*, 1997), the relative efficacy of CBT and medication, alone and in combination, remains uncertain. Thus, well-designed comparative treatment outcome studies are necessary in both adults and children. Of particular importance then, the authors will shortly complete an NIMH-funded comparative treatment outcome study of initial treatments in OCD (Franklin *et al.*, 2003). Using a volunteer sample of 120 (60 per site) youths aged 8–16 years with a DSM-IV diagnosis of OCD, this 5-year treatment outcome study contrasts the degree and durability of improvement obtained across four treatment conditions: medication with sertraline (MED), OCD-specific CBT, both MED and CBT (COMB) and two control conditions (pill PBO and educational support (ES)). The experimental design covers two phases. Phase I compares the outcome of MED, CBT, COMB and control conditions. In phase II, responders advance to a 16-week discontinuation study to assess treatment durability. The primary outcome measure is the Y-BOCS. Assessments blind to treatment status take place at: week 0 (pretreatment); weeks 1, 4, 8 and 12 (phase I treatment); and weeks 16, 20, 24 and 28 (phase II discontinuation). Besides addressing comparative efficacy and durability of the specified treatments, this study also examines: time–action effects; differential effects of treatment on specific aspects of OCD, including functional impairment; and predictors of response to treatment. Once completed, this study will be followed by an augmentation trial of CBT versus an atypical neuroleptic in SSRI partial responders.

17.6 Summary

Despite limitations in the research literature, cognitive behavioural psychotherapy, alone or in combination with pharmacotherapy, has currently established itself as the psychotherapeutic treatment of choice for OCD in children and adolescents. Ideally, young persons with OCD should first receive CBT that has been optimized for treating childhood-onset OCD and, if not rapidly responsive, either intensive CBT or concurrent pharmacotherapy with an SSRI. Moreover, since cognitive behavioural psychotherapy, including booster treatments during medication discontinuation, may improve both short- and long-term outcome in drug-treated patients, all patients who receive medication also should receive concomitant CBT. In this regard, arguments advanced against CBT for OCD, such as symptom substitution, danger of interrupting rituals, uniformity of learned symptoms and incompatibility with pharmacotherapy, have all proven unfounded. Perhaps the most insidious myth is that CBT is a simplistic treatment that ignores 'real problems'. The authors believe that the opposite is true. Helping patients make rapid and difficult behaviour change over short time intervals takes both clinical knowledge and focused treatment. Currently, state-of-the-art treatments for paediatric OCD are best delivered by a multidisciplinary team usually, but not always, located in a subspecialty clinic setting. Translation of specialty practice to community settings is essential if demonstrably effective treatments, such as CBT for OCD, are to be made available to the children and adolescents suffering from this disorder on a wider scale.

17.7   Acknowledgements

This manuscript, which was adapted from March *et al.* (2001), was supported in part by NIMH Grants 1 R10 MH55121 (Drs March and Foa) and 1 K24 MHO1557 (Dr March) and by the Robert and Sarah Gorrell family.

17.8   REFERENCES

American Psychiatric Association (1994). *Diagnostic and Statistical Manual of Mental Disorders*, 4th edn. Washington, DC: American Psychiatric Association.

Amir, N., Freshman, M. and Foa, E. B. (2000). Family distress and involvement in relatives of obsessive-compulsive disorder patients. *Journal of Anxiety Disorders*, **14**, 209–17.

Baer, L., Jenike, M. A., Black, D. W., Treece, C., Rosenfeld, R. and Greist, J. (1992). Effect of axis II diagnoses on treatment outcome with clomipramine in 55 patients with obsessive-compulsive disorder. *Archives of General Psychiatry*, **49**, 862–6.

Clarke, G. N. (1995). Improving the transition from basic efficacy research to effectiveness studies: methodological issues and procedures. *Journal of Consulting and Clinical Psychology*, **63**, 718–25.

de Haan, E., Hoogduin, K. A., Buitelaar, J. K. and Keijsers, G. P. (1998). Behavior therapy versus clomipramine for the treatment of obsessive-compulsive disorder in children and adolescents. *Journal of the American Academy of Child and Adolescent Psychiatry*, **37**, 1022–9.

Fals-Stewart, W., Marks, A. P. and Schafer, J. (1993). A comparison of behavioral group therapy and individual behavior therapy in treating obsessive-compulsive disorder. *Journal of Nervous and Mental Disease*, **181**, 189–93.

Flament, M. F., Koby, E., Rapoport, J. L. *et al.* (1990). Childhood obsessive-compulsive disorder: a prospective follow-up study. *Journal of Child Psychology and Psychiatry and Allied Disciplines*, **31**, 363–80.

Flament, M. F., Whitaker, A., Rapoport, J. L. *et al.* (1988). Obsessive compulsive disorder in adolescence: an epidemiological study. *Journal of the American Academy of Child and Adolescent Psychiatry*, **27**, 764–71.

Foa, E. and Emmelkamp, P. (1983). *Failures in Behavior Therapy*. New York: Wiley and Sons.

Foa, E. B. and Kozak, M. J. (1991). Emotional processing: theory, research, and clinical implications for anxiety disorders. In J. Safran and L. Greenberg (eds.), *Emotion, Psychotherapy and Change*, Volume 372. New York: Guilford Press, pp. 21–49.

(1996). Obsessive-compulsive disorder. In C. G. Lindemann (ed.), *Handbook of the Treatment of the Anxiety Disorders*. Northvale: Jason Aronson, pp. 139–71.

Foa, E. B., Steketee, G., Grayson, B., Turner, M. and Latimer, P. (1984). Deliberate exposure and blocking of obsessive-compulsive rituals: immediate and long-term effects. *Behavior Therapy*, **15**, 450–72.

Franklin, M., Foa, E. and March, J. S. (2003). The pediatric obsessive-compulsive disorder treatment study: rationale, design and methods. *Journal of Child and Adolescent Psychopharmacology*, **13** (Suppl 1): S39–51.

Franklin, M. E., Kozak, M. J., Cashman, L. A., Coles, M. E., Rheingold, A. A. and Foa, E. B. (1998). Cognitive-behavioral treatment of pediatric obsessive-compulsive disorder: an open clinical trial. *Journal of the American Academy of Child and Adolescent Psychiatry*, **37**, 412–19.

Franklin, M. E., Rynn, M., March, J. S. and Foa, E. B. (2002). Obsessive-compulsive disorder. In M. Hersen (ed.), *Clinical Behavior Therapy: Adults and Children*. New York: John Wiley and Sons, Inc, pp. 276–303.

Franklin, M. E., Tolin, D. F., March, J. S. and Foa, E. B. (2001). Treatment of pediatric obsessive-compulsive disorder: a case example of intensive cognitive-behavioral therapy involving exposure and ritual prevention. *Cognitive and Behavioral Practice*, **8**, 297–304.

Giulino, L., Gammon, P., Sullivan, K. *et al.* (2002). Is parental report of upper respiratory infection at the onset of obsessive-compulsive disorder suggestive of pediatric autoimmune neuropsychiatric disorder associated with streptococcal infection? *Journal of Child and Adolescent Psychopharmacology*, **12**, 157–64.

Goodman, W., Rasmussen, S., Foa, E. and Price, L. (1994). Obsessive-compulsive disorder. In R. Prien and D. Robinson (eds.), *Clinical Evaluation of Psychotropic Drugs: Principles and Guidelines*. New York: Raven Press, pp. 431–66.

King, R., Leonard, H. and March, J. (1998). Practice parameters for the assessment and treatment of children and adolescents with obsessive-compulsive disorder. *Journal of the American Academy of Child and Adolescent Psychiatry*, **37** (Suppl 10), 27S–45S.

Kovacs, M. (1996). *The Children's Depression Inventory*. Toronto: MultiHealth Systems.

Leonard, H. L., Swedo, S. E., Lenane, M. C. *et al.* (1993). A 2- to 7-year follow-up study of 54 obsessive-compulsive children and adolescents. *Archives of General Psychiatry*, **50**, 429–39.

March, J. (1998a). Cognitive behavioral psychotherapy for pediatric OCD. In M. Jenike, L. Baer and Minichello (eds.), *Obsessive-Compulsive Disorders*, 3rd edn. Philadelphia: Mosby, pp. 400–20.

(1998b). *Manual for the Multidimensional Anxiety Scale for Children (MASC)*. Toronto: MultiHealth Systems.

March, J. and Leonard, H. (1996). Obsessive-compulsive disorder in children and adolescents: a review of the past 10 years. *Journal of the American Academy of Child and Adolescent Psychiatry*, **35**, 1265–73.

March, J. and Mulle, K. (1995). Manualized cognitive-behavioral psychotherapy for obsessive-compulsive disorder in childhood: a preliminary single case study. *Journal of Anxiety Disorders*, **9**, 175–84.

(1998). *OCD in Children and Adolescents: A Cognitive-Behavioral Treatment Manual*. New York: Guilford Press.

March, J., Frances, A., Kahn, D. and Carpenter, D. (1997). Expert consensus guidelines: treatment of obsessive-compulsive disorder. *Journal of Clinical Psychiatry*, **58** (Suppl 4), 1–72.

March, J. S., Franklin, M., Nelson, A. and Foa, E. (2001). Cognitive-behavioral psychotherapy for pediatric obsessive-compulsive disorder. *Journal of Clinical Child Psychology*, **30**, 8–18.

March, J. S., Mulle, K. and Herbel, B. (1994). Behavioral psychotherapy for children and adolescents with obsessive-compulsive disorder: an open trial of a new protocol-driven treatment package. *Journal of the American Academy of Child and Adolescent Psychiatry*, **33**, 333–41.

McDougle, C. J., Goodman, W. K., Leckman, J. F., Barr, L. C., Heninger, G. R. and Price, L. H. (1993). The efficacy of fluvoxamine in obsessive-compulsive disorder: effects of comorbid chronic tic disorder. *Journal of Clinical Psychopharmacology*, **13**, 354–8.

Piacentini, J., Jaffer, M., Bergman, R. L., McCracken, J. and Keller, M. (2001). *Measuring Impairment in Childhood OCD: Psychometric Properties of the COIS*. Paper presented at the Annual Meeting of the American Academy of Child and Adolescent Psychiatry, Honolulu.

Rasmussen, S. A. and Eisen, J. L. (1990). Epidemiology of obsessive compulsive disorder. *Journal of Clinical Psychiatry*, **53** (Suppl), pp. 10–13; discussion, p. 14.

Scahill, L., Riddle, M. A., McSwiggin-Hardin, M. *et al.* (1997). Children's Yale-Brown Obsessive Compulsive Scale: reliability and validity. *Journal of the American Academy of Child and Adolescent Psychiatry*, **36**, 844–52.

Silverman, W. and Albano, A. (1996). *The Anxiety Disorders Interview Schedule for DSM-IV: Child and Parent Versions*. San Antonio, TX: The Psychological Corporation.

Soechting, I. and March, J. (2002). Cognitive aspects of obsessive compulsive disorder in children. In R. Frost and G. Steketee (eds.), *Cognitive Approaches to Obsessions and Compulsions: Theory, Assessment, and Treatment*. Amsterdam: Pergamon/Elsevier Science Inc, pp. 299–314.

Swedo, S. E., Leonard, H. L., Garvey, M. *et al.* (1998). Pediatric autoimmune neuropsychiatric disorders associated with streptococcal infections: clinical description of the first 50 cases. *American Journal of Psychiatry*, **155**, 264–71.

van Oppen, P., de Haan, E., van Balkom, A. J., Spinhoven, P., Hoogduin, K. and van Dyck, R. (1995). Cognitive therapy and exposure in vivo in the treatment of obsessive compulsive disorder. *Behaviour Research and Therapy*, **33**, 379–90.

Wever, C. (1994). *Combined medication and behavioral treatment of OCD in adolescents*. Proceedings of the Second Annual Australian Conference on OCD, Sydney, Australia.

Wever, C. and Rey, J. M. (1997). Juvenile obsessive-compulsive disorder. *Australia New Zealand Journal of Psychiatry*, **31**, 105–13.

18

Anxiety disorders

Jennifer L. Allen and Ronald M. Rapee

Macquarie University, Sydney, New South Wales, Australia

Anxiety is a normal human reaction, but becomes a problem when it begins to interfere with a child's education, family and peer relationships, self-esteem, general happiness or ability to participate in everyday activities. Factors that need to be considered when deciding whether or not a child's fear is 'abnormal' include the degree of distress experienced and the age-appropriateness of the fear. There is no set-point at which anxiety goes from being 'normal' to 'maladaptive'. Rather, anxiety is best conceptualized as a continuum, with anxiety disorders towards the severe end (Schniering et al., 2000). The need for intervention in children who are impaired by their level of anxiety is highlighted by research showing that children and adolescents who do not receive treatment have a significantly poorer prognosis than those who obtain help (Dadds et al., 1997).

18.1 Diagnosis

The fourth edition of the *Diagnostic and Statistical Manual of Mental Disorders* (DSM-IV; American Psychiatric Association, 1994) includes the following categories of anxiety disorders that can be found in children: separation anxiety disorder (SAD), panic disorder–agoraphobia, obsessive compulsive disorder (OCD), post-traumatic stress disorder (PTSD), acute stress disorder, specific phobia, social phobia and generalized anxiety disorder (GAD). While there is no category specifically for childhood anxiety disorders, DSM-IV does take into account differences in the manifestation of anxiety in children due to cognitive and developmental differences. For example, criteria note that, unlike adults, children and adolescents may not necessarily recognize their fears or anxious behaviours as excessive or unreasonable. In addition, symptoms such as crying, tantrums and clinging are cited as behavioural indicators for anxiety in children. Given that

Cognitive Behaviour Therapy for Children and Families, ed. Philip J. Graham.
Published by Cambridge University Press. © Cambridge University Press 2004.

anxiety is a common and often transient feature of childhood, DSM-IV also stipulates that symptoms of the anxiety disorder must be present for 6 months before a diagnosis can be given.

18.2   Description of disorders and prevalence

SAD is characterized by developmentally inappropriate and excessive anxiety about separation from home or attachment figures, while social phobia is characterized by a fear of one or more situations in which there is the possibility of negative evaluation by others. Children with social phobia fear that they will act in a way that is humiliating or embarrassing – therefore, social situations may be avoided to prevent this possibility from occurring.

The primary feature of GAD is excessive and uncontrollable worry. Children with GAD may worry about any number of areas including health, schoolwork (e.g. tests and homework), family finances, world affairs (e.g. war and natural disasters), new situations, sports performance, as well as social and interpersonal concerns. Symptoms accompanying GAD include restlessness, fatigue, difficulty concentrating, irritability, muscle tension and sleep disturbance. OCD (see Chapter 17) is identified by the presence of thoughts, images or impulses that are perceived as intrusive and distressing (i.e. obsessions), as well as repetitive behaviours that are aimed at reducing the likelihood of a feared event (i.e. compulsions).

PTSD (see Chapter 20) may occur after experiencing, witnessing or being confronted by an event that threatened or caused death or serious injury to self or others. Panic disorder is identified by frequent unexpected panic attacks that are accompanied by physiological (e.g. racing heart and dizziness) and cognitive symptoms (e.g. fear of dying, having a heart attack or losing control), while agoraphobia refers to avoidance of situations due to fear of being unable to escape or get help in the event of having a panic attack.

18.3   Aetiology and maintenance of child anxiety

An understanding of the factors involved in the aetiology and maintenance of child anxiety is important in assisting therapists to apply and modify interventions to suit the needs of children and families. Studies examining the aetiology of child anxiety have focused on three main areas: genetics, temperament and environmental factors. For a more detailed review of these factors, refer to Chorpita and Barlow (1998), Hudson and Rapee (in press), Manassis and Bradley (1994) and Rapee (2001).

There is strong evidence supporting a genetic basis to anxiety, with genes accounting for approximately 30–40% of the variance (Andrews *et al.*, 1990). Hudson and Rapee (in press) have suggested that this genetic vulnerability manifests itself through the child's temperament. Temperament refers to the inborn behavioural style of a child, which is partly mediated by genetics and expressed through both nervous system reactivity and regulation (Prior *et al.*, 2000). Although temperament appears to play a role in the development of anxiety, not all children who possess this temperamental vulnerability go on to develop an anxiety disorder. Therefore, other factors besides genetics and its temperamental manifestations must contribute to the development of anxiety.

Twin studies in children have shown that shared environmental factors make a large contribution towards the development of anxiety symptoms and disorder (e.g. Topolski *et al.*, 1997; Eley and Stevenson, 2000). The way in which the family environment might influence the development and maintenance of anxiety has been the focus of much investigation. Family environmental factors implicated in the development of child anxiety include parenting style, parental support of avoidance and observational learning.

A review of the literature on parenting style and anxiety revealed a consistent relationship between anxiety and a more involved and controlling parenting style (Rapee, 1997). Research indicates that parents may play a role in promoting their child's anxious behaviours. Barrett and colleagues (1996b) asked anxious children and controls to interpret and provide plans of action concerning ambiguous scenarios. Anxious children were more likely than controls to interpret these situations as threatening and to select avoidant plans of action. After a discussion with their parents about the situation, the likelihood of an anxious child selecting a threatening interpretation and an avoidant plan of action increased dramatically. Examination of the content of family discussions revealed that parents of anxious children promoted avoidant child behaviour by modelling avoidance, verbalizing doubts in their child's abilities and providing acceptance and comfort when their child displayed avoidant behaviour (Dadds *et al.*, 1996). It remains to be determined whether parents of anxious children promote anxious behaviours or whether it is the child's anxious behaviour which is responsible for eliciting overprotective responses from parents. It is possible that both of these factors contribute to the development of anxiety (Rapee, 2001). Others in the child's environment (e.g. teachers, peers and siblings) may also support anxious or avoidant behaviours.

External environmental stressors may also contribute to the development of an anxiety disorder. PTSD is an extreme example of how exposure to an external event can cause anxiety. Finally, anxious children have been shown to experience

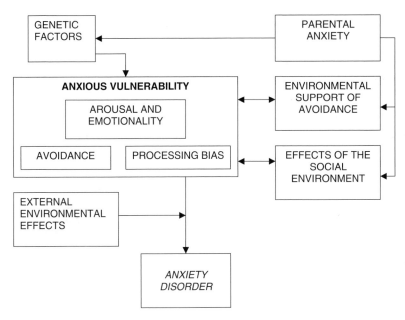

Figure 18.1   A model of the development of anxiety (Rapee, 2001; Hudson and Rapee, in press).

a greater number of stressful life events in the 12 months preceding the onset of their problems than non-anxious children (Goodyer and Altham, 1991).

18.4   Integrative model for the development of anxiety

Based on the preceding evidence, Rapee (2001) and Hudson and Rapee (in press) have proposed a broad model that elucidates the many possible pathways to the development of an anxiety disorder (see Figure 18.1). In this model, some children are born with a genetic vulnerability to anxiety. This vulnerability is manifested through the child's temperament, evidenced by high levels of arousal, emotionality and an avoidant coping style. In turn, the child's temperament may guide them to select environments that support and maintain their avoidance and, in particular, may elicit protective behaviours from others such as parents. Reciprocally, this 'overprotection' may increase the child's perceptions of threat and decrease their perceptions of control over danger (Rapee, 1997). Parents of anxious children are likely to be anxious themselves and this anxiety makes a parent especially vulnerable to falling into an overprotective cycle.

The model also draws attention to the potential role of social learning in the development of anxiety. Observational learning and the provision of information from significant others may increase a child's avoidance and threat perception and reduce perceptions of control over threat. These experiences may occur independently of the child's temperament or interact with an anxious vulnerability. However, anxious children may choose environments that increase the likelihood of encountering anxious modelling of behaviour. For example, inhibited children may be more likely to have friends who are also inhibited. Finally, an inhibited temperament may progress to disorder through moderation with external environmental events. This can include major life events or more subtle learning experiences. While some events may be capable of producing anxiety independent of vulnerability, they are more likely to have a greater impact on those who already possess a vulnerability to anxiety.

18.5   Treatment outcome

A growing body of evidence indicates that relatively brief CBT interventions are effective in both reducing children's anxiety and improving general functioning. In general, randomized controlled studies of CBT for child anxiety have included components such as psychoeducation concerning the nature of anxiety, relaxation, cognitive restructuring and graded exposure in their treatment programmes. These skills are then consolidated through the assignment of practice tasks between sessions.

Kendall (1994) conducted the first randomized trial examining the efficacy of CBT with anxious children using his 'Coping Cat' programme. This programme addressed both cognitive and behavioural components of anxiety. Children aged 9–13 years ($n = 47$) with broad-based anxiety disorders participated in the 16-session individual treatment programme. At post-treatment, 64% of children who participated in this research trial were anxiety diagnosis free, compared with 5% of children in the waiting list control group. Children showed significant improvement on parental and self-report measures of distress, parent-reported coping as well as measures of behavioural observation. Change in diagnostic status and improvement on self-report measures were maintained at 1-year follow-up. These findings were replicated in a second randomized trial (Kendall et al., 1997).

Studies have also investigated the efficacy of group treatment for child anxiety. Group treatment offers several advantages, including greater cost-effectiveness and faster reduction of waiting lists. Flannery-Schroeder and Kendall (2000) randomly allocated 37 children aged 8–14 years with broad-based anxiety diagnoses to group treatment, individual treatment or to a waiting list control condition. Intervention consisted of 18 sessions based on Kendall's 'Coping Cat' workbook. As in Kendall's previous treatment studies (Kendall, 1994; Kendall et al., 1997), there was minimal parental involvement. Both the individual and group conditions resulted in clinically significant gains. In comparison with 8% of waiting list controls, 73% of children who received individual treatment and 50% of children who received group treatment did not meet diagnostic criteria for their pretreatment diagnosis at post-treatment. Children in the two treatment conditions also showed greater improvement on child and parent reports of anxiety and coping at post-treatment and 3-month follow-up relative to waiting list controls. Flannery-Schroeder and Kendall (2000) concluded that there was no overall difference between treatment groups, with comparable treatment gains for both individual and group treatment. Therefore, it appears that it is possible to substitute cost-effective group treatments while still ensuring that children receive optimum treatment.

18.5.1   Parents in treatment

Given research and theory concerning the role of parental anxiety and observational learning in the maintenance and development of child anxiety, several studies have investigated the possibility of improving outcome by including parents in the treatment process. Parental involvement has been expanded from the minimal contact present in Kendall's 'Coping Cat' programme (Kendall, 1994; Kendall *et al.*, 1997) to concurrent treatment sessions for parents and children (e.g. Rapee, 2000). Dadds *et al.* (1992) conducted the first study to include a significant parent component (Family Anxiety Management; FAM), designed to run in parallel with a child-focused CBT programme. This component educated parents about child management techniques such as rewarding children's courageous behaviour and dealing with children's anxious behaviours. Parents were also taught how to deal with their own emotional upsets, to identify their own anxious behaviours and how to model problem-solving and proactive responses to feared situations. At post-treatment, 70% of the CBT + FAM group were anxiety diagnosis free. Children also showed improvement on parent and child measures.

Barrett *et al.* (1996a) extended this study by comparing three conditions: child-only CBT ($n = 28$), CBT plus family component (CBT + FAM; $n = 25$) and a waiting list control group ($n = 26$). Although children in both CBT and CBT + FAM conditions performed better than waiting list control, the CBT + FAM group showed greater improvement to the CBT-only group on several parent and child measures. Follow-up analyses showed that the additional benefit obtained with FAM was found mainly in younger children and not in adolescents. Mendlowitz and colleagues (1999) also compared a parent and child CBT group ($n = 18$) with child-only ($n = 23$) and parent-only treatment groups ($n = 21$). While all groups showed improvement pre- to post-treatment in comparison with a waiting list control group, children in the parent–child treatment showed greater improvement on measures of anxiety, depression and use of adaptive coping strategies. Therefore, it appears that including parents in treatment enhances the efficacy of CBT for younger anxious children. Further, the inclusion of an anxiety management component for anxious parents may also enhance effects (Cobham *et al.*, 1998).

Rapee (2000) investigated whether the gains reported by individual family treatment would also be evident if children and parents were treated in a brief group format. Children aged 7–16 years ($n = 95$) with various different anxiety diagnoses participated in the nine-session 'Cool Kids' programme, which is similar to the treatment package of Barrett *et al.* (1996a). Children who received treatment showed significantly greater improvement on measures of anxiety than waiting list controls. These gains were maintained and, in some cases, increased at 12-month follow-up. Despite the change to a group format and a reduced number of sessions, effect sizes were similar to those found in individual treatment studies (e.g. Kendall, 1994; Barrett *et al.*, 1996a).

A recent study conducted by Manassis and colleagues (2002) compared the efficacy of group family versus individual family treatment for childhood anxiety disorders. Children in both conditions showed improvement; however, clinician ratings of general functioning showed greater improvement for children in the group condition. There were no differences between individual or group treatment with regard to child and parent measures. Contrary to expectations, children with high social anxiety showed greater improvement if they received individual treatment. Manassis and colleagues suggested that perhaps the group situation is too overwhelming for highly socially anxious children, interfering with the learning of new skills.

In line with the move to group treatment, recent research has begun to focus on improvements in the cost-effectiveness of treatment delivery. One method by which this might be achieved is through self-help methods. In a current study in the authors' clinic, treatment delivered via parents in the form of bibliotherapy materials was compared with the usual group treatment. Preliminary data indicated approximately 20% of children are diagnosis free following bibliotherapy compared with 60% in clinician-led group treatment and 5% of waiting list (Abbott *et al.*, 2002). In a further development, it has been shown that the effects of bibliotherapy can be increased by occasional clinician contact via telephone or email (Lyneham and Rapee, 2002).

18.5.2   Are CBT interventions for child anxiety effective in the long term?

Several studies have demonstrated that relatively brief CBT interventions maintain their effectiveness in the longer term. Kendall and Southam-Gerow (1996) conducted a 2–5-year follow-up with the children who participated in Kendall's 1994 study. Findings indicated that gains made by these children were maintained, in terms of diagnostic status and parent-report and child self-report measures. A 6-year follow-up of the child-only CBT and CBT + FAM treatments in the original Barrett et al. (1996a) study found that 85.7% of children no longer met diagnostic criteria for an anxiety disorder (Barrett et al., 2001). Gains made at the 12-month follow-up assessed via clinician ratings, parent-report and child self-report measures were maintained. Furthermore, CBT and CBT plus family management were equally effective. A long-term follow-up of brief family group CBT found that children continued to show improvement over time, with 91% of participants anxiety diagnosis free at 3-year follow-up in comparison with 71% anxiety diagnosis free at post-treatment (Toren et al., 2000).

18.5.3   Conclusion

In summary, the evidence suggests that most children can be successfully treated with relatively brief individual or group CBT interventions. Success may be further enhanced with the inclusion of parents in treatment, especially with younger children. Treatment gains are enhanced for children with anxious parents if their parents also receive anxiety management. Importantly, gains made during treatment appear to be maintained in the long term. Treatment studies examining the effectiveness of CBT for child anxiety in differing modalities (e.g. bibliotherapy and email-assisted programmes) provide options for those working with children living in remote or rural areas, or for whom attendance at therapy is difficult due to financial or personal reasons.

18.6   Treatment

This section will provide an overview of the treatment programme currently in use at the Macquarie University Child and Adolescent Anxiety Clinic, Sydney, Australia. This programme has shown great success with children diagnosed with broad-based anxiety disorders (see Rapee, 2000). Components of this programme are described in detail in Rapee et al. (2000). A copy of the ten-session 'Cool Kids' treatment manual and workbooks are available from the clinic (www.psy.mq.edu.au/MUARU).

18.6.1   Programme structure

The 'Cool Kids' programme used at the authors' clinic is based on a cognitive behavioural model developed from Kendall's 'Coping Cat' programme and the 'Coping Koala' programme of Barrett et al. (1996a). The authors' programme is designed for families utilizing a small group format, but good results have also been achieved with individual family treatment of children and adolescents. Therefore, therapists who are unable to run a group can adapt this programme for individual families. 'Cool Kids' groups consist of five to seven families, consisting of the child and, where possible, both parents. The programme consists of ten 2-hour sessions conducted over a 16-week period. The first seven sessions are held weekly, with the last three sessions staggered at intervals. This tapering of treatment contact gives families time to practise skills and gradually decreases the amount of therapist contact. In the programme, children and parents are also assigned tasks to complete at home each week. These tasks help parents and children to consolidate material learned in-session and to practise the skills they have learned. Each session begins by welcoming group members and review (10–15 minutes). Children are encouraged to discuss their week, using their practice task as a guide. The therapist then spends time with young people alone (40–60 minutes), followed by therapist time with parents alone (40–60 minutes). At the end of each session, the entire group rejoins for a review of the session and practice tasks (10–25 minutes).

18.6.2   Components of the 'Cool Kids' programme

The primary goals of Cool Kids are: (1) to learn skills to manage anxiety; (2) reduce avoidance of feared situations; and (3) for children eventually to become independent of their parents and the therapist by using the skills and knowledge gained through the programme. Specific components of this programme include psychoeducation, cognitive restructuring ('realistic' or 'detective' thinking), graded exposure ('stepladders') and parent management. There are also optional modules addressing issues often relevant to anxious children, such as social skills, teasing and assertiveness. This enables therapists to modify the programme according to group/individual client needs. The following section discusses the main components of Cool Kids.

18.6.2.1   Psychoeducation

Information concerning the nature, causes and maintenance of anxiety is presented to parents. This covers differences between 'healthy' and 'unhealthy' anxiety and physiological, cognitive and behavioural aspects of anxiety and how these will be addressed by different components of treatment. Children discuss emotions and the different ways in which they experience anxiety.

18.6.2.2   Realistic or detective thinking

In the authors' programme, the cognitive restructuring component is termed 'realistic thinking' for adolescents and 'detective thinking' for children. Children pick their favourite superhero or detective, who will help them look for 'clues' or 'evidence' against their anxious thoughts or predictions that something bad will happen when in the presence of feared situations or stimuli. The term 'realistic thinking' is used with parents and adolescents to illustrate that the aim is to modify extreme unrealistic beliefs rather than changing all their negative beliefs to positive ones. Young people are encouraged to weigh up *all* the evidence for and against their negative prediction, in order to generate 'calm thoughts' that are believable to them. Parents are also taught cognitive restructuring so that they can assist their child with the technique and address their own fears if necessary.

Explanation of cognitive restructuring starts by introducing parents and young people to the link between situations, thoughts and feelings using examples. At the beginning of treatment, young people are asked to monitor situations, thoughts and level of anxiety (on a 'worry' scale). The aim of this exercise is to practise identifying anxious thoughts so that they can be challenged. Therapists then discuss (with parents and adolescents) the two main cognitive biases displayed by anxious individuals: overestimating the likelihood of unpleasant events happening and overestimating how bad the consequences would be if the event did happen. Group members are taught different techniques to gather evidence against the likelihood of their prediction that something bad will happen, based on their past experience and general knowledge. Adolescents take cognitive restructuring a step further, by learning to identify and challenge the consequences of the feared event. Young people are asked to complete forms recording situations where they felt anxious, their negative prediction about this situation and evidence against this prediction. Young people then generate a 'calm thought' which is based on their realistic appraisal of the anxiety-provoking event.

Cognitive restructuring can be a powerful tool in the reduction of anxiety; however, those who try to educate children about this technique often come up against some common hurdles. For example, some children become so anxious in a feared situation that they are unable to remember their detective thinking. In this situation, cue cards can be used to remind children of their calm thought for that situation. If families are aware that a situation is coming up that will prove difficult, the child can practise detective thinking before the event occurs. Another common problem is that some children have difficulty grasping the concepts behind cognitive restructuring. It is, therefore, important to work through examples both in and out of session, and for the child to practise regularly with the help of both therapists and their parents. It is important that children are able to identify their anxious thoughts and understand the link between thoughts and feelings before moving on to challenging anxious thoughts. For children experiencing difficulties with cognitive restructuring, alternative anxiety management techniques may include self-instructional training (see Meichenbaum, 1977) or relaxation (see Rapee *et al.*, 2000).

18.6.2.3   Graded exposure ('stepladders')

The aim of exposure is to encourage children to face situations they fear and avoid. This in done in a graded or 'stepped' manner with the least feared situations faced first to encourage compliance. Graded exposure enables children to learn that: (1) the situation is not threatening and (2) that they have the ability to cope with the situation (Foa and McNally, 1996; Williams, 1996). Exposure is arguably the most effective treatment strategy for the reduction of anxiety in both children and adults (Rapee *et al.*, 2000). In the authors' programme, cognitive restructuring is taught before the introduction to graded exposure – this is so that generating evidence that certain events are not so bad and that one can cope with the situation can be reinforced by directly experiencing the event. Therapists may wish to combine exposure with relaxation to help children to master excessive anxiety in feared situations.

Parents and children will need a careful explanation of the graded exposure rationale and process, given that exposure requires children to face situations that are likely to have caused distress in the past. Parents may be reluctant for their child to face certain fears due to concerns for their child's capacity to tolerate anxiety or they may step in to rescue the child from the situation. It is important to discuss understandable feelings of helplessness and guilt that parents may have when encouraging their child to face situations they are afraid of. If a parent also fears the situation, they can attempt exposure to provide a model of courage for their child. Children's anxiety about exposure can be addressed by giving them some control over the process. Children choose the fears they would like to overcome together with their parents. They are told that they will begin with easy situations at first, and that they will only progress to the next step when they feel ready to do so. Adolescents are usually able to generate their own stepladder with therapist assistance; however, at the very least, parents need to be aware of what their adolescent is doing so that they can provide encouragement and rewards.

After working through some examples of stepladders in-session, parents and children are encouraged to create a list of feared situations together. Families are instructed to generate a list of fears that are divided into high, medium and low worry categories and to help their child assign a worry rating to each situation listed. The list of fears and worries is then used to develop specific exposure hierarchies or 'stepladders'. Children and parents select a feared situation they would like to work on and begin building a stepladder, with steps gradually increasing in difficulty. The group format can be used to advantage here, with other group members assisting in brainstorming possible steps. It is important that children begin with steps that are small so that they can begin to build confidence in both themselves and the technique. Steps may need to be repeated several times before progressing to the next level of difficulty. The stepladder process should be supervised to ensure that children are not attempting steps that are too difficult (or not difficult enough). Therapists need to ensure that the family goes away with a clear concrete and specific plan of what step is to be done, and when and where, and what reward the young person will receive on completion of the task. The inclusion of parents in the development of graded stepladders ensures that parents have the time and resources to assist their child with each step. The use of everyday activities is encouraged, as steps that require an excessive amount of effort, time or resources are less likely to be completed. Children should be encouraged to complete a detective thinking form about the exposure task both before and after the exercise to challenge their underlying anxious beliefs.

Children will need encouragement and motivation in order to face feared situations. The authors' programme addresses these issues through the use of praise, rewards and introducing young people to the concept of 'self-reward'. Young people are encouraged to praise themselves using positive self-talk about their efforts. Often, anxious children have unrealistically high standards about performance, which contributes to their reluctance to try new or difficult activities. Children are set several exercises to encourage them to praise themselves for facing their fears. Parents are also educated about the importance of providing clear and specific praise with regard to the behaviour. Rewards should be used to reinforce children's attempts at facing their fears. Rewards can take the form of activities, praise, material things or points which can be traded for rewards once a certain number have been collected. It is stressed to parents that rewards must be proportional to the achievement. If a child has made a serious attempt at facing a fear, they should be rewarded; however, they should be given a better reward for successfully completing the step. It is also important that reward and praise is given as soon as possible after exposure, particularly with younger children.

Over the course of treatment, therapists need to address any difficulties with exposure and brainstorm solutions with group members. One common reason why a task is not completed may be that it was too anxiety provoking for the child. In this case, the child may need to drop back a 'step' or two or choose a task lower on their stepladder to build confidence before re-attempting the task. It is also vital to stress to families that children need to stay in the feared situation for long enough for their belief to be proved false and for their level of anxiety to come down in order for exposure to be effective. If a child pulls out of a task before her belief is proved false, her anxiety will not be reduced and may even increase. Therapists will also need to check that rewards are being awarded in a way that is consistent with the parent–child agreement.

18.6.2.4   Parent management

The management component of the programme focuses on strategies parents can use to build up courageous behaviours in their child, as well as strategies to reduce anxious behaviours. Strategies to help build up courageous behaviour include attention, modelling, encouraging independence, praise and rewards, as discussed earlier. Parents are encouraged to give time and attention to their children when they are being courageous or well-behaved as opposed to when they are anxious or disruptive. Modelling of courageous behaviour is another important issue for therapists to address. Parents are asked to think about any anxieties they have in common with their child and to address these fears by completing their own detective thinking forms and creating their own stepladder. Parents need to encourage their child to be independent by providing guidance, rather than 'taking over' for their child or allowing them to avoid feared situations. For example, when a child is feeling anxious, a parent could encourage him or her practise their detective thinking rather than allowing their child to avoid the situation.

Strategies to reduce anxious behaviours include consistency, avoidance of excessive reassurance and keeping emotions under control. Therapists need to stress to parents the importance of consistency with regard to both rewards and punishment. Parents need to carry through on their stated intentions with regard to both rewards and punishments. Parents also need to beware of accidentally rewarding a child's anxious or naughty behaviour by giving into their demands (e.g. when whining or crying). Both parents need to discuss which behaviours they consider appropriate and which they do not, and come to an agreement so that parenting is consistent. Providing children with excessive reassurance should be avoided, as children need to learn that the feared situation is safe, rather than only believing that the situation is safe or that they are able to cope because their parents have reassured them of this. However, reassurance *is* helpful when it is given with regard to the child's ability to handle the situation. Techniques to keep emotions under control are also discussed, as parenting tends to become less consistent when parents are feeling very emotional. At times such as this, it is a good idea for the parent to withdraw from the situation and ask their partner, grandparents, friends or other social supports to spend time with their child.

18.7   Case examples

The following vignettes are based on cases seen by Jennifer Allen at the Macquarie University Child and Adolescent Anxiety Clinic.

18.7.1   Alison (separation anxiety, specific phobia)

Alison, a 9-year-old child, was referred by her mother and school counsellor. Alison's mother, Kathy, reported that Alison would often feel sick, throw tantrums or cry in the morning before going to school. Several times this year, Alison had visited the school nurse, complaining of stomach pains, so Kathy had been called into school to take her home. Alison said that she was scared that something bad might happen to her mother when they were apart, such as her mother having a car accident. Alison often slept with her parents at night because she was scared about burglars. Alison would also often turn down invitations from other children to play or attend slumber parties due to these fears. Her separation anxiety was also having an impact on her parents, as her mother was finding dealing with Alison's tantrums stressful and her parents were unable to go out by themselves. Alison met criteria for a primary diagnosis of SAD and the additional diagnosis of specific phobia for her fear of the dark.

Initial sessions with Alison focused on identifying physical symptoms of anxiety, on identifying her anxious thoughts and gaining an understanding of the link between situations, thoughts and feelings. When she began feeling anxious, Alison reminded herself of the 'evidence' that nothing bad had ever happened to herself or her mother when they are apart, and, therefore, that it was unlikely to happen in future. Alison chose Jennifer Lopez (J-Lo) as her superhero to help her find clues or evidence against her anxious thoughts. One of Alison's calm thoughts was to think of J-Lo's song 'I'm gonna be allright'.

Alison's worries list included going to school, going to friends' houses or parties and sleeping in bed by herself. Stepladders were drawn up for each of these situations. Together with her parents, rewards for each step were agreed on. Often, opportunities for exposure present themselves during treatment. For example, Alison knew she would be invited to a slumber party for her best friend Annette in 1 month's time. Therefore Alison and her parents decided to make this one of her goals. Alison rated this task at an 8 on the 10-point worry scale.

Alison's goal was: to be able to go to a friend's slumber party without worrying about her mother (Table 18.1).

Table 18.1 Alison's exposure stepladder and worry scale ratings

(1)	While at a friend's house, her mother leaves for 10 minutes	(3)
(2)	While at a friend's house, her mother leaves for 30 minutes	(4)
(3)	Kathy drops Alison off at Annette's house to play for 1 hour and then leaves	(5)
(4)	Repeat the previous step at a different friend's house	(5)
(5)	Kathy drops Alison off at Annette's house to play for 2 hours	(6)
(6)	Going over to another friend's house for dinner	(6)
(7)	Staying over at Grandma's for one night	(7)
(8)	Staying over at Annette's for one night	(7)
(9)	Going to Annette's slumber party	(8)

The authors' programme also advocates use of in-session exposure. In-session, Alison and other group members played some games in the dark, a fun way of gaining exposure to this feared situation. Alison and her family were asked to play these games at home in the dark as one practise task. In the sixth session, the group made an excursion to a local shopping centre. The session before parents and children were asked to generate some exposure tasks they could do. Parents were instructed to assist their child with detective thinking before and after each task. This gives therapists an opportunity to see how parents assist their child with cognitive restructuring and provide feedback. Alison's task was to walk to the other end of the shopping centre without her parents. Here, the therapist noticed that Alison was 'rushing' through the task. Therefore, Alison was asked to repeat the step, but this time to walk more slowly and to stop and play the free video game at the electrical store for 5 minutes before returning to her parents. Before attempting these in-sessions tasks, the therapist discussed with Kathy her own anxiety about Alison's safety while parted from her in the shopping centre and assisted her in filling out her own 'detective thinking' sheet about this concern.

Alison's parents found the parent management component helpful, especially with regard to dealing with her tantrums and school attendance. Her parents no longer allowed her to stay home from school or come home if she was anxious. A 'star chart' which gave Alison stars for when she went to school or slept on her own without a tantrum was implemented. Alison traded these points in for rewards negotiated with her parents. The school counsellor and teacher were also enlisted as 'coaches' in therapy, instituting a system of social reward for Alison's attendance at school.

By the end of therapy, Alison was happily staying over at friends' houses and her parents were able to go out together for dinner without Alison becoming upset.

She was still throwing some tantrums before school, but these had considerably lessened since the commencement of the group programme. Alison's goals for the future were to be able to cope with her parents going away for a weekend and to be able to attend a 1-week school camp the next year. Alison and her parents prepared some steps leading up to these goals which they intended to work on after the end of the programme.

18.7.2   Michael (generalized anxiety disorder and social phobia)

Michael, a 16-year-old adolescent, was referred by his parents, who described him as a 'worry wart'. Michael reported worrying about things such as his grades at school, 'getting into trouble' from teachers and parents, world events (e.g. war and terrorism), making friends, his future (e.g. coping with senior high school and future career) and things being 'perfect' (e.g. being on time and making mistakes on school assignments). As a result of this worry, Michael had trouble sleeping, experienced headaches and often felt irritable. As well as these more general worries, Michael reported anxiety and avoidance of several social situations (e.g. public speaking, parties and situations requiring assertiveness). Michael met criteria for a primary diagnosis of GAD and an additional diagnosis of social phobia. Michael also reported some symptoms of depression, such as low self-esteem but symptoms were not of the frequency or severity to warrant a diagnosis. During assessment, Michael's father Stan disclosed that he was currently seeing a psychiatrist for depression.

Early in therapy, Michael's self-monitoring thought forms revealed an extensive list of worries triggering his anxiety. Michael had difficulty with cognitive restructuring, especially when evaluating the 'cost' of his prediction that something bad was going to happen realistically. For example, for Michael, the cost of failing a test was catastrophic and attempts by the therapist or other group members to encourage Michael to examine alternative views on this had little impact on his evaluation of consequences. Michael's father reinforced these fears around his schoolwork, repeatedly stressing the importance of good grades and the impact that failure to obtain his expected results might have on Michael's future. The therapist addressed this by working with Michael and his parents integrating issues concerning perfectionism into a stepladder (Table 18.2). Michael's goal was not to be upset by making mistakes at school. Attempts by the therapist to encourage Stan to apply realistic thinking techniques to his own fears about his son's academic performance were resisted.

Although in-session Michael had generated the stepladder, it soon became apparent that he found it difficult to complete the steps. It is possible that Michael may have generated these steps and made a commitment to tackling these

Table 18.2 Michael's stepladder and worry scale ratings

(1)	Deliberately hand in an essay with an ink stain on it	(3)
(2)	Deliberately arrive 5 minutes late for class	(4)
(3)	Doodle on a page of homework that will be handed in	(4
(4)	Deliberately make a mistake in a class maths exercise	(5)
(5)	Hand in an essay with two spelling mistakes	(6)
(6)	Forget to bring a textbook needed for class	(6)
(7)	Answer a question in class without being certain of the answer	(7)
(8)	Deliberately give the wrong answer in class	(8)
(9)	Deliberately write the wrong answer on the board in maths class	(9)

steps in order to 'fake good' for his parents and the therapist, especially given his perfectionism and fear of authority figures. As a result, the stepladder was redrafted to include more steps at lower worry ratings, and several steps were to be repeated before progressing to the next step.

Michael's parents also found the management component of the programme difficult, as Michael's father appeared to be very defensive and viewed any education about strategies parents could use to promote courageous behaviour in their child as a personal attack on his own abilities as a father. Any strategies suggested by therapists or other parents in the group to assist Michael's parents in reducing their son's anxiety were greeted with rejection. Stan repeatedly made comments throughout therapy such as 'there's no point' and 'we've tried everything, nothing works'. Michael's difficulty completing the steps of the first stepladder provided further fuel to these beliefs.

In-session exposure included group members giving an impromptu speech while being videotaped. Before giving his speech, Michael was asked what symptoms of anxiety he thought the others would notice (e.g. blushing, shaking and avoiding eye contact) and to rate on a scale of 0–10 how noticeable each symptom would be. The other adolescents in the group agreed to provide honest feedback concerning these symptoms, using the same rating scale. Feedback from group members indicated that Michael was overestimating how obvious these symptoms of anxiety were. This feedback was then incorporated into his realistic thinking as further evidence against his anxious thoughts. Michael also chose to complete several tasks during the group shopping centre excursion to address his fear of being assertive, such as buying a CD and then asking to exchange it for another one.

Although Michael made some progress with regards to social fears, his worry, especially with regard to issues around schoolwork and perfectionism, did not shift markedly during the programme. Michael and his family provide an example of a situation in which individual therapy might be the preferable approach, while allowing more time for rapport and for dealing with family issues, such as the father's depression, to be addressed.

18.8　REFERENCES

Abbott, M. J., Gaston, J. and Rapee, R. M. (2002). *Bibliotherapy in the treatment of children with anxiety disorders*. Paper presented at the 3rd International Child and Adolescent Mental Health Conference, Brisbane, June 11–15.

American Psychiatric Association (1994). *Diagnostic and Statistical Manual of Mental Disorders*, 4th edn. Washington DC: American Psychiatric Association.

Andrews, G., Stewart, G. W., Allen, R. and Henderson, A. S. (1990). The genetics of six neurotic disorders. *British Journal of Psychiatry*, **157**, 6–12.

Barrett, P. M., Dadds, M. R. and Rapee, R. M. (1996a). Family treatment of childhood anxiety: a controlled trial. *Journal of Consulting and Clinical Psychology*, **64**, 333–42.

Barrett, P. M., Duffy, A. L., Dadds, M. R. and Rapee, R. M. (2001). Cognitive-behavioural treatment of anxiety disorders in children: long-term (6 year) follow-up. *Journal of Consulting and Clinical Psychology*, **69**, 135–41.

Barrett, P. M., Rapee, R. M., Dadds, M. R. and Ryan, S. M. (1996b). Family enhancement of cognitive style in anxious and aggressive children. *Journal of Abnormal Child Psychology*, **24**, 187–203.

Chorpita, B. F. and Barlow, D. H. (1998). The development of anxiety: the role of control in the early environment. *Psychological Bulletin*, **124**, 3–21.

Cobham, V. E., Dadds, M. R. and Spence, S. H. (1998). The role of parental anxiety in the treatment of childhood anxiety. *Journal of Consulting and Clinical Psychology*, **66**, 893–905.

Dadds, M. R., Heard, P. M. and Rapee, R. M. (1992). The role of family intervention in the treatment of child anxiety disorders: some preliminary findings. *Behaviour Change*, **9**, 171–7.

Dadds, M. R., Heard, P. M. and Rapee, R. M. (1996). Family process and child anxiety and aggression: an observational analysis. *Journal of Abnormal Child Psychology*, **24**, 715–34.

Dadds, M. R., Spence, S. H., Holland, D. E., Barrett, P. M. and Laurens, K. R. (1997). Prevention and early intervention for anxiety disorders: a controlled trial. *Journal of Consulting and Clinical Psychology*, **65**, 627–35.

Eley, T. C. and Stevenson, J. (2000). Specific life events and chronic experiences differentially associated with depression and anxiety in young twins. *Journal of Abnormal Child Psychology*, **28**, 383–94.

Flannery-Schroeder, E. C. and Kendall, P. C. (2000). Group and individual cognitive-behavioral treatments for youth with anxiety disorders. *Cognitive Therapy and Research*, **24**, 251–78.

Foa, E. B. and McNally, R. J. (1996). Mechanisms of change in exposure therapy. In R. M. Rapee (ed.), *Current Controversies in the Anxiety Disorders*. New York: Guilford Press, pp. 329–43.

Goodyer, I. M. and Altham, P. M. E. (1991). Lifetime exit events and recent social and family adversities in anxious and depressed school-age children and adolescents II. *Journal of Affective Disorders*, **21**, 229–38.

Hudson, J. L. and Rapee, R. M. (in press). From anxious temperament to disorder: an etiological model of generalized anxiety disorder. In R. G. Heimberg, C. L. Turk and D. S. Mennin (eds.), *The Etiology and Development of Generalised Anxiety Disorder*. New York: Guilford Press.

Kendall, P. C. (1994). Treating anxiety disorders in children: results of a randomised clinical trial. *Journal of Consulting and Clinical Psychology*, **65**, 724–30.

Kendall, P. C. and Southam-Gerow, M. A. (1996). Long-term follow-up of a cognitive-behavioral therapy for anxiety-disordered youth. *Journal of Consulting and Clinical Psychology*, **64**, 724–30.

Kendall, P. C., Flannery-Schroeder, E. C., Panichelli-Mindel, S. M., Southam-Gerow, M., Henin, A. and Warman, M. J. (1997). Therapy for youths with anxiety disorders: a second randomized clinical trial. *Journal of Consulting and Clinical Psychology*, **65**, 366–80.

Lyneham, H. J. and Rapee, R. M. (2002, June). *Evaluation of Tele-psychology treatment approaches for children with anxiety disorders*. Paper presented at the 3rd International Conference on Child and Adolescent Mental Health, Brisbane, Australia.

Manassis, K. and Bradley, S. J. (1994). The development of childhood anxiety disorders: towards an integrated model. *Journal of Applied Developmental Psychology*, **15**, 345–66.

Manassis, K., Mendlowitz, S. L., Scapillato, D. *et al.* (2002). Group and individual cognitive-behavioral therapy for childhood anxiety disorders: a randomized trial. *American Academy of Child and Adolescent Psychiatry*, **41**, 1423–30.

Meichenbaum, D. (1977). *Cognitive-behaviour modification: An Integrative Approach*. New York: Plenum.

Mendlowitz, S. L., Manassis, K., Bradley, S., Scapillato, D., Mietzitis, S. and Shaw, B. F. (1999). Cognitive-behavioral group treatments in childhood anxiety disorders: the role of parental involvement. *Journal of the American Academy of Child and Adolescent Psychiatry*, **38**, 1223–9.

Prior, M., Sanson, A., Smart, D. and Overklaid, F. (2000). *Pathways from Infancy to Adolescence: Australian Temperament Project 1983–2000*. Melbourne: Australian Institute of Family Studies.

Rapee, R. M. (1997). Potential role of childrearing practices in the development of anxiety and depression. *Clinical Psychology Review*, **17**, 47–67.

  (2000). Group treatment of children with anxiety disorders: outcome and predictors of treatment response. *Australian Journal of Psychology*, **52**, 125–30.

  (2001). The development of generalized anxiety. In M. W. Vasey and M. R. Dadds (eds.), *The Developmental Psychopathology of Anxiety*. Oxford: Oxford University Press, pp. 481–503.

Rapee, R. M., Wignall, A. M., Hudson, J. L. and Schniering, C. A. (2000). *Treating Anxious Children and Adolescents: An Evidence-Based Approach*. Oakland, CA: New Harbinger Publications.

Schniering, C. A., Hudson, J. L. and Rapee, R. M. (2000). Issues in the diagnosis and assessment of anxiety disorders in children and adolescents. *Clinical Psychology Review*, **20**, 453–78.

Topolski, T. D., Hewitt, J. K., Eaves, L. J. *et al.* (1997). Genetic and environment influences on child reports of manifest anxiety and symptoms of separation anxiety and overanxious disorders: a community-based twin study. *Behaviour Genetics*, **27**, 15–28.

Toren, P., Wolmer, L., Rosental, B. *et al.* (2000). Case series: brief parent-child group therapy for childhood anxiety disorders using a manual-based cognitive-behavioural technique. *Journal of the American Academy of Child and Adolescent Psychiatry*, **39**, 1309–12.

Williams, S. L. (1996). Therapeutic changes in phobic behavior are mediated by changes in perceived self-efficacy. In R. M. Rapee (ed.), *Current Controversies in the Anxiety Disorders*. New York: Guilford Press, pp. 344–68.

19

School refusal

David Heyne

Leiden University, Leiden, The Netherlands

Neville King

Monash University, Clayton, Victoria, Australia

Thomas H. Ollendick

Virginia Polytechnic University, Blacksbury, Virginia, USA

19.1 Introduction

School refusal is a persistent school attendance problem that: jeopardizes a young person's social, emotional, academic and vocational development; contributes to distress for concerned parents and school staff; and often presents a real challenge to education and mental health professionals (Kahn *et al.*, 1996). Some authors (e.g. Kearney and Silverman, 1996) use the term *school refusal behaviour* to refer to a range of attendance problems, including truancy. Others draw a distinction between school refusal as one type of attendance problem and truancy as another, using the term *school refusal* to refer to cases where difficulty attending school is associated with emotional distress (e.g. King and Bernstein, 2001), is not associated with serious antisocial behaviour (e.g. Honjo *et al.*, 2001) and involves the child usually staying at home versus being absent from home (e.g. Kameguchi and Murphy-Shigematsu, 2001). Like these authors, the authors of this chapter also prefer to distinguish between school refusal and truancy, as these often require different approaches to intervention (Berg, 2002).

Following the work of Berg and colleagues (Berg *et al.*, 1969; Bools *et al.*, 1990; Berg, 2002), school refusal is defined by: (1) reluctance or refusal to attend school; (2) the child usually remaining at home during school hours, rather than concealing the problem from parents; (3) displays of emotional upset at the prospect of attending school, which may be reflected in excessive fearfulness, temper tantrums, misery or possibly unexplained physical symptoms; (4) an

Cognitive Behaviour Therapy for Children and Families, ed. Philip J. Graham.
Published by Cambridge University Press. © Cambridge University Press 2004.

absence of severe antisocial tendencies, beyond the child's resistance to parental attempts to get them to school; and (5) reasonable parental efforts to secure the child's attendance at school, at some stage in the history of the problem. As well as differentiating between school refusal and truancy, these criteria help to distinguish between school refusal and *school withdrawal*, the latter type of attendance problem being associated with overt or covert parental support for the young person's non-attendance (cf. Blagg, 1987; Kahn and Nursten, 1962).

19.2   Phenomenology

School refusal can appear suddenly (e.g. immediately after a legitimate absence due to illness) or may develop slowly (e.g. progressing from vague complaints of dislike of school, through slowness in getting ready for school to outright refusal to attend). Absenteeism may be extensive (e.g. consistent absence for months or years at a time), sporadic (e.g. on days involving specific subjects) or non-existent (e.g. daily distress in going to school during periods of regular attendance). The emotional distress associated with school refusal may manifest in a wide variety of ways, with varying degrees of severity, at varying times and in various settings.

Behaviourally, there may be whining and temper tantrums when the young person is pressured to attend school. To avoid the distress associated with attendance, he or she may refuse to get out of bed or refuse to get into the car or bus to travel to school. Some young people threaten to run away from home or to harm themselves (Coulter, 1995; Berg, 2002). Others head towards school and then rush home in a state of anxiety before arriving there, or, having settled in well after arrival at school, re-experience distress and resist attendance when it is time for school again the following day (Berg, 2002). Somatic symptoms are frequently associated with school refusal. Common complaints include gastrointestinal symptoms (e.g. diarrhoea, nausea and vomiting), pain symptoms (e.g. headaches and back pain), cardiopulmonary symptoms (e.g. palpitation and shortness of breath) and other autonomic symptoms (e.g. fever and vertigo) (Honjo *et al.*, 2001). The cognitive component of school refusal involves distorted thinking associated with school attendance. Young people may, for example, overestimate the likelihood of anxiety-provoking situations occurring at school or harm befalling their parents, underestimate their ability to cope with situations, magnify or selectively attend to the unpleasant aspects of school attendance or misinterpret the thoughts and actions of others at school (e.g. King *et al.*, 1998a; Kearney, 2001).

Over time, the young person may become progressively withdrawn, disengaging from usual activities and refusing to have any contact with peers. Mood problems may intensify, and anxiety may generalize across situations (Torma and Halsti, 1975; Berg, 2002). The young person's self-worth can deteriorate as he or she labels him/herself as being different from peers and as he or she falls further behind academically. Through all of this, family tension and parental distress are prone to mount.

Although diagnoses are not applicable in all cases of school refusal (e.g. Berg *et al.*, 1993; Bernstein and Borchardt, 1996), many school refusers meet criteria for anxiety disorders, mood disorders or both (e.g. Last and Strauss, 1990; Bernstein, 1991). In cases where disorder-level criteria are not met, young people are still prone to experience problematic anxiety symptoms (cf. Bools *et al.*, 1990) and/or depressive symptoms (cf. Kearney, 1993). Diagnostic comorbidity is common (e.g. Bernstein and Garfinkel, 1986; Last *et al.*, 1987; Last and Strauss, 1990) and expectable age-related trends in diagnoses and symptoms are observed. For example, separation anxiety disorder is more common among younger school refusers (e.g. Last and Strauss, 1990), and adolescent school refusers are more likely to experience social phobia and possibly panic disorder (e.g. Last and Strauss, 1990; Bernstein and Borchardt, 1991) as well as depressive symptoms (e.g. Baker and Wills, 1978).

School refusal is also associated with externalizing behaviours. School refusers may become stubborn, argumentative and display aggressive behaviours when their parents attempt to get them to go to school (Berg, 2002), although more severe antisocial behaviours such as stealing and destructiveness are not characteristically shown (Berg, 2002). School refusers who consistently display multiple externalizing behaviours over time may be diagnosed with oppositional defiant disorder.

19.3   Aetiology

The aetiology of school refusal is often complex, and a helpful way to organize the array of potentially relevant factors is to consider the domains of predisposing, precipitating and perpetuating factors. Within each domain, there is likely to be a confluence of individual, family, school and community factors. Table 19.1 presents some of the factors that may be involved in the development and maintenance of school refusal.

19.4   Assessment

The heterogeneous nature of school refusal, with its varied presentations and numerous aetiological factors, points to the importance of a multi-source and

Table 19.1 Factors potentially contributing to the development and maintenance of school refusal

Development of school refusal (predisposing and precipitating factors)

Individual factors

    e.g. vulnerability to stress, anxious temperament, onset of depression

    e.g. initial absences due to health problems

    e.g. academic difficulties

Home and family factors

    e.g. illness in a parent

    e.g. marital distress or other family distress (e.g. financial difficulties, work pressures, social disconnection)

    e.g. school refusal in a sibling

    e.g. mother commencing work

School factors

    e.g. aversive experiences at school (e.g. bullying by peers, clash with teacher, social isolation)

    e.g. tests, class presentations, physical education class, etc.

    e.g. change of school/class/teacher

    e.g. insufficient experience of success/enjoyment at school

Community factors

    e.g. increased academic competitiveness

    e.g. economic factors impacting school effectiveness

    e.g. violence/traumatic events in the vicinity of the school

Maintenance of school refusal (perpetuating factors)

Individual factors

    e.g. negative reinforcement through the young person's avoidance of stressful aspects of school (e.g. being in the classroom, mixing with friends again, explaining absences, catching up with school work)

    e.g. low self-efficacy

    e.g. development or exacerbation of depression

Home and family factors

    e.g. positive reinforcement through inadvertent access to home-based items and experiences (e.g. television, computer, pets, toys, foods, outings, parental attention)

    e.g. parents' inconsistent approaches to managing non-attendance

    e.g. reduced parental effectiveness (e.g. insufficient attention to the young person's progress, ineffective use of instructions), perhaps as a result of parental distress and/or low self-efficacy

    e.g. parental attitudes reflecting relinquished responsibility, waiting until the young person chooses to return

School factors

    e.g. minimal/problematic communication between family and school

    e.g. unresponsiveness to the value of a graded approach to the young person's return to school

    e.g. uninformed and inadvertently unsupportive staff drawing attention to the young person's prior absence

Community factors

    e.g. minimal support for parents/families in addressing school refusal

    e.g. professionals' inconsistent advice/approach regarding the management of non-attendance

multi-method approach to assessment. Below, a range of assessment methods reflecting a cognitive behavioural conceptualization of school refusal are presented. Arising data are used to form and test hypotheses about the development and maintenance of the school refusal. Some of the data will be particularly useful in evaluating the effectiveness of specific interventions.

During assessment, a medical examination should first be conducted to rule out physical aetiologies, given that school refusal is often associated with somatic complaints and sometimes follows a genuine physical illness. Consultation should occur with any professionals who have already been involved in the case (e.g. general practitioner, paediatrician and school guidance officer). As well as eliciting useful assessment information, this process ultimately facilitates the implementation of a consistent management plan.

19.4.1   Clinical behavioural interviews and behavioural observations

Clinical behavioural interviews yield detailed information about target behaviours (e.g. the young person refusing to get out of bed and parental responses to the young person's tantrums) and the variables that occasion and maintain the behaviours. They also help the clinician to select from among the range of assessment procedures and instruments as presented below, and they inform the selection of additional assessment methods as required (e.g. psychoeducational testing). Guidelines for conducting interviews with school-refusing young people and their parents have been provided by Blagg (1987) and Heyne and Rollings (2002). Given that young people and their parents will often have different perspectives on the problem, the authors spend considerable time conducting separate interviews so that each may freely discuss their views (cf. Blagg, 1987). All too frequently, young people are unable or unwilling to identify reasons for their difficulties (e.g. Coulter, 1995), and so to avoid jeopardizing the establishment of a working relationship the authors refrain from asking about non-attendance too early in the assessment process, lest it exacerbate their frustration or resistance. The authors also visit the school to interview relevant staff about the young person's social, emotional, behavioural and academic functioning. Efforts are made to determine whether any of the child's fears and anxieties are reality based, such as the experience of recurrent bullying at school.

Stemming from the work of Mansdorf and Lukens (1987), the clinical behavioural interviews are supplemented with self-statement assessments, conducted separately with the school refuser and his or her parents (see Heyne and Rollings, 2002). This form of assessment helps to identify child and parent cognitions which may be associated with the development and maintenance of school refusal, and which may warrant attention during treatment. When feasible, direct observations of the young person and parents are conducted in the home and school settings, providing a source of detailed information about the antecedents and consequences of the young person's reluctance and resistance. Alternatively, parents and school staff are supported in the process of making and recording behavioural observations, using tailored monitoring diaries (see Kearney (2001) for a discussion of direct behavioural observation procedures).

19.4.2   Diagnostic interviews

Diagnostic interviews assist in developing a profile of the range and severity of difficulties experienced by the young person, and then in planning differential treatments. Silverman and Albano's (1996) Anxiety Disorders Interview Schedule for Children (ADIS-C) facilitates differential diagnosis among major disorders in the *Diagnostic and Statistical Manual of Mental Disorders* (DSM-IV; American Psychiatric Association, 1994). Designed around anxiety-related disorders in children and adolescents, it also includes sections on mood disorders and behaviour disorders. Separate interview schedules are available for use with the child (ADIS-C) and with the parents (ADIS-P), and composite diagnoses are developed based on the reports of both parties. The benefits of employing this method for diagnostic assessment need to be weighed up against the time required for use of a diagnostic interview schedule and the clinician's competence in diagnosis (see Grills and Ollendick, 2002).

19.4.3   Self-report measures and self-monitoring

A wide range of psychometrically sound self-report measures may be used to assess levels of fear, anxiety and depression experienced by young people with school refusal. Measures of fear and anxiety include: the Fear Survey Schedule for Children-Revised (FSSC-R; Ollendick, 1983) and its later version, the Fear Survey Schedule for Children-II (FSSC-II; Gullone and King, 1992); the Revised Children's Manifest Anxiety Scale (RCMAS; Reynolds and Richmond, 1978) and a newer measure of anxiety, the Spence Children's Anxiety Scale (SCAS; Spence, 1998); and more focused measures such as the Social Anxiety Scale for Children-Revised (SASC-R; La Greca and Stone, 1993). The Children's Depression Inventory (CDI; Kovacs, 1992) is commonly employed to assess depression. The Self-Efficacy Questionnaire for School Situations (SEQ-SS; Heyne *et al.*, 1998) is a self-report measure specifically designed to assess school refusers' cognitions regarding the ability to cope with potential anxiety-provoking situations like doing school work and handling peers' questions about absence from school.

Recent reviews provide detailed discussion of self-report measures for use in the assessment of school refusal (see Ollendick and King, 1998; Kearney, 2001).

Self-monitoring facilitates a more focused assessment by asking the young person to report on clinically relevant target behaviours as they occur, helping to identify the antecedents and consequences that maintain school refusal (Ollendick and King, 1998). Depending on the young person's age and compliance, self-monitoring diaries can be used for recording levels of emotional distress on school mornings, and in specific situations such as attending certain subjects or being in the school yard during lunch-times.

19.4.4   Parent- and teacher-completed measures

A variety of parent- and teacher-completed measures have been used in the assessment of school refusal. For example, the Child Behavior Checklist (CBCL; Achenbach, 1991a) assesses parent perceptions of the competencies and behaviour problems of children aged 4–18 years; the Teacher's Report Form (TRF; Achenbach, 1991b) is a corresponding measure for gaining the perspective of school staff. There is much research support for the psychometric properties of these measures, and their clinical utility is enhanced by the extensive normative data for boys and girls of varying ages, including scores for subscales such as withdrawal, social problems, anxiety/depression, somatic complaints and aggressive behaviours. Often, parents are also asked to monitor behaviours specific to the school refusal situation (e.g. the young person's daily attendance, emotional distress and levels of cooperation and resistance). Additional monitoring may occur around aspects such as parental responses to the young person's behaviour and levels of stress experienced by the family (cf. Kearney and Albano, 2000a,b).

Assessment of parent and family functioning is important in understanding the situation surrounding the young person's school refusal (cf. Kearney, 2001). When indicated by the clinical interviews, the authors ask parents to complete the Beck Depression Inventory (Beck *et al.*, 1996), the Brief Symptom Inventory (Derogatis, 1993) and the Abbreviated Dyadic Adjustment Scale (Sharpley and Rogers, 1984). Parents and adolescent school refusers are also invited to complete the general functioning subscale of the McMaster Family Assessment Device (Epstein *et al.*, 1983). (See Kearney (2001) for a review of additional parent and family measures that might be employed in the assessment of school refusal.)

19.4.5   Review of attendance record

A review of the school's attendance record provides useful information about the extent and pattern of non-attendance. Regular absences associated with certain activities (e.g. school excursions), classes (e.g. physical education classes or language classes) or days of the week (e.g. following paternal access visits) may shed light on the factors maintaining the school refusal. In chronic cases, parents may become fully cognisant of the overall extent of their child's non-attendance only when presented with the attendance record from the past months or years.

19.4.6   Systematic functional analysis

A rapid, systematic functional analysis for school refusal may be facilitated via the School Refusal Assessment Scale (SRAS; Kearney and Silverman, 1993), a child self-report measure (SRAS-C) with a corresponding parent-completed measure (SRAS-P). The SRAS-C and SRAS-P each contain 16 items assessing four functions hypothesized to maintain school refusal behaviour (as outlined in the introduction, the term 'school refusal behaviour' is used by some authors to encompass a range of attendance problems, including school refusal and truancy; however, the assessment of 'school refusal' *per se* is also facilitated by the use of the SRAS): (1) avoidance of stimuli that provoke a sense of general negative affectivity; (2) escape from aversive social or evaluative situations; (3) attention-seeking behaviour; and (4) pursuit of tangible reinforcement outside of school. The functional condition with the highest score (based on combined child and parent reports) is deemed to be the primary factor maintaining the school refusal behaviour. Prescribed treatments are indicated for each of the functional conditions (see Kearney and Albano, 2000a,b). However, to determine the most appropriate form of treatment, hypotheses arising from this functional analysis system ought to be further developed in the light of other information gathered during the assessment (cf. Kearney, 2001).

19.4.7   Integration of assessment information

The assessment information is drawn together to develop a diagnostic profile of the young person and a case formulation. The case formulation identifies the individual factors (e.g. learning history, cognitions, somatic symptoms, social skills, academic difficulties and comorbid mood problems), family factors (e.g. parental anxiety/depression and response to non-attendance) and school fac-tors (e.g. teacher support and isolation in the playground) associated with the development and maintenance of the young person's refusal to attend school, together with the strengths of the individual, the family and the school setting. This information informs the targets and process for the intervention plan which is aimed at the resumption of regular and voluntary attendance and the reduction of emotional distress. A myriad of other complexities must also be considered during assessment and treatment planning, such as the impact of socioeconomic disadvantage, single parent households and ethnocultural diversity.

Between assessment and treatment, a feedback session is conducted with the young person and the parents, often separately. The authors explain the findings of the assessment, relate these to the plans for treatment and invite comment, clarification and questions. By consulting with the young person and parents, the aim is to develop a shared understanding of the problem and to foster a collaborative problem-solving approach to treatment. Relevant school staff are also contacted and briefed on the assessment findings.

19.5   Treatment

Of the psychosocial treatment approaches used with school refusal (e.g. play therapy, pychodynamic psychotherapy, family therapy and cognitive behaviour therapy (CBT)), only CBT has been subjected to rigorous evaluation in randomized controlled clinical trials and it is currently regarded as having encouraging empirical support (King and Bernstein, 2001). CBT was found to be superior to a wait-list control condition (King *et al.*, 1998b) and at least as effective as an educational support therapy (Last *et al.*, 1998). A study evaluating the relative benefits of child-focused CBT and caregiver-focused CBT (Heyne *et al.*, 2002) lends further support to the efficacy of CBT for school refusal. An earlier clinical trial (Kennedy, 1965) and a non-randomized comparative study (Blagg and Yule, 1984) are also supportive (albeit to a lesser extent) of the more strictly behavioural approaches to treating school refusal.

The aim of early return to school is usually emphasized in behavioural and cognitive behavioural treatments (Blagg, 1987; Mansdorf and Lukens, 1987; King *et al.*, 1995; Heyne *et al.*, 2002), just as it may be in family-focused approaches (Place *et al.*, 2000) or a psychodynamic approach (see review by Want, 1983). Thus, temporary home tuition is usually contraindicated (King and Bernstein, 2001). Early return aims to curb the escalation of problems associated with further missed schoolwork, increased social isolation, lowered self-confidence and self-worth and the intensification of avoidance behaviours.

Below, the authors' CBT programme for school refusal will be outlined, comprising child therapy and work with caregivers (King *et al.*, 1998b; Heyne *et al.*, 2002). Child therapy involves the use of behavioural and cognitive procedures directly with the young person, helping them to acquire and then employ the necessary skills for coping with school return and regular attendance. Work with caregivers focuses on the role that parents and teachers can play in managing environmental contingencies at home and school – contingencies that are maintaining the school refusal problem and those that facilitate the young person's regular and voluntary school attendance. The child-, parent- and school-based interventions involve the judicious selection of and emphasis on intervention components as indicated by the diagnostic profile and case formulation. This individualized approach rests on the complex array of possible factors involved in the development and maintenance of school refusal, together with the need to be sensitive to the individuality of each child, family and school situation (cf. Barrett *et al.*, 1996).

Treatment is often conducted intensely across 4 weeks, including between six and eight sessions with the young person, five and eight sessions with the parents and one consultation and regular telephone contact with school staff. The young person and the parents are encouraged to engage in specially tailored between-session practice tasks to reinforce and generalize skills beyond the clinical setting and to effect change in the young person's behaviour in the home and school environments.

19.5.1   Child therapy

19.5.1.1   Initial phase with the young person

Typically, young people refusing to attend school are unlikely to work willingly towards school return, and the task of engaging them in an intervention programme can be challenging. The clinician may foster engagement by consistently offering empathic acknowledgement of the difficulty faced by the young person, cultivating a positive expectation that things will improve and modelling confidence in the young person and the strategies recommended. Other considerations for engaging school refusers are presented elsewhere (Heyne and Rollings, 2002; see also Chapter 5). From the outset of the intervention, the clinician models, provides instruction in and fosters the young person's use of problem-solving. Guided 'brainstorming' activities focus on anticipating challenging situations which might realistically arise, generating possible solutions for handling the situations, considering the likely outcomes of the solutions, deciding on a particular solution and planning for use of the solution (cf. Kendall *et al.*, 1992).

Training in relaxation provides the young person with an efficient means of managing and reducing anxious arousal associated with school attendance (e.g. when approaching the school grounds on the day of school return and giving class talks). In learning to identify and manage discomforting feelings, young people are better placed to confront challenging situations and to employ other skills and strategies in the process of coping with school attendance. Indications for relaxation training include elevated scores on the subscales of selected measures (e.g. the physiological subscale of the RCMAS and the somatic complaints subscales of the CBCL and TRF), together with reports of somatic complaints during clinical behavioural and diagnostic interviews. Relaxation training may

Table 19.2   Relaxation training procedures

Procedure	Description	Reference
Progressive Muscle Relaxation (PMR) Training for Older Children	Modified version of adult-based PMR script for use with young people. PMR is a process of systematically relaxing the various muscle groups in the body.	Ollendick and Cerny (1981)
Progressive Muscle Relaxation (PMR) Training for Younger Children	Uses visual imagery to engage younger children in PMR.	Koeppen (1974)
Robot–Ragdoll Technique	A variation on PMR which is useful for active children who have difficulty sitting still and engaging in the PMR routine.	Kendall *et al.* (1992)
Autogenic relaxation training	The client covertly repeats a series of physiologically orientated phrases read by the therapist, enabling the client to induce a state of mental and physical calm.	Davis *et al.* (1995)
Guided Imagery	The practitioner guides the client through a series of imagined scenes (standardized or personalized) which evoke a sense of calm and relaxation.	Examples of standardized scenes in Bourne (1990) and Rapee *et al.* (2000)
Breathing Retraining	The client learns to control their rate and depth of breathing in order to manage tension and anxiety. This is a more inconspicuous form of relaxation.	Andrews *et al.* (1994)

From Heyne *et al.* (2002).

also occur as a stress management procedure for a young person with generalized anxiety disorder, or in preparation for desensitization procedures to be employed with the young person (see below). In order to engage the young person sufficiently to help them ultimately acquire some form of cue-controlled relaxation, the clinician should identify a procedure that is both acceptable and effective for the young person (see Table 19.2).

Social skills training aimed at enhancing the young person's social competence is employed in two predominant situations. First, many school refusers report uncertainty and anxiety about handling questions from peers or teachers regarding their absence from school. Such reports are elicited via the SEQ-SS or arise through the clinical behavioural interview. Secondly, some children's skills in making and maintaining friendships or handling teasing and bullying may be underdeveloped, leaving them vulnerable to isolation and seeking to avoid the school situation. Social competencies, social withdrawal and social problems are assessed via subscales on the CBCL, TRF, SRAS and RCMAS, through interviews with parents, children and school staff and through observation in the clinical setting. More specific measures such as the SASC-R may also be used to assess aspects of social functioning. The enhancement of social competence is discussed in Chapter 23.

A vital aspect of treatment for school refusal is a focus on the young person's cognitions. Emotionally distressed school refusers may, for example, process events in a distorted manner (e.g. 'I know the teacher doesn't like me because she raises her voice'), overestimate the probability of negative events occurring (e.g. 'Mum will fall ill while I'm at school'), underestimate coping resources (e.g. 'I won't know what to do if the teacher asks me a question') and engage in negative self-evaluations (e.g. 'I'm hopeless at sport'). During assessment, indicators of the importance of cognitive therapy may come from the clinical behavioural interview with the child (including the adjunctive self-statement assessment), the diagnostic interview, self-efficacy expectations assessed via the SEQ-SS, the worry / oversensitivity subscale of the RCMAS and items in the CDI. Of course, many more indications will arise through the course of intervention with the young person.

Cognitive therapy with school refusers is aimed at modifying maladaptive cognitions in order to effect a change in the young person's emotions and behaviour, mobilizing them towards school attendance. The 'Seven Ds' is an aid in the process of conducting cognitive therapy, emphasizing key components involved in *describing* the cognitive therapy model, *detecting* cognitions, *determining* which cognitions to address, *disputing* maladaptive cognitions, *discovering* adaptive cognitions or coping statements, *doing* between-session practice tasks and *discussing* the outcome of the tasks (Heyne and Rollings, 2002). Cartoon materials are often useful in helping younger children understand the connection between thoughts, feelings and actions, and in engaging them in the process of detecting their maladaptive cognitions and discovering more adaptive cognitions (e.g. Kendall *et al.*, 1992; Barrett *et al.*, 2000). Disputational procedures more suited to the cognitive ability of many adolescents are presented elsewhere (e.g. Zarb, 1992; Beck, 1995).

19.5.1.2   Implementation phase with the young person

Naturally, exposure to school attendance constitutes a key component of CBT for school refusal. In conjunction with the above preparatory strategies, school return arrangements must be negotiated with the young person, parents and school staff. When young people have been fully absent from school (as opposed to attending sporadically), the authors aim for school return to occur midway through the intervention. This allows sufficient time for the young person to develop the above-mentioned skills during the lead up to the exposure associated with school return, and it allows opportunities for collaboratively trouble-shooting difficulties that arise during and after the return to school. With patience and persistence, it is often necessary to monitor progress and revise plans for the young person's return to school.

For many school refusers exhibiting high levels of anxiety, a graduated return to school is usually negotiated, constituting *in vivo* desensitization via exposure. This involves a step-by-step approach to conquering the anxiety elicited by school return (e.g. attending for one class on the first day, two classes the next day, etc.). The young person draws on his or her relaxation skills and cognitive coping statements to manage the anxiety associated with the successive steps. The young person's input into the development of the graded *attendance plan* is very important (see Heyne and Rollings, 2002). When the child's anxiety is very high, imaginal desensitization may need to occur prior to planned school return, perhaps incorporating emotive imagery with younger children (cf. King *et al.*, 2001).

Some young people and their families prefer that the process of school return involve full-time attendance as soon as attendance is resumed. This is usually more stressful than a graduated return to school, but it is intended to prevent or minimize the embarrassment for young people of having to explain why they are leaving school part way through the day. Rapid school return is probably more appropriate for young children with mild or recent onset school refusal.

19.5.1.3   Concluding sessions with the young person

In an effort to prevent relapse, the young person may participate in a 'Secrets to Success' activity towards the end of treatment (cf. 'My Commercial', Kendall *et al.*, 1992). The young person is given an opportunity to share their ideas about how to respond effectively to school refusal, which may be in the form of a poster, playing the 'expert in the field' during an audiotaped or videotaped mock interview or commercial or conducting a 'motivational talk' for another clinician or family members. This activity helps reinforce what the child has learned, celebrates the achievements and builds up a coping template (Kendall *et al.*, 1992) and self-esteem (Kearney and Hugelshofer, 2000). In the future, the poster or tape may serve as a prompt for the young person's successful management of setbacks.

19.5.2　Work with caregivers

19.5.2.1　Initial phase with the parents

Parents are encouraged to discuss any doubts about their child's current school or classroom placement, in order to reduce the likelihood that plans for facilitating school return become unstuck because of their ambivalence about such matters. When doubts do emerge, a problem-solving discussion takes place to consider all of the advantages and disadvantages of making changes. Anxious, indifferent or sceptical parents may also benefit, in the initial phase, from educational hand-outs describing the development and nature of school refusal (see Table 19.1 for example), emotional problems and behaviour problems, together with information about the effectiveness of current approaches to treatment. This underscores the role that parents may play in addressing school refusal and builds hope for change. Within the framework of a return to school approximately midway through treatment, parents are helped to make a decision about the best day for school return. Important factors include the availability of two adults to facilitate the young person's attendance and knowledge of the young person's timetable at school. To help create a positive experience for the child on the first day of school return, it is helpful to plan for return on a day with, for example, the least number of disliked subjects or teachers.

In the lead up to school return, the clinician helps parents to plan and institute smooth morning routines for the young person (e.g. waking up and getting showered and dressed) and to manage the young person's access to reinforcing items and experiences when at home during school hours. This reduces the secondary gain that may otherwise strengthen the young person's resolve not to attend school. Assessment of secondary gain occurs through clinical behavioural interviews and via subscale 4 on the SRAS. Parents who may give vague and imprecise instructions about school-related issues receive training in command giving, with emphasis on gaining the young person's attention and using clear and specific instructions (cf. Forehand and McMahon, 1981). Consistent with operant principles, parents are instructed in the recognition and reinforcement of the young person's appropriate coping behaviours and school attendance, and in the planned ignoring of inappropriate behaviours such as tantrums, negotiating alternative dates for attendance and somatic complaints without known organic cause (Blagg, 1987; Kearney and Roblek, 1998). Performance-based methods of modelling, rehearsal and feedback are employed during training in these behaviour management strategies, providing parents with opportunities to gain confidence and increase their competence in the use of the strategies. In time, the calm and consistent use of planned ignoring can lead to a reduction in inappropriate behaviours, while naturally occurring reinforcers in the school environment and in the broader experience of the young person supplant the need for contrived reinforcers.

Parents' use of exposure-based principles and behaviour management strategies can be applied to related problem areas in the lead up to school return. For example, the young person with separation anxiety may be exposed to progressively longer periods of separation from parents before a school return is attempted. The parents of a socially anxious child may facilitate an increase in their child's social involvement during the first half of treatment, prior to school return.

19.5.2.2   Implementation phase with the parents

During intervention, if the child has not come to the point of attending school voluntarily, parents are encouraged to consider employing a firmer approach. Having issued clear expectations and instructions regarding attendance, parents may need to escort their child to school, a role that necessitates very good planning and support (Kennedy, 1965; Kearney and Roblek, 1998). This process of 'professionally informed parental pressure' (cf. Gittelman-Klein and Klein, 1971) allows parents to block the young person's entrenched avoidance of school, and the ensuing exposure to school attendance can ultimately lead to a reduction in emotional distress and to the experience of naturally occurring positive events at school. Drawing on the clinical behavioural interview, the clinician and parents target and develop plans for handling potentially problematic situations (i.e. helping the child get out of bed and ready for school, escorting the child to school and dealing with running away). Parents often benefit from cognitive and behavioural strategies aimed at helping themselves remain calm and committed during the management of their child's non-attendance, and allowing them to model confidence in the child's ability to cope with school return. Unhelpful parental attitudes and beliefs to be addressed during cognitive therapy may include: 'my child is incapable of coping with school attendance' (e.g. Coulter, 1995); 'I shouldn't push' (e.g. Mansdorf and Lukens, 1987); and 'something has

to change in my child's mind in order for him to be able to attend school'
(e.g. Anderson *et al.*, 1998). Parental cognitions may be systematically assessed
through the parent self-statement assessment process.

19.5.2.3   Concluding sessions with the parents

Attention to relapse prevention occurs in the final session(s) via a review of
the components of intervention. Particular attention is given to those strategies found to be most useful, together with discussion about high-risk times,
indications of impending relapse and appropriate responses. The clinician may
conduct booster sessions or telephone follow-ups with the parents and young
person at those times known to be difficult, such as the return to school after a
holiday period or genuine illness, a change of school or re-arrangements at school
and examinations (cf. Blagg and Yule, 1984; Kearney and Hugelshofer, 2000).

19.5.2.4   School-based strategies for facilitating attendance

School-based strategies focus on preparatory work and behaviour management
strategies that support the young person's reintegration into the school system.
Depending on the young person's preference, classmates may be advised of the
school return and encouraged to be supportive and to refrain from probing about
non-attendance. The clinician and school staff can also explore arrangements to
accommodate the young person's special needs (e.g. reduced homework requirements, academic remediation, change of classroom and modified curriculum)
on a temporary or permanent basis. The authors have often found it critical
to ensure school staff are fully informed about the special needs of the young
person and the arrangements which have been made to accommodate them. A
memo to relevant staff reduces the possibility that, for example, the distressed
young person is questioned about prior absences or pressured to stay at school
for longer than the arranged time.

A supportive staff member is identified who might help the young person settle
in on arrival at school and familiarize them with the routine for the day, and who
can closely monitor their attendance and emotional well-being while settling
back into school. It may also be helpful to have the young person or school staff
select one or two students to act as 'buddies' who will provide peer support
during the early stages of school re-entry, and who could make contact with the
young person during subsequent absences. Engineering positive experiences for
the young person helps to make the school environment a more reinforcing
place to be, and specific reinforcement of the young person's attendance and
efforts at coping is also desirable. Staff have often been creative in constructing

Table 19.3 Possible reinforcing experiences and items in the school setting

Type of reinforcer	Examples from real-life applications
Increased access to current positives	Sports equipment
	Time on the computer
	Time in the garden
	Extra playtime with friends
	Attending extra art classes
Social and success	One-to-one support with a staff member/favourite teacher
	Special mentor lunches
	Praise
	A party with friends and year-level coordinator
	Student-centred lunch-time activities (e.g. video watching)
	Stars and stamps
	Rotating the wheels on the teacher's car
	Principal's award
Privileges	Choosing a class activity
	Feeding the fish
	Pinning up art work
	Being the stationery monitor or lunch monitor
	Being the teacher's secretary (e.g. clean/tidy teacher's desk)
Tangibles	Canteen vouchers
	Chocolate bars at the end of the day
	Magazines
	Fish and chips for the whole class for lunch
	Sparkle pens

menus of reinforcing experiences and items differentially employed in primary and secondary school settings (see Table 19.3). Staff are also encouraged to use planned ignoring of inappropriate behaviours such as pleading to go home or tantrums, employing the same supportive yet consistent approach as outlined for parents.

Just as parents may harbour unhelpful attitudes and beliefs that reduce the effectiveness of their management of school refusal, so too may school staff and other professionals (cf. Coulter, 1995). This situation necessitates a patient and sensitive approach to addressing such cognitions. Conversely, some schools readily initiate and embrace creative approaches to supporting the young person (e.g. classroom seating plans which include the absent child, class notes to the non-attending student and describing what the other students miss about them). School staff and parents are encouraged to develop close communication during intervention. This ensures clear understanding and consistency during the implementation of plans such as graded return to school or graded reintroduction to the completion of homework, it can reduce parent anxiety about how the young person is coping through the day and it allows for prompt responses to events such as the young person running away from school or signs of a setback.

19.6 Closing comments

CBT for school refusal is a brief intervention that is regarded as an acceptable approach by families and school staff (King *et al.*, 1998b; Heyne, 1999). While it is often instrumental in reducing young people's emotional distress and helping them to attend school regularly and voluntarily, adjunctive or alternative treatments are sometimes required, especially for adolescents aged 14 years and older (Heyne, 1999). Following a *stages of treatment* model (cf. Heyne *et al.*, in press), intervention might begin with CBT and, if there is only a partial response, CBT may be continued in modified form (e.g. greater attention to parental psychopathology and further adaptation to the specific needs of the depressed young person) or pharmacological intervention may be added. The combined use of CBT and pharmacological intervention may be a helpful first stage of treatment for some school refusers with comorbid severe depressive and anxiety disorders, although it is sometimes ineffective for this group (e.g. Bernstein *et al.*, 2001).

If following reasonable trials (in dose, duration and delivery) of CBT or CBT plus routinely employed pharmacological interventions there is still no response, other interventions need to be considered such as family therapy (cf. Kearney and Albano, 2000b), alternative pharmacological agents (cf. Heyne *et al.*, in press) and alternative educational settings (cf. Place *et al.*, 2000). Greater emphasis may also need to be given to wider systems beyond the family, especially when family systems are allied to the child to the extent that parental management of attendance is inhibited (see Coulter, 1995).

19.7 Acknowledgements

The authors acknowledge the support of Ms Wendy Bristow, librarian in the Victorian Child Psychiatry Training Department, for her consistently enthusiastic work in helping to access relevant literature.

This chapter is an adaptation of Heyne and King (in press).

19.8   REFERENCES

Achenbach, T. M. (1991a). *Manual for the Child Behavior Checklist/4–18 and 1991 Profile*. Burlington, VT: University of Vermont Department of Psychiatry.

(1991b). *Manual for the Teacher's Report Form and 1991 Profile*. Burlington, VT: University of Vermont Department of Psychiatry.

American Psychiatric Association (1994). *Diagnostic and Statistical Manual of Mental Disorders*, 4th edn. Washington, DC: American Psychiatric Association.

Anderson, J., King, N., Tonge, B., Rollings, S., Young, D. and Heyne, D. (1998). Cognitive-behavioural intervention for an adolescent school refuser: a comprehensive approach. *Behaviour Change*, **15**, 67–73.

Andrews, G., Crino, R., Hunt, C., Lampe, L.and Page, A. (1994). *The Treatment of Anxiety Disorders: Clinician's Guide and Patient Manuals*. Melbourne: Cambridge University Press.

Baker, H. and Wills, U. (1978). School phobia: classification and treatment. *British Journal of Psychiatry*, **132**, 492–9.

Barrett, P. M., Dadds, M. R. and Rapee, R. M. (1996). Family treatment of childhood anxiety disorders: a controlled trial. *Journal of Consulting and Clinical Psychology*, **64**, 333–42.

Barrett, P. M., Lowry, H. and Turner, C. (2000). *FRIENDS Program: Participant Workbook for Children*. Brisbane: Australian Academic Press.

Beck, J. (1995). *Cognitive Therapy: Basics and Beyond*. New York: Guilford Press.

Beck, A. T., Steer, R. A. and Brown, G. K. (1996). *Beck Depression Inventory*, 2nd edn. New York: Psychological Corporation.

Berg, I. (2002). School avoidance, school phobia, and truancy. In M. Lewis (ed.), *Child and Adolescent Psychiatry: A Comprehensive Textbook*, 3rd edn. Sydney: Lippincott Williams and Wilkins, pp. 1260–6.

Berg, I., Butler, A., Franklin, J., Hayes, H., Lucas, C. and Sims, R. (1993). DSM-III-R disorders, social factors and management of school attendance problems in the normal population. *Journal of Child Psychology and Psychiatry*, **34**, 1187–203.

Berg, I., Nichols, K. and Pritchard, C. (1969). School phobia: its classification and relationship to dependency. *Journal of Child Psychology and Psychiatry*, **10**, 123–41.

Bernstein, G. A. (1991). Comorbidity and severity of anxiety and depressive disorders in a clinic sample. *Journal of the American Academy of Child and Adolescent Psychiatry*, **30**, 43–50.

Bernstein, G. A. and Borchardt, C. M. (1991). Anxiety disorders of childhood and adolescence: a critical review. *Journal of the American Academy of Child and Adolescent Psychiatry*, **30**, 519–32.

(1996). School refusal: family constellation and family functioning. *Journal of Anxiety Disorders*, **10**, 1–19.

Bernstein, G. and Garfinkel, B. D. (1986). School phobia: the overlap of affective and anxiety disorders. *Journal of the American Academy of Child Psychiatry*, **25**, 235–41.

Bernstein, G. A., Hektner, J. M., Borchardt, C. M. and McMillan M. H. (2001). Treatment of school refusal: one-year follow-up. *Journal of the American Academy Child and Adolescent Psychiatry*, **40**, 206–13.

Blagg, N. (1987). *School Phobia and Its Treatment*. New York: Croom Helm.

Blagg, N. and Yule, W. (1984). The behavioural treatment of school refusal: a comparative study. *Behaviour Research and Therapy*, **22**, 119–27.

Bools, C., Foster, J., Brown, I. and Berg, I. (1990). The identification of psychiatric disorders in children who fail to attend school: a cluster analysis of a non-clinical population. *Psychological Medicine*, **20**, 171–81.

Bourne, E. J. (1990). *The Anxiety and Phobia Workbook*. Oakland, CA: New Harbinger Publications Inc.

Coulter, S. (1995). School refusal, parental control and wider systems: lessons from the management of two cases. *Irish Journal of Psychological Medicine*, **12**, 146–9.

Davis, M., Eshelman, E. and McKay, M. (1995). *The Relaxation and Stress Reduction Workbook*. Oakland, CA: New Harbinger Publications.

Derogatis, L. R. (1993). *The Brief Symptom Inventory*, 2nd edn. Riderwood, MD: Clinical Psychometric Research.

Epstein, N. B., Baldwin, L. M. and Bishop, D. S. (1983). The McMaster Family Assessment Device. *Journal of Marital and Family Therapy*, **9**, 171–80.

Forehand, R. L. and McMahon, R. J. (1981). *Helping the Noncompliant Child: A Clinician's Guide to Parent Training*. New York: Guilford Press.

Gittelman-Klein, R. and Klein, D. F. (1971). Controlled imipramine treatment of school phobia. *Archives of General Psychiatry*, **25**, 204–7.

Grills, A. E. and Ollendick, T. H. (2002). Issues in parent-child agreement: the case of structured diagnostic interviews. *Clinical Child and Family Psychology Review*, **5**, 57–83.

Gullone, E. and King, N. J. (1992). Psychometric evaluation of a revised fear survey schedule for children and adolescents. *Journal of Child Psychology and Psychiatry*, **33**, 987–98.

Heyne, D. (1999). *Evaluation of Child Therapy and Caregiver Training in the Treatment of School Refusal*, PhD dissertation. Melbourne: Monash University.

Heyne, D. and King, N. J. (in press). Treatment of school refusal. In P. Barrett and T. H. Ollendick (eds.), *Handbook of Interventions that Work with Children and Adolescents: From Prevention to Treatment*. London: John Wiley and Sons.

Heyne, D. and Rollings, S. (2002). *School Refusal*. Oxford: BPS Blackwell.

Heyne, D., King, N. J. and Tonge, B. (in press). School refusal. In T. H. Ollendick and J. March (eds.), *Phobic and Anxiety Disorders in Children and Adolescents: A Clinician's Guide to Effective Psychosocial and Pharmacological Interventions*. Oxford: Oxford University Press.

Heyne, D., King, N. J., Tonge, B. J. and Cooper, H. (2002). School refusal: description and management. *New Ethicals Journal*, **5**, 63–9.

Heyne, D., King, N. J., Tonge, B. *et al.* (1998). The Self-Efficacy Questionnaire for School Situations: development and psychometric evaluation. *Behaviour Change*, **15**, 31–40.

(2002). Evaluation of child therapy and caregiver training in the treatment of school refusal. *Journal of the American Academy of Child and Adolescent Psychiatry*, **41**, 687–95.

Honjo, S., Nishide, T., Niwa, S. *et al.* (2001). School refusal and depression with school inattendance in children and adolescents: comparative assessment between the Children's Depression Inventory and somatic complaints. *Psychiatry and Clinical Neurosciences*, **55**, 629–34.

Kahn, J. and Nursten, J. (1962). School refusal: a comprehensive view of school phobia and other failures of school attendance. *American Journal of Orthopsychiatry*, **32**, 707–18.

Kahn, J., Nursten, J. and Carroll, H. C. M. (1996). An overview. In I. Berg and J. Nursten (eds.), *Unwillingly to School*. London: Gaskell, pp. 159–73.

Kameguchi, K. and Murphy-Shigematsu, S. (2001). Family psychology and family therapy in Japan. *American Psychologist*, **56**, 65–70.

Kearney, C. A. (1993). Depression and school refusal behavior: a review with comments on classification and treatment. *Journal of School Psychology*, **31**, 267–79.

(2001). *School Refusal Behavior in Youth: A Functional Approach to Assessment and Treatment*. Washington, DC: American Psychological Association.

Kearney, C. A. and Albano, A. M. (2000a). *When Children Refuse School: A Cognitive-Behavioral Therapy Approach – Parent Workbook*. San Antonio, TX: The Psychological Corporation.

(2000b). *When Children Refuse School: A Cognitive-Behavioral Therapy Approach – Therapist Guide*. San Antonio, TX: The Psychological Corporation.

Kearney, C. A. and Hugelshofer, D. S. (2000). Systemic and clinical strategies for preventing school refusal behavior in youth. *Journal of Cognitive Psychotherapy*, **14**, 51–65.

Kearney, C. A. and Roblek, T. L. (1998). Parent training in the treatment of school refusal behavior. In J. M. Briesmeister and C. E. Schaefer (eds.), *Handbook of Parent Training: Parents as Co-therapists for Children's Behavior Problems*. New York: John Wiley and Sons, Inc., pp. 225–56.

Kearney, C. A. and Silverman, W. K. (1993). Measuring the function of school refusal behavior: the School Refusal Assessment Scale. *Journal of Clinical Child Psychology*, **22**, 85–96.

(1996). The evolution and reconciliation of taxonomic strategies for school refusal behavior. *Clinical Psychology: Science and Practice*, **3**, 339–54.

Kendall, P. C., Chansky, T. E., Kane, M. T. *et al.* (1992). *Anxiety Disorders in Youth: Cognitive-Behavioral Interventions*. Boston: Allyn and Bacon.

Kennedy, W. A. (1965). School phobia: rapid treatment of fifty cases. *Journal of Abnormal Psychology*, **70**, 285–9.

King, N. J. and Bernstein, G. A. (2001). School refusal in children and adolescents: a review of the past ten years. *Journal of the American Academy of Child and Adolescent Psychiatry*, **40**, 197–205.

King, N. J., Heyne, D., Gullone, E. and Molloy, G. N. (2001). Usefulness of emotive imagery in the treatment of childhood phobias: clinical guidelines, case examples and issues. *Counselling Psychology Quarterly*, **14**, 95–101.

King, N. J., Ollendick, T. H. and Tonge, B. J. (1995). *School Refusal: Assessment and Treatment*. Boston: Allyn and Bacon.

King, N. J., Ollendick, T. H., Tonge, B. J. *et al.* (1998a). School refusal: an overview. *Behaviour Change*, **15**, 5–15.

King, N. J., Tonge, B. J., Heyne, D. *et al.* (1998b). Cognitive-behavioral treatment of school-refusing children: a controlled evaluation. *Journal of the American Academy of Child and Adolescent Psychiatry*, **37**, 375–403.

Koeppen, A. S. (1974). Relaxation training for children. *Elementary School Guidance and Counseling*, 14–21.

Kovacs, M. (1992). *Children's Depression Inventory*. New York: Multi-Health Systems, Inc.

La Greca, A. M. and Stone, W. L. (1993). Social Anxiety Scale for Children – Revised: factor structure and concurrent validity. *Journal of Clinical Child Psychology*, **22**, 17–27.

Last, C. G. and Strauss, C. C. (1990). School refusal in anxiety-disordered children and adolescents. *Journal of the American Academy of Child and Adolescent Psychiatry*, **29**, 31–5.

Last, C. G., Hansen, C. and Franco, N. (1998). Cognitive-behavioral treatment of school phobia. *Journal of the American Academy of Child and Adolescent Psychiatry*, **37**, 404–11.

Last, C. G., Strauss, C. C. and Francis, G. (1987). Comorbidity among childhood anxiety disorders. *Journal of Nervous and Mental Disease*, **175**, 726–30.

Mansdorf, I. J. and Lukens, E. (1987). Cognitive-behavioral psychotherapy for separation anxious children exhibiting school phobia. *Journal of the American Academy of Child and Adolescent Psychiatry*, **26**, 222–5.

Ollendick, T. H. (1983). Reliability and validity of the Revised Fear Survey Schedule for Children (FSSC-R). *Behaviour Research and Therapy*, **21**, 685–92.

Ollendick, T. H. and Cerny, J. A. (1981). *Clinical Behavior Therapy with Children*. New York: Plenum Press.

Ollendick, T. H. and King, N. J. (1998). Assessment practices and issues with school-refusing children. *Behaviour Change*, **15**, 16–30.

Place, M., Hulsmeier, J., Davis, S. and Taylor, E. (2000). School refusal: a changing problem which requires a change of approach? *Clinical Child Psychology and Psychiatry*, **5**, 345–55.

Rapee, R., Spence, S., Cobham, V. and Wignall, A. (2000). *Helping your Anxious Child: A Step-By-Step Guide for Parents*. Oakland, CA: New Harbinger Publications.

Reynolds, C. R. and Richmond, B. O. (1978). What I think and feel: a revised measure of children's manifest anxiety. *Journal of Abnormal Child Psychology*, **6**, 271–80.

Sharpley, C. F. and Rogers, H. J. (1984). Preliminary validation of the abbreviated Spanier Dyadic Adjustment Scale: some psychometric data regarding a screening test of marital adjustment. *Educational and Psychological Measurement*, **44**, 1045–50.

Silverman, W. K. and Albano, A. M. (1996). *Anxiety Disorders Interview Schedule for DSM-IV, Child and Parent Versions*. San Antonio, TX: Psychological Corporation.

Spence, S. (1998). A measure of anxiety symptoms among children. *Behaviour Research and Therapy*, **36**, 545–66.

Torma, S. and Halsti, A. (1975). Factors contributing to school phobia and truancy. *Psychiatria Fennica*, **76**, 209–20.

Want, J. H. (1983). School-based intervention strategies for school phobia: a ten-step 'common sense' approach. *The Pointer*, **27**, 27–32.

Zarb, J. (1992). *Cognitive-Behavioral Assessment and Therapy with Adolescents*. New York: Brunner/Mazel.

20

Post-traumatic stress disorders

William Yule, Patrick Smith and Sean Perrin

Institute of Psychiatry, London, UK

Research over the last three decades has shown that children and adolescents who have been exposed to extreme stressors manifest a range of short- and long-term reactions, including anxiety, fears and depression, as well as post-traumatic stress disorder (PTSD). The diagnosis was initially controversial, particularly as applied to children, but has proven to be a useful framework for describing and understanding children's reactions to a variety of life-threatening experiences. This in turn has led to the refinement of interventions for children; broadly based cognitive behavioural therapies (CBTs) within a multi-modal, family-based approach are the treatment of choice.

20.1 Post-traumatic stress reactions in children and adolescents

PTSD was first recognized by the American Psychiatric Association in the third edition of the *Diagnostic and Statistical Manual* (American Psychiatric Association, 1980); and in the 1987 revision it was acknowledged that it can also occur in children. The most recent edition, DSM-IV (American Psychiatric Association, 1994), describes in more detail the way in which a number of symptoms may manifest in children. PTSD is defined as: (1) exposure to an event in which the person experienced, witnessed or was confronted with the actual or threatened death or serious injury, or a threat to the physical integrity of self or others, and in which the person's response involved intense fear, helplessness or horror; (2) persistent re-experiencing of the event; (3) persistent avoidance of related stimuli or numbing of responsiveness; and (4) persistent symptoms of increased arousal.

The World Health Organization's *International Classification of Diseases (10th Edition)* (ICD-10) (World Health Organization, 1992) now also recognizes PTSD as a disorder, but places different emphasis on the symptoms required to meet the criteria for a diagnosis. Specifically, ICD-10 states that symptoms of emotional numbing are not necessary for the diagnosis of PTSD, although it can be a frequent accompaniment to the disorder. Both DSM and ICD are very adult orientated, but given the wide recognition that symptoms of emotional numbing are both rare and difficult to determine in children and adolescents, then the ICD criteria are somewhat more appropriate for children.

Work with children who have survived a variety of life-threatening experiences has demonstrated that they do indeed show this tripartite grouping of symptoms – re-experiencing, avoidance and increased arousal. Cardinal symptoms manifest differently at different ages, and a range of other reactions is also common (e.g. Terr, 1979; Kinzie *et al.*, 1986; McFarlane, 1987; Yule and Williams, 1990; Pynoos *et al.*, 1993; Vogel and Vernberg, 1993; La Greca *et al.*, 2002).

Most children are troubled by repetitive, intrusive thoughts about the trauma. Such thoughts can occur at any time, but particularly when trying to fall asleep. At other times, intrusive thoughts and images are triggered off by reminders in the environment. Bad dreams and nightmares are common. Younger children may show repetitive play and drawing involving themes related to the traumatic event. Many children develop fears associated with specific aspects of the traumatic event, with phobic levels of avoidance to trauma-related stimuli and reminders. Children may avoid thinking about the event because it is overwhelmingly distressing. Survivors often experience a pressure to talk about their experiences, but find it very difficult to talk with parents and peers. Child survivors can become very alert to danger in their environment, being adversely affected by reports of other related traumatic events. Sleep disturbances are very common, particularly within the first few weeks of the event, and children often wake through the sleep cycle. Separation difficulties are frequent, even among teenagers. Many children become much more irritable and angry with both parents and peers, and younger children are likely to show regressive and anti-social behaviours. Children commonly experience difficulties in concentration, especially in school work.

Children also report a number of cognitive changes. Post-trauma, many feel that the world is a much more dangerous place. Survivors learn that life is fragile and may not see themselves as living to adulthood. Life priorities frequently change in response to trauma. Some children feel that they should live each day to the full and not make any plans for the future. Others realize that they have been over-concerned with materialistic or petty matters and resolve to rethink their values, frequently taking on the image of themselves as a helper to others. Many experience 'survivor guilt', attributing blame to themselves about others dying or being seriously injured and thinking that they should have done more to help others to survive. In addition, a range of other reactions is also common, including depression, anxiety, oppositional behaviour and prolonged grief reactions.

Scheeringa and colleagues (Scheeringa and Zeanah, 1995; Scheeringa *et al.*, 1995) have developed an alternate set of criteria based on DSM-IV for diagnosing PTSD in infants and young children (those <4 years of age). While currently under investigation and not in widespread use, they may prove useful in guiding the reader towards some of the developmental issues of importance to traumatized children (see also Vernberg and Varela, 2001). Further consideration of developmental aspects of PTSD are to be found in Salmon and Bryant (2002) and Meiser-Stedman (2002).

20.2   The incidence and prevalence of PTSD in children

Following initial scepticism that children develop PTSD, many studies of survivors of specific disasters appeared (see reviews in Vogel and Vernberg, 1993; Shannon *et al.*, 1994; Pfefferbaum, 1997; Yule *et al.*, 1999). These indicated that, where reasonably standard assessment had been undertaken, the incidence of PTSD in survivors was often in the range of 30–60%. More recently, studies of child survivors of road traffic accidents, again using standardized methods, report that around 25–30% develop PTSD (Yule, 2000). Thus, a substantial minority of children develop PTSD; at the same time, a majority are resilient and do not develop PTSD. Thus, the experience of a traumatic event is necessary but not sufficient to cause PTSD.

One of the largest studies of adolescents following a disaster has been the study of survivors of the sinking of the cruise ship, *Jupiter*, in 1988. Out of nearly 400 children on board, 200 were traced and systematically assessed some 5–8 years later (Yule *et al.*, 2000). Fifty-two per cent were found to have developed PTSD, mainly in the first few weeks after the sinking. In keeping with Meichenbaum's (1994) view, there were very few cases of late-onset PTSD. About one-third recovered within 1 year of onset, but one-quarter still suffered from the disorder for over 5 years, with 34% still meeting criteria 5–8 years after the sinking. Thus, not only did the survivors of this disaster develop higher rates of PTSD than had previously been recorded, the problems remained over many years in a substantial minority of cases. Even so, it has to be stressed that many children did not develop PTSD and, of those who did, most appear to have recovered spontaneously.

The follow-up study of *Jupiter* survivors established that the adolescents also developed a wide range of other psychiatric disorders (Bolton *et al.*, 2000). They showed considerably raised rates of anxiety and affective disorders compared with controls; rates of diagnosis were higher in females than males. The disorders were especially raised among those children who had also developed PTSD.

20.3   Behavioural and cognitive accounts of PTSD

It is apparent from the above description that children can and do develop PTSD, but it is becoming clearer that: (1) children's reactions range more broadly than the narrow confines prescribed in DSM (American Psychiatric Association, 1994); (2) far from all exposed children go on to develop PTSD (e.g. Schwarz and Kowalski, 1991; Yule *et al.*, 2000); and (3) most recover without treatment.

Research over the past decade has cast light on the risk, protective and maintaining factors in childhood PTSD, indicating that the aetiology and course of PTSD in childhood are complex functions of developmental stage, pre-exposure history (e.g. Udwin *et al.*, 2000), temperament, family functioning (McFarlane, 1987; Bryce *et al.*, 1989; Smith *et al.*, 2001), objective trauma severity (Pynoos *et al.*, 1987; Kuterovac *et al.*, 1994), post-trauma coping style and social support (Vernberg *et al.*, 1996), nature of the trauma memory laid down (Ehlers *et al.*, 2003), attributional style and misappraisals of the event (Joseph *et al.*, 1993), appraisals of the symptoms (Ehlers *et al.*, 2003; R. Meiser-Stedman, unpublished data), thought control strategies (Aaron *et al.*, 1999; Ehlers *et al.*, 2003) and reactions to secondary adversity (cf. Pynoos, 1994). With this broad context in mind, several classes of model have been proposed to account for the development and maintenance of PTSD symptomatology. Most relevant to CBTs are those derived from learning theory (e.g. Keane *et al.*, 1985), and those based on information processing theory (e.g. Foa *et al.*, 1989), particularly the recent emphasis on appraisal and attitude to the event.

Learning theory has been fundamental in formulating interventions for PTSD (see below), but cannot help in explaining individual differences in reactions (Foa *et al.*, 1989). Information processing models seek to do this; recognizing that stressors cannot be completely defined in objective terms (Rachman, 1980), these models take into account individual differences in threat appraisal, attributions and the meaning ascribed to trauma. Common to most cognitive conceptualizations is the notion that individuals bring to the traumatic event a set of beliefs and models of the world, themselves and others (Janoff-Bulman, 1985, 1992). Exposure to trauma provides information which is incompatible with these models and yet is highly salient. Post-traumatic reactions result when there is a failure to integrate this new information into pre-existing meaning structures (see Dalgliesh, 1999). Foa and Kozak (1986) give an example of one such model.

Although developed from work with traumatized adults, there is emerging evidence that the role of threat appraisal, attributional processes and attitudinal changes central to cognitive accounts of PTSD in adults are also important factors which mediate the re-integration of traumatic memories in children. In line with adult work (e.g. Foa *et al.*, 1991; Thrasher *et al.*, 1994), Moradi (1996) has reported a specific attentional bias to trauma-related material in children with PTSD, using a modified Stroop task. This finding has recently been replicated by Ribchester (2001) in a study of children who developed PTSD following a road traffic accident. Indeed, scores on the Stroop task proved better predictors of the development of PTSD than did more traditional measures of severity of the accident. Attributional processes can also mediate symptoms. In young survivors of a shipping accident, Joseph *et al.* (1993) found that more internal and controllable attributions were associated with intrusive thoughts and depressive feelings 1 year after the accident. Consistent with the adult literature regarding the 'shattering' of pre-trauma assumptions (Janoff-Bulman, 1992), Johnson *et al.* (1996) report evidence of attitudinal changes in children who survived an earthquake, which were related specifically to PTSD symptomatology.

By far and away the most important development as far as theoretical models are concerned in the past decade has been the publication of the more explicitly cognitive models of Brewin (2001) and Ehlers and Clark (2000). Brewin emphasizes different memory processes, and in particular notes that, whereas most normal memories are verbally encoded and accessible, traumatic memories are more often laid down in unprocessed ways and are largely situationally accessible. This distinction between SAMs (situationally accessible memories) and VAMs (verbally accessible memories) implies that, in order to alter the vivid SAMs, it is necessary in treatment to have them verbally encoded so that more normal patterns of memory decay can occur.

Ehlers and Clark (2000) point to an important puzzle in how PTSD is conceptualized and classified. DSM classifies PTSD as an anxiety disorder and yet, unlike other anxiety disorders that are characterized by faulty appraisals of an impending threat, PTSD is more accurately described as a disorder in which there is a problem with the *memory* of an event that has already happened. This formulation emphasizes both the original appraisal of the traumatic event and the subsequent disturbances in autobiographical memory. Various associated reactions prevent normal resolution of these difficulties so that cognitive therapy targets both the faulty appraisals and the poor elaboration and contextualization of the memory.

Three factors are seen in the Ehlers and Clark model as influencing the development and the maintenance of PTSD. These are, first, *trauma memory deficits*.

The memory is poorly elaborated and not well integrated into autobiographical memory. Both incomplete cognitive processing at the time and later cognitive avoidance result in the fragmented memory remaining unchanged. 'Data driven processing' – concentrating on the sensory aspects of the event rather than its meaning – is a significant indicator of incomplete cognitive processing of the emotional reaction. Secondly, there are *appraisals*, in which excessively negative appraisals of the event lead to a sense of current threat that is not justified. Thirdly, there are *maintaining behaviours and cognitive strategies.* Thought suppression, avoidance, rumination and persistent dissociation are all examples of dysfunctional strategies that aim to control the reactions to the traumatic event but which only serve to maintain them. Indices of these cognitive variables were found to increase the accuracy of predicting which children would develop and continue to have PTSD following road traffic accidents (Ehlers *et al.*, 2003). The maintaining factors are, therefore, prime targets in CBT with children.

Behavioural and cognitive accounts of PTSD are broadly compatible. Both imply that exposure to trauma-related cues and memories in tolerable doses is necessary to reduce PTSD symptoms, and this forms the basis for cognitive behavioural interventions. Cognitive therapies therefore target the fragmentation of the trauma memory. Children are encouraged to relate what happened and assisted not only to fill in any gaps but, more importantly, to put the memory in a time-coded context (among other things to tell themselves that it happened in the past and is no longer a current threat). Children's misappraisals are challenged and they are helped to realize (when true) that they were not to blame. Symptoms are clearly identified, labelled, normalized and explained. Dysfunctional coping strategies such as cognitive or behavioural avoidance are identified and alternatives developed. Finally, it is important to help parents reconstrue their beliefs about the traumatic event and its possible consequences. As far as practicable, parents should be involved as co-therapists in any treatment.

20.4 Assessing PTSD in children and adolescents

Because PTSD overlaps several domains of functioning, assessment is necessarily broad and incorporates direct interview with the child, information gathering from family and teachers and the use of self-report inventories and diaries.

When interviewing children, it is important to remember that often this will be the first time they have discussed the event in detail. In some senses, then, the first interview comprises imaginal exposure (see below) and must be handled with care. Pynoos and Eth (1986) describe in detail a broadly applicable technique for interviewing young children shortly after they have witnessed a traumatic event. The therapist must be skilled in balancing the needs of obtaining accurate information while at the same time ensuring that the first interview is a therapeutic one.

A number of standardized self-report measures and semi-structured interviews are now available (see McNally, 1991; Nader et al., 1994; Saylor and DeRoma, 2002 for comprehensive reviews). Probably the most widely used measure of PTSD symptomatology is the 'impact of event scale' (IES) (Horowitz et al., 1979) which assesses symptoms of intrusion and avoidance, and this has been used with children as young as 8 years old (Yule and Williams, 1990; Yule and Udwin, 1991). However, the 15-item version had some items that were too difficult for children to use so that, following various factor analytical studies, a new child-friendly, 13-item version has been developed (Children and War Foundation, 2002; Smith et al., 2002). The Post-Traumatic Diagnostic Scale (PDS) (Foa et al., 1997) not only covers all 17 DSM items listed as the major symptoms of PTSD as present in children and adolescents but it also provides a continuous scale that is intended to be sensitive to change and thus useful during therapy.

It is usual to screen for comorbidity, and commonly used measures of childhood depression, anxiety and fears include the Birleson Depression Inventory (Birleson, 1981), the Children's Manifest Anxiety Scale (Reynolds and Richmond, 1978) and the Fear Survey Schedule for Children (Ollendick, 1983). Semi-structured interviews based on DSM criteria can aid the interviewer in diagnosing PTSD. The Clinician Administered PTSD Scale for Children (CAPS-C; Nader et al., 1994), the Diagnostic Interview Schedule for Children (DISC; Shaffer et al., 1996), the Diagnostic Interview for Children and Adolescents Revised (DICA; Reich et al., 1991) and the Anxiety Disorders Interview Schedule (ADIS-C, Silverman and Albano, 1996) all require the interviewer to be trained in the administration of the scale and have been shown to possess adequate validity and reliability. Unfortunately, there has been a dearth of standardized approaches to the assessment of stress reactions in children under 8 years of age. While children aged between 3 and 8 years can often give adequate verbal responses to questions from standardized measures used with older children, there is a need to develop measures particularly suited to young children.

Given the finding that in both adults (Ehlers and Steil, 1995) and children (Ehlers et al., 2003) measures of cognitive distortion have been shown to account for a very large proportion of the variance in predicting who develops PTSD, then a children's version of the Post-traumatic Cognitions Inventory (PCTI) (Foa et al., 1999) should become a very useful process measure to include, but it is still being developed. The modified Stroop task (Moradi et al., 1999; Ribchester, 2001) shows considerable promise as a way of monitoring cognitive processing and predicting response to treatment, but is still too specialized for routine clinical use.

Comprehensive interview with the child's carers is necessary if treatment formulation and planning is to be successful. Most semi-structured diagnostic interviews include both child and parent versions which allow the interviewer to cover all symptoms systematically with carers. This is particularly important where the symptom may be of a particularly embarrassing nature or where the child may be unaware of their behaviour. Beyond coverage of current symptom state, a full pretrauma history from carers will help in understanding: the child's usual reactions to stress and his or her ways of coping; whether current symptomatology is in part a function of prior temperament; what changes in behaviour the traumatic event precipitated; and the appropriate treatment goals to set. Taking the child's developmental level into account will allow one to assess which, if any, of the presenting complaints are normal age-appropriate behaviours (for example, separation anxiety), as well as guiding the choice of treatment strategies. Given the important mediating role of parental reactions and fears (e.g. McFarlane, 1987), assessment of all family members is usually necessary to determine whether adults or siblings also require intervention and to advise carers on management of their children.

Finally, effective intervention will depend also on a thorough assessment of the child or family's living situation. In cases where the traumatic event is relatively discrete and the family remains intact (such as in some road traffic accidents), crucial family resources will still be available to the child. In cases where other family members have been involved in the traumatic event, work with them will probably be necessary in order to assist them to help their children more effectively. In yet other cases – e.g. where the child has suffered a parental bereavement – very practical issues of social welfare will arise. In situations of ongoing community violence or armed conflict, taking account of the context in which the child is living will allow judgement as to whether, when and what kind of intervention is most appropriate.

20.5 Treatment

Derived from behavioural and cognitive models of PTSD, at the core of CBT treatment is the use of imaginal and *in vivo* exposure techniques within a safe therapeutic environment (Keane *et al.*, 1985) to allow adequate emotional processing of traumatic memories (Rachman, 1980). The problem for the clinician is how to help the survivor remember and re-experience the event and the emotions that it engenders in such a way that the distress can be mastered rather than magnified. This will depend foremost on the establishment of a safe and trusting environment in which the traumatic event can be remembered and discussed. Therapists must be prepared to ask children about the most difficult aspects of the traumatic experience, but at the same time ensure that exposure to traumatic memories is paced in such a way that the child does not experience overwhelming anxiety. For many children, talking directly about the traumatic event may be too difficult and other means of accessing traumatic memories must be found. Asking children to draw their experiences often assists in the recall of both the event and the accompanying emotions (Pynoos and Eth, 1986) and, with younger children, play may be similarly used (Misch et al., 1993).

Imaginal and *in vivo* exposure remain core components of CBT. Children are asked to recount what happened to them and to rate how upset they feel during this. Therapists watch the child closely to note when they might be blocking on particular 'hot spots' in the narrative and will then return to those parts of the memory. Saigh (1987a) was the first to show that, as Rachman (1980) had predicted, longer exposure sessions than normal are needed if desensitization and symptom reduction is to occur. Saigh (1992) has subsequently summarized a five-stage intervention process involving education, imagery training, relaxation training, the presentation of anxiety-provoking scenes and debriefing, and Saigh *et al.* (1996) have discussed the use of flooding treatment for PTSD in children in greater detail.

The most recent developments have elaborated on the cognitive processing of the emotional reactions, informed by findings from experimental cognitive psychology of memory and emotions. P. Smith and colleagues (unpublished data) have developed a ten-session, CBT treatment manual for children and adolescents with PTSD This manual is currently undergoing evaluation as part of a randomized controlled trial by the authors and is broadly based on the cognitive behavioural model of PTSD set forth by Ehlers and Clark (2000). The treatment has five main goals: (1) trauma memories need to be elaborated and integrated into autobiographical memory so that re-experiencing symptoms are reduced; (2) misappraisals of the trauma and/or of PTSD symptoms need to be modified so that the sense of current threat is reduced; (3) dysfunctional coping strategies that prevent memory elaboration, exacerbate symptoms or hinder a reassessment of problematic appraisals need to be eliminated; (4) maladaptive beliefs of the parents with respect to the traumatic event and its sequelae need to be identified and modified; and (5) parents need to be recruited as co-therapists.

Very often, as part of the traumatic reaction and of avoidance of reminders of the event, children will have restricted their previous activities. Throughout treatment, they will be encouraged to 'reclaim their lives' by participating in enjoyable activities. These activities may be set as part of the weekly home-work. The exposure part of treatment will usually take the form of imaginal reliving. The child is encouraged to tell what happened but also to concentrate on how they felt at the time, what they were thinking and what other sensa-tions they experienced. As their accounts are developed, so the accounts will be more elaborated and the memories put in a correct time context. The session is audiotaped and the child is given a copy to listen to as part of between-session homework. In part of each session, progress is reviewed with the parents and they are given the rationale for each stage of therapy.

In summary, therapeutic exposure in the context of a safe and trusting rela-tionship is at the heart of CBT for treating PTSD in children. Care must be taken that exposure sessions are sufficiently long for desensitization to occur and for emotional processing to be promoted – repetitive retelling is not enough alone. In addition, depending on the age of the child, the time since the traumatic event and the pattern of symptom presentation, a variety of other techniques are commonly used, both to target particularly distressing symptoms and to bolster coping strategies for the future. We have concentrated in this chapter on individual work within a family context, but it should be noted that a variety of other cognitive behaviourally derived interventions, such as critical incident stress debriefing, a preventative intervention (Dyregrov, 1991) and group therapy (e.g. Galante and Foa, 1986; Yule and Udwin, 1991) are advocated, with the choice of treatment strategy depending mainly on the nature of the traumatic event and the time since its occurrence. Moreover, a manual has been developed to provide basic help to children affected by wars and natural disasters (Smith *et al.*, 1999; Smith *et al.*, 2002; cf. www.childrenandwar.org). Initial results from using this in the field have been very positive.

20.6 Efficacy of treatment

CBT involving prolonged exposure to traumatic cues and treatments aimed at anxiety management were reported to be effective in reducing PTSD symptoms in rigorously controlled investigations of PTSD in adults (see Foa and Meadows, 1997 and Olasov-Rothbaum *et al.*, 2000 for reviews). Research on CBT in children with PTSD has lagged behind its adult counterpart (see Vernberg and Vogel, 1993; Cohen *et al.*, 2000).

Some of the most rigorously controlled investigations of CBT published to date have been carried out with sexually abused children. Berliner and Saunders (1996) found that the addition of CBT interventions did not improve the effectiveness of the more traditional group therapy. By way of contrast, Deblinger *et al.* (1996)

found group-administered CBT to be superior to traditional group therapy, particularly when it involved the parents.

Cohen and Mannarino (1996, 1997, 1998) conducted two randomized controlled trials of CBT in sexually abused children with mixed results. In the first study with 68 sexually abused preschoolers, a trauma-focused CBT intervention for the child and parent together produced better results than a non-directive supportive therapy condition involving the preschooler only, and these results were maintained at 6- and 12-month follow-ups (Cohen and Mannarino, 1997). In a subsequent randomized trial with 49 older children aged 7–14 years, while CBT was superior to non-directive supportive therapy in reducing depression and improving social competence, no group differences were found on the measure of PTSD (Cohen and Mannarino, 1998). Similarly, Celeano et al. (1996) randomly assigned 32 sexually abused, school-age children to an eight-session CBT group or treatment as usual, and found no group differences in PTSD symptoms. King et al. (2000) treated 36 sexually abused children aged 5–17 years in one of three conditions: CBT with child alone; a family CBT; wait list control. Active treatment proved better than wait list and improvements were maintained at 12 weeks, but the involvement of parents did not increase the efficacy of treatment. For a review of less well-controlled and case studies, see King et al. (1999).

Goenjian et al. (1997) compared CBT with no treatment for traumatized children following an earthquake in Armenia. School-based intervention involved group discussion about the trauma, relaxation and desensitization, grief work and normalization of responses, and was found to be superior to no-treatment on self-report measures of PTSD and distress. The intervention did not reduce depression in the treated group but children in the no-treatment, comparison schools became more depressed over the period of study.

March et al. (1998) tested the efficacy of an 18-week, group-administered CBT package for PTSD in 17 older children and adolescents who had suffered a single incident trauma. Eight of the 14 subjects who completed the treatment (57%) were free of PTSD at the end of treatment and another four were free of PTSD at 6-month follow-up (an overall recovery rate of 86%). Saigh (1987a,b, 1989) has produced a series of single-case, multiple-baseline studies demonstrating the effectiveness of prolonged imaginal exposure for children with PTSD arising from interpersonal violence and war.

On the premise that prevention is better than cure, there have been a number of studies of adults exposed to traumatic events in which early, crisis-oriented interventions were used. The most clearly described intervention has been Mitchell's Critical Incident Stress Debriefing, but there has been considerable debate about the overall efficacy of that and other early interventions that have employed radically different models and yet also been termed 'debriefing' (see Raphael and Wilson, 2000; Dyregrov, 2001 for a discussion of the issues). Few outcome studies of early intervention have been conducted with children. Yule (1992) observed that children who attended debriefing meetings after a shipping accident fared better on a range of outcome measures than children who were not offered such help. Inferences from this uncontrolled study must be limited, however, since the debriefing group also received additional treatment. Better evidence comes from Stallard and Law's (1993) uncontrolled trial of debriefing showing significant improvements on standardized self-report measures in a small group of young children involved in a road traffic accident. At present, it is not known whether all survivors benefit or when is best to offer such debriefing (Yule, 2001).

20.7 Future research

Further research is needed in a number of areas. Refinement of the phenomenology and long-term course of post-traumatic stress reactions by age and type of trauma is needed, but hampered at present by the lack of age-appropriate standardized measures for younger children. Analysis of the way that children explain and ascribe meaning to traumatic events, descriptions of their post-traumatic attitudes towards the world and themselves and investigation of changes in (preconscious) information processing will contribute to a fuller understanding of traumatic stress reactions. Most importantly, there is a need for treatment outcome studies of PTSD in children and adolescents. Studies of both referred and non-referred children with PTSD, and carefully selected control groups, are necessary before firm conclusions can be reached about the chronicity of symptoms and the effectiveness of current treatments.

20.8 REFERENCES

Aaron, J., Zaglul, H. and Emery, R. E. (1999). Posttraumatic stress in children following physical injury. *Journal of Pediatric Psychology*, **24**, 335–45.

American Psychiatric Association (1980). *Diagnostic and Statistical Manual of Mental Disorders*, 3rd edn. Washington, DC: APA.

  (1994). *Diagnostic and Statistical Manual of Mental Disorders*, 4th edn. Washington, DC: APA.

Berliner, L. and Saunders, B. E. (1996). Treating fear and anxiety in sexually abused children: results of controlled 2-year follow-up study. *Child Maltreatment*, **1**, 294–309.

Birleson, P. (1981). The validity of depressive disorder in childhood and the development of a self-rating scale: a research report. *Journal of Child Psychology and Psychiatry*, **22**, 73–88.

Bolton, D., O'Ryan, D., Udwin, O., Boyle, S. and Yule, W. (2000). The long-term psychological effects of a disaster experienced in adolescence. II: General psychopathology. *Journal of Child Psychology and Psychiatry*, **41**, 513–23.

Brewin, C. R. (2001). A cognitive neuroscience account of posttraumatic stress disorder and its treatment. *Behaviour Research and Therapy*, **39**, 373–93.

Bryce, J., Walker, N., Ghorayeb, F. and Kanj, M. (1989). Life experiences, response styles, and mental health among mothers in Beirut, Lebanon. *Social Science and Medicine*, **28**, 685–95.

Celano, M., Hazzard, A., Webb, C. and McCall, C. (1996). Treatment of traumagenic beliefs among sexually abused girls and their mothers: an evaluation study. *Journal of Abnormal Child Psychology*, **24**, 1–16.

Children and War Foundation (2002). www.childrenandwar.org.

Cohen, J. A. and Mannarino, A. P. (1996). A treatment outcome study for sexually abused preschool children: initial findings. *Journal of the American Academy of Child and Adolescent Psychiatry*, **35**, 42–50.

   (1997). A treatment study for sexually abused children: Outcome during a one-year followup. *Journal of the American Academy of Child and Adolescent Psychiatry*, **36**, 1228–35.

   (1998). Interventions for sexually abused children: Initial treatment outcome findings. *Child Maltreatment*, **3**, 17–26.

Cohen, J. A., Berliner, L. and March, J. S. (2002). Treatment of children and adolescents. In E. Foa, T. Keane and M. Freidman (eds.), *Effective Treatments for PTSD: Practice Guidelines from the International Society for Traumatic Stress Studies*. New York: Guilford, pp. 106–38.

Dalgleish, T. (1999). Cognitive theories of posttraumatic stress disorder. In W. Yule (ed.), *Posttraumatic Stress Disorders*. Chichester, Wiley, pp. 193–220.

Deblinger, E., Lippman, J. and Steer, R. (1996). Sexually abused children suffering posttraumatic stress symptoms: initial treatment findings. *Child Maltreatment*, **1**, 310–21.

Dyregrov, A. (1991). *Grief in Children: A Handbook for Adults*. London: Jessica Kingsley Publishers.
   (2001). Early intervention – a family perspective. *Advances in Mind-Body Medicine*, **17**, 168–74.

Ehlers, A. and Clark, D. M. (2000). A cognitive model of posttraumatic stress disorder. *Behaviour Research and Therapy*, **38**, 319–45.

Ehlers, A. and Steil, R. (1995). Maintenance of intrusive memories in posttraumatic stress disorder: a cognitive approach. *Behavioural and Cognitive Psychotherapy*, **23**, 217–49.

Ehlers, A., Mayou, R. A. and Bryant, B. (2003). Cognitive predictors of posttraumatic stress disorder in children: results of a prospective longitudinal study. *Behaviour Research and Therapy*, **41**, 1–10.

Foa, E. B. and Kozak, M. J. (1986). Emotional processing of fear: exposure to corrective information. *Psychological Bulletin*, **99**, 220–35.

Foa, E. B. and Meadows, E. A. (1997). Psychosocial treatments for posttraumatic stress disorder: a critical review. *Annual Review of Psychology*, **48**, 449–80.

Foa, E. B., Cashman, L., Jaycox, L. and Perry, K. (1997). The validation of a self-report measure of posttraumatic stress disorder: the Posttraumatic Diagnostic Scale. *Psychological Assessment*, **9**, 445–51.

Foa, E. B., Ehlers, A., Clark, D. M., Tolin, D. and Orsillo, S. M. (1999). The posttraumatic cognitions inventory (PCTI): development and validation. *Psychological Assessment*, **11**, 303–14.

Foa, E. B., Feske, U. and Murdock, T. B. (1991). Processing of threat related information in rape victims. *Journal of Abnormal Psychology*, **100**, 156–62.

Foa, E. B., Steketee, G. and Olasov-Rothbaum, B. (1989). Behavioral/cognitive conceptualizations of post-traumatic stress disorder. *Behavior Therapy*, **20**, 155–76.

Galante, R. and Foa, D. (1986). An epidemiological study of psychic trauma and treatment effectiveness after a natural disaster. *Journal of the American Academy of Child Psychiatry*, **25**, 357–63.

Goenjian, A. K., Karayan, I., Pynoos, R. *et al.* (1997). Outcome of psychotherapy among early adolescents after trauma. *American Journal of Psychiatry*, **154**, 536–42.

Horowitz, M. J., Wilner, N. and Alvarez, W. (1979). Impact of event scale: a measure of subjective stress. *Psychosomatic Medicine*, **41**, 209–18.

Janoff-Bulman, R. (1985). The aftermath of victimization: rebuilding shattered assumptions. In C. R. Figley (ed.), *Trauma and Its Wake*. New York: Brunner/Mazel, pp. 15–35.

(1992). *Shattered Assumptions: Towards a New Psychology of Trauma*. New York: The Free Press.

Johnson, K. M., Foa, E. B., Jaycox, L. H. and Rescorla, L. (1996). Post trauma attitudes in traumatised children. Poster presented at the XIIth ISTSS Annual Meeting, San Fransisco.

Joseph, S., Brewin, C., Yule, W. and Williams, R. (1993). Causal attributions and psychiatric symptoms in adolescent survivors of disaster. *Journal of Child Psychology and Psychiatry*, **34**, 247–53.

Keane, T. M., Zimmering, R. T. and Caddell, J. M. (1985). A behavioral formulation of PTSD in Vietnam veterans. *Behavior Therapist*, **8**, 9–12.

King, N. J., Tonge, B. J., Mullen, P., Myerson, N., Heyne, D. and Ollendick, T. H. (1999). Cognitive-behavioural treatment of sexually abused children: a review of research. *Behavioural and Cognitive Psychotherapy*, **27**, 295–309.

King, N. J., Tonge, B. J., Mullen, P. *et al.* (2000). Treating sexually abused children with posttraumatic stress symptoms: a randomized clinical trial. *Journal of the American Academy of Child and Adolescent Psychiatry*, **39**, 1347–55.

Kinzie, J. D., Sack, W. H., Angell, R. H., Manson, S. and Rath, B. (1986). The psychiatric effects of massive trauma on Cambodian children. I. The children. *Journal of the American Academy of Child and Adolescent Psychiatry*, **25**, 370–6.

Kuterovac, G., Dyregrov, A. and Stuvland, R. (1994). Children in war: a silent majority under stress. *British Journal of Medical Psychology*, **67**, 363–75.

LaGreca, A. M., Silverman, W. K., Vernberg, E. M. and Roberts, M. C. (eds.) (2002). *Helping Children Cope with Disasters and Terrorism*. Washington, DC: American Psychological Association.

March, J. S., Amaya-Jackson, L., Murray, M. C. and Schulte, A. (1998). Cognitive-behavioral psychotherapy for children and adolescents with posttraumatic stress disorder after a single-incident stressor. *Journal of the American Academy of Child and Adolescent Psychiatry*, **37**, 585–93.

McFarlane, A. C. (1987). Family functioning and overprotection following a natural disaster: the longitudinal effects of post-traumatic morbidity. *Australia and New Zealand Journal of Psychiatry*, **21**, 210–18.

McNally, R. J. (1991). Assessment of posttraumatic stress disorder in children. *Psychological Assessment*, **3**, 531–7.

Meichenbaum, D. (1994). *A Clinical Handbook/Practical Therapist Manual for Assessing and Treating Adults with Post-Traumatic Stress Disorder (PTSD)*. Ontario: Institute Press.

Meiser-Stedman, R. (2002). Towards a cognitive-behavioral model of PTSD in children and adolescents. *Clinical Child and Family Psychology Review*, **5**, 217–32.

Misch, P., Phillips, M., Evans, P. and Berekowitz, M. (1993). Trauma in preschool children: a clinical account. *Association of Child Psychology and Psychiatry: Occasional Papers*, **8**, 11–18.

Moradi, A. R. (1996). *Cognitive Characteristics of Children and Adolescents with PTSD and Children and Adolescents of Adults with PTSD*. PhD thesis, University of London.

Moradi, A. R., Neshat-Doost, H. T., Taghavi, R., Yule, W. and Dalgleish, T. (1999). Performance of children and adolescents with PTSD on the Stroop colour-naming task. *Psychological Medicine*, **29**, 415–19.

Nader, K. O., Kreigler, J., Keane, T., Blake, D. and Pynoos, R. (1994). *Clinician Administered PTSD Scale: Child and Adolescent Version (CAPS-C)*. White River Junction, VT: National Centre for PTSD.

Olasov-Rothbaum, B., Meadows, E. A., Resick, P. and Foy, D. W. (2002). Cognitive-behavioral therapy. In E. Foa, T. Keane and M. Freidman (eds.), *Effective Treatments for PTSD: Practice Guidelines from the International Society for Traumatic Stress Studies*, New York: Guilford, pp. 60–83.

Ollendick, T. H. (1983). Reliability and validity of the Revised Fear Survey Schedule for Children (FSSC-R). *Behavior Therapy*, **21**, 685–92.

Pfefferbaum, B. (1997). Posttraumatic stress disorder in children: a review of the past 10 years. *Journal of the American Academy of Child and Adolescent Psychiatry*, **36**, 1503–11.

Pynoos, R. S. (1994). Traumatic stress and developmental psychopathology in children and adolescents. In R. S. Pynoos (ed.), *Posttraumatic Stress Disorder: A Clinical Review*. Lutherville, MD: Sidran Press.

Pynoos, R. S. and Eth, S. (1986). Witness to violence: the child interview. *Journal of the American Academy of Child and Adolescent Psychiatry*, **25**, 306–19.

Pynoos, R. S., Frederick, C., Nader, K. *et al.* (1987). Life threat and posttraumatic stress symptoms in school-age children. *Archives of General Psychiatry*, **44**, 1057–63.

Pynoos, R. S., Goenjian, A., Karakashian, M. *et al.* (1993). Posttraumatic stress reactions in children after the 1988 Armenian earthquake. *British Journal of Psychiatry*, **163**, 239–47.

Rachman, S. (1980). Emotional processing. *Behaviour Research and Therapy*, **18**, 51–60.

Raphael, B. and Wilson, J. P. (eds.) (2000). *Psychological Debriefing: Theory, Practice and Evidence*. Cambridge: Cambridge University Press.

Reich, W., Shakya, J. J. and Taibelson, C. (1991). *Diagnostic Interview for Children and Adolescents (DICA)*. St Louis, MO: Washington University.

Reynolds, C. R. and Richmond, B. O. (1978). What I think and feel: a revised measure of children's manifest anxiety. *Journal of Abnormal Child Psychology*, **6**, 271–80.

Ribchester, T. (2001). *Examining the Efficacy of EMDR as a Treatment for PTSD in Children and Adolescents*. DClin Psychol thesis, University of London.

Saigh, P. A. (1987a). In-vitro flooding of an adolescent's posttraumatic stress disorder. *Journal of Clinical Child Psychology*, **16**, 147–50.

(1987b). In-vitro flooding of a childhood posttraumatic stress disorder. *School Psychology Review*, **16**, 203–11.

(1989). The use of in-vitro flooding in the treatment of a traumatized adolescent. *Journal of Behavioural and Developmental Paediatrics*, **10**, 17–21.

(1992). The behavioral treatment of child and adolescent posttraumatic stress disorder. *Advances in Behaviour Research and Therapy*, **14**, 247–75.

Saigh, P. A., Yule, W. and Inamdar, S. C. (1996). Imaginal flooding of traumatized children and adolescents. *Journal of School Psychology*, **34**, 163–83.

Salmon K. and Bryant, R. A. (2002). Posttraumatic stress disorder in children: the influence of developmental factors. *Clinical Psychology Review*, **22**, 163–88.

Saylor, C. and DeRoma, V. (2002). Assessment of children and adolescents exposed to disaster. In A. M. LaGreca, W. K. Silverman, E. M. Vernberg and M. C. Roberts (eds.), *Helping Children Cope with Disasters and Terrorism*. Washington, DC: American Psychological Association, pp. 35–53.

Scheeringa, M. S. and Zeanah, C. H. (1995). Symptom expression and trauma variables in children under 48 months of age. *Infant Mental Health Journal*, **16**, 259–70.

Scheeringa, M. S., Zeanah, C. H., Drell, M. J. and Larrieu, J. A. (1995). Two approaches to diagnosing posttraumatic stress disorder in infancy and early childhood. *Journal of the American Academy of Child and Adolescent Psychiatry*, **34**, 191–200.

Schwarz, E. D. and Kowalski, J. M. (1991). Posttraumatic stress disorder after a school shooting: effects of symptom threshold selection and diagnosis by DSM-III, DSM-III-R, or proposed DSM-IV. *American Journal of Psychiatry*, **148**, 592–7.

Shaffer, D., Fisher, P., Dulcan, M. *et al.* (1996). The NIMH diagnostic interview schedule for children (DISC-2.3): description, acceptibility, prevalences, and performance in the MECA study. *Journal of the America Academy of Child and Adolescent Psychiatry*, **35**, 865–77

Shannon, M. P., Lonigan, C. J., Finch, A. J. and Taylor, C. M. (1994). Children exposed to disaster. I: Epidemiology of posttraumatic symptoms and symptom profiles. *Journal of the American Academy of Child and Adolescent Psychiatry*, **33**, 80–93.

Silverman, W. and Albano, A. M. (1996). *Anxiety Disorders Interview Schedule for DSM IV: Child Version (ADIS-C)*. New York: The Psychological Corporation.

Smith, P., Dyregrov, A., Yule, W., Perrin, S., Gupta. L. and Gjestad, R. (1999). *A Manual for Teaching Survival Techniques to Child Survivors of Wars and Major Disasters*. Bergen, Norway: Foundation for Children and War (see www.childrenandwar.org).

Smith, P., Perrin, S., Dyregov, A. and Yule, W. (2002). Cross-cultural validity of the impact of event scale in a sample of Bosnian children. *Personality and Individual Differences*, **34**, 315–22.

Smith, P., Perrin, S., Yule, W. and Rabe-Hesketh, S. (2001). War exposure and maternal reactions in the psychological adjustment of children from Bosnia-Hercegovina. *Journal of Child Psychology and Psychiatry*, **42**, 395–404.

Stallard, P. and Law, F. (1993). Screening and psychological debriefing of adolescent survivors of life threatening events. *British Journal of Psychiatry*, **163**, 660–5.

Terr, L. C. (1979). The children of Chowchilla. *Psychoanalytic Study of the Child*, **34**, 547–623.

Thrasher, S. M., Dalgleish, T. and Yule, W. (1994). Information processing in posttraumatic stress disorder. *Behaviour Research and Therapy*, **32**, 247–54.

Udwin, O., Boyle, S., Yule, W., Bolton, D. and O'Ryan, D. (2000). Risk factors for long-term psychological effects of a disaster experienced in adolescence: predictors of posttraumatic stress disorder. *Journal of Child Psychology and Psychiatry*, **41**, 969–79.

Vernberg, E. M. and Varela, R. E. (2001). PTSD: a developmental perspective. In M. Vasey and M. R. Dadds (eds.), *The Developmental Psychopathology of Anxiety*. New York: Oxford University Press, pp. 386–406.

Vernberg, E. M. and Vogel, J. M. (1993). Task Force Report Part 2: Interventions with children after disasters. *Journal of Clinical Child Psychology*, **22**, 485–98.

Vogel, J. M. and Vernberg, E. M. (1993). Task Force Report Part 1: Children's psychological responses to disasters. *Journal of Clinical Child Psychology*, **22**, 464–84.

Vernberg, E. M., LaGreca, A. M., Silverman, W. K. and Prinstein, M. J. (1996). Prediction of posttraumatic stress symptoms in children after Hurricane Andrew. *Journal of Abnormal Psychology*, **105**, 237–48.

World Health Organization (1992). *International Classification of Diseases*, 10th edn. Geneva: World Health Organization.

Yule, W. (1992). Post traumatic stress disorder in child survivors of shipping disasters: the sinking of the 'Jupiter'. *Psychotherapy and Psychosomatics*, **57**, 200–5.

   (2000). Treatment of PTSD in children following RTAs. In E. Blanchard and E. Hickling (eds.), *The International Handbook of Road Traffic Accidents and Psychological Trauma: Current Understanding, Treatment and Law*. Oxford: Elsevier, pp. 375–87.

   (2001). When disaster strikes – the need to be 'wise before the event': crisis intervention with children and adolescents. *Advances in Mind-Body Medicine*, **17**, 191–6.

Yule, W. and Udwin, O. (1991). Screening child survivors for post-traumatic stress disorders: experiences from the 'Jupiter' sinking. *British Journal of Clinical Psychology*, **30**, 131–8.

Yule, W. and Williams, R. (1990). Post traumatic stress reactions in children. *Journal of Traumatic Stress*, **3**, 279–95.

Yule, W., Bolton, D., Udwin, O., Boyle, S., O'Ryan, D. and Nurrish, J. (2000). The long-term psychological effects of a disaster experienced in adolescence. I: The incidence and course of post traumatic stress disorder. *Journal of Child Psychology and Psychiatry*, **41**, 503–11.

Yule, W., Perrin, S. and Smith, P. (1999). PTSD in children and adolescents. In Yule, W. (ed.), *Post Traumatic Stress Disorder*. Chichester: Wiley, pp. 25–50.

21

Disorders of eating control

Anne Stewart

Warneford Hospital, Oxford, UK

21.1 Introduction

Eating disorders are common in teenage girls, with prevalence rates for anorexia nervosa and bulimia nervosa being 0.3%–0.6% and approximately 1%, respectively (Fairburn and Beglin, 1990; Whitaker *et al.*, 1990; Rathner and Messner, 1993; Van Hoeken *et al.*, 1998). Disorders of eating control not reaching diagnostic criteria are considerably more common (Childress *et al.*, 1993). Many adolescents have negative cognitions about their shape and weight, commonly leading to dieting as a way of improving self-image (Killen *et al.*, 1994; Smolak and Levine, 1994). Dieting is an established risk factor for eating disorders (Patton *et al.*, 1990) and, for those adolescents who go on to develop an eating disorder, negative cognitions may become established. Even those who regain their weight may continue to hold negative cognitions about their body and, therefore, are vulnerable to further weight loss (Fairburn *et al.*, 1993a). Low self-esteem is frequently present in adolescents who develop these difficulties (Button *et al.*, 1996). Cognitive behaviour therapy (CBT) can provide a useful therapeutic approach to address negative cognitions about shape and weight and underlying core beliefs as well as promoting behavioural change (Garner *et al.*, 1997; Wilson *et al.*, 1997). However, the models developed for adults require adaptation for use with adolescents (Lock, 2002).

This chapter explores the use of CBT in adolescents with eating disorders, focusing on anorexia nervosa and bulimia nervosa. First, the diagnostic and clinical features of these disorders will be described, followed by the research basis for the use of CBT. A cognitive model for the development and maintenance of eating disorders will be presented and CBT based on this model described in detail.

Cognitive Behaviour Therapy for Children and Families, ed. Philip J. Graham.
Published by Cambridge University Press. © Cambridge University Press 2004.

21.2   Diagnostic and clinical features of eating disorders

Diagnostic criteria of anorexia nervosa are as follows: low weight (more than 15% weight deficit), fear of weight gain, abnormal perceptions of body weight and shape, refusal to gain weight and hormonal changes. Diagnostic criteria of bulimia nervosa are: binge eating, purging the body (e.g. by vomiting, laxatives, restrictive eating or overexercise) and overconcern about shape and weight. In practice, many adolescents have mixed features or atypical presentations. Common clinical features accompanying a number of different presentations include low self-esteem, poor body image, overconcern about shape and weight, lack of cohesive identity, preoccupation with food and dieting, social withdrawal, relationship difficulties, need for self-control and denial of pleasure. In anorexia nervosa, symptoms of starvation complicate the picture and, in bulimia nervosa, bingeing and vomiting may be accompanied by other impulsive behaviours such as drug and alcohol abuse or self-harm. These features are incorporated within the cognitive model described later.

21.3   Evidence basis for CBT in eating disorders

21.3.1   Bulimia nervosa

For bulimia nervosa, CBT is considered the treatment of choice. Since the article by Fairburn (1981) describing the use of CBT for bulimia nervosa, there have been more than 30 comparative trials (e.g. Fairburn *et al.*, 1986a; Agras *et al.*, 1989; Fairburn *et al.*, 1991; Agras *et al.*, 1992; Fairburn *et al.*, 1993a; Thackwray *et al.*, 1993; Fairburn *et al.*, 1995; Walsh *et al.*, 1997). In each instance, CBT is equal or superior to every modality against which it has been compared (both active treatments and control). Those studies with long-term follow-up have found that gains have been maintained (Agras *et al.*, 1994; Fairburn *et al.*, 1995). Interpersonal therapy has been shown to be as effective as CBT in the long term (Fairburn *et al.*, 1991, 1995) and may be a useful alternative for patients for whom CBT is either not acceptable or not effective.

Despite its proven efficacy in the short and long term, a significant number of patients only make a partial response to CBT and some do not respond at all (Fairburn *et al.*, 1992). Fairburn *et al.* (2003) suggest that the scope of CBT should be extended to include a focus on interpersonal issues, self-esteem, perfectionism and mood intolerance, where relevant, as well as standard elements of CBT.

There is interest in self-help treatment for bulimia nervosa, and several manuals are available (Schmidt and Treasure, 1993; Cooper, 1995; Fairburn, 1995). Controlled evaluations indicate the effectiveness of self-help in less severe cases, particularly if a limited number of therapist-guided sessions are held alongside (Treasure *et al.*, 1994; Carter and Fairburn, 1998; Cooper *et al.*, 1996).

To date, there are no published controlled trials of CBT with adolescents with bulimia nervosa, although adolescents have been included in some of the adult studies. There is also little research evaluating other forms of therapy. Dodge *et al.* (1995) reported a case series on the use of the Maudsley family therapy approach in bulimia nervosa in adolescents, noting significant improvements in eating behaviour at the end of treatment. Lock (2002) has reported a case series of adolescents with bulimia nervosa who received a modified family-based cognitive behavioural approach with good outcome.

21.3.2   Anorexia nervosa

CBT is beginning to be used more widely in anorexia nervosa, although there is no compelling evidence for its efficacy as yet. A case report by Cooper and Fairburn (1984) suggested a positive effect of CBT. However, only a handful of controlled studies of psychotherapy have been undertaken. Channon *et al.* (1989) compared CBT with behavioural treatment and 'treatment as usual' and found all groups significantly improved at 6-month follow-up, although CBT emerged as a more acceptable form of therapy. However, there were methodological limitations to this study. Serfaty *et al.* (1999) conducted a randomized controlled trial comparing dietary advice with CBT in the outpatient treatment of anorexia nervosa. At 6-month follow-up, 23 out of 25 patients in the CBT group remained engaged in treatment, whereas the entire dietary control group had dropped out. The CBT group showed significant changes in BMI and scores on the Eating Disorder Inventory (EDI).

There have, to date, been no controlled trials of CBT in anorexia nervosa with adolescents. There is, however, evidence for the efficacy of a family approach in adolescents with anorexia nervosa (Russell *et al.*, 1992; Dare *et al.*, 1995; Robin *et al.*, 1999; Eisler *et al.*, 2000), although none of the studies has used a no-treatment control.

The model of working with adolescents with bulimia nervosa and anorexia nervosa described in this chapter draws on existing research. However, there is an inadequate evidence basis for CBT in adolescents with eating disorders, and an urgent need for well-designed controlled trials to investigate this approach.

21.4   A cognitive model of eating disorders in adolescence

A number of cognitive behavioural models of bulimia nervosa and anorexia nervosa have been developed in relation to presentation in adult life (Fairburn, 1981;

Vitousek and Orimoto, 1993; Cooper, 1997; Wolff and Serpell, 1998; Fairburn *et al.*, 1999b; Fairburn *et al.*, 2003). A cognitive model relevant to adolescent disorders needs to include developmental issues of adolescence, as well as the role of family and peer relationships.

Most existing models focus on the maintenance of eating disorders. Indeed, an understanding of how an eating disorder can be self-reinforcing is essential for both patient and therapist throughout treatment. Additionally, for some patients, an understanding of how their problems developed may be helpful in the later stages of treatment. The following models of development and maintenance of eating disorders are based on existing models, while taking into account systemic and developmental factors.

21.4.1   Development of eating disorders

The cognitive model for emotional disorders, as developed by Beck (1976), is used as a basis for understanding the development of eating disorders (Figure 21.1).

Early individual experience is shaped by a number of genetic and environmental influences. Risk factor studies have begun to clarify the relevant early experiences in eating disorders (Fairburn *et al.*, 1997, 1999b; see Figure 21.1). A combination of these early factors may operate together leading to the development of core beliefs in some people such as: *I am unlovable, I am no good, I am vulnerable, I am defective, I am controlled by others, I deserve to be punished.*

A number of conditional assumptions may arise from core beliefs that relate to shape and weight, and to more general issues, e.g. *to be attractive, I have to be thin, to be successful I have to be thin, I must be in control, I must do everything perfectly for people to love me, I must not allow myself to enjoy anything.*

These beliefs and assumptions develop during childhood and adolescence; however, their strength and importance may not be obvious until they are activated by a critical incident(s). Puberty itself may be a critical incident for many young girls. Following puberty, girls' body image often deteriorates and an overconcern about physical appearance, including feelings of fatness, becomes common (Shore and Porter, 1990). A number of studies have found that eating problems substantially increase at puberty (Koff and Rierdan, 1993; Levine *et al.*, 1994). Indeed, early puberty is a risk factor for later eating disorders (Fairburn *et al.*, 1997). During puberty, there are a number of developmental changes which can be problematic for some girls, particularly if they are already vulnerable. These include adjusting to the biological changes, developing relationships, becoming independent, coping with work pressures and developing an identity.

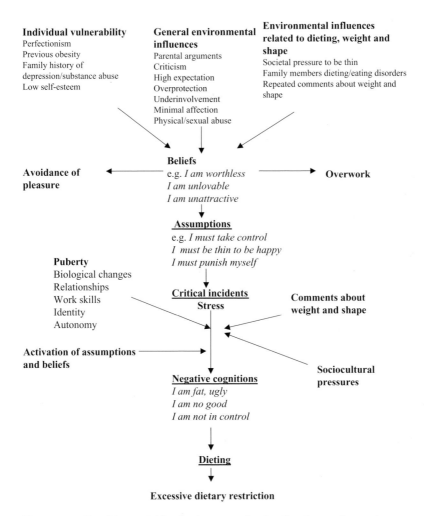

Figure 21.1   Cognitive model for development of eating disorders: early experience.

Current stresses/life events such as marital dysharmony, an abusive environment or comments about weight and shape can act as triggers. Underlying assumptions and beliefs may be activated and negative automatic thoughts emerge, compounding feelings of low self-esteem and loss of control. The adolescent may diet to feel more in control and better about herself.

This developmental model is particularly relevant for those adolescents who have strongly held negative beliefs that predate the development of the eating disorder. However, for some adolescents, low self-esteem arises secondary to the eating disorder, rather than being an underlying risk factor.

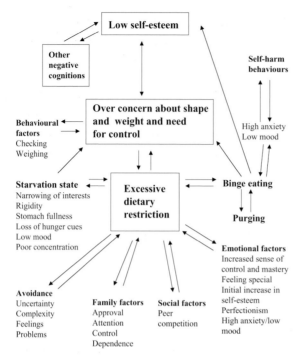

Figure 21.2   Maintaining factors in adolescent eating disorders.

21.4.2   Maintenance of eating disorders

Once the young person has developed abnormal eating attitudes and behaviour, a number of factors can maintain this behaviour. The following model of maintenance is adapted from the cognitive models for the maintenance of bulimia nervosa and anorexia nervosa developed by Fairburn (1981) and Fairburn *et al.* (1999b). Issues relating to control, as described by Fairburn *et al.* (1999a), are highly relevant for adolescent girls, many of whom are trying to find a way of taking control of their lives, when many aspects appear out of control. Family, peer and developmental aspects are also prominent in this model (Figure 21.2).

At the core of this model are the unhelpful cognitions about shape and weight and the need for control that drive the disorder. These concerns may trigger excessive dietary restriction, which can either lead to a starvation state (as in anorexia nervosa) or to binge eating and purging (as in bulimia nervosa). A number of factors help to maintain this process, as discussed below.

21.4.2.1   Individual emotional factors

As the young person restricts her eating with consequent weight loss, she can initially feel a sense of increased control and mastery. This leads to a temporary increase in self-esteem. The young person feels that, if only she could lose even more weight or be even more careful with her diet, self-esteem will increase again. Young people who have perfectionist traits are driven to develop highly effective and rigid dietary restriction that reinforces their sense of achievement. Additionally, the process of weight loss can lead to a feeling of being special and different, which the young person may be fearful of losing if they gain weight. In some adolescents, dietary restriction or binge eating can also be a way of coping with unpleasant emotional states, such as high anxiety or low mood.

21.4.2.2 Behavioural factors
Commonly, young people with eating disorders engage in behaviours such as frequent weighing or checking of various parts of their body. This results in a preoccupation with perceived deficits, which reinforces their concern about shape and weight.

21.4.2.3 Family factors
The effect of the eating disorder on the family may maintain the behaviour in a number of ways. First, the initial weight loss may attract approval from parents, although as the weight loss continues this approval may turn to concern. Serious weight loss generally increases parental attention, which can be experienced as positive; there is often fear of losing this once weight gain starts. Secondly, the sense of control often experienced with dietary restriction may be seen as the only way to take control in a family where, perhaps, they have little control. Thirdly, many young people with eating disorders seek reassurance from parents, particularly mothers, that they look attractive. This reassurance may work in the short term, but when excessive can maintain the problem, in a similar way to reassurance in health anxiety. Fourthly, some young people find it hard to grow up and gain independence. Losing weight may be a way of staying dependent on their families, thus avoiding the problems of growing up. Finally, at the time that their daughter is developing anorexia, parents may be going through their own midlife difficulties, making it harder for them to be aware of and give attention to their daughter's problems.

21.4.2.4 Social factors
Dieting is very common in adolescent girls (Hill *et al.*, 1992). Losing weight can be a way of gaining peer approval, at least in the short term. As further weight is lost, this may elicit concern from peers, which can also be reinforcing.

21.4.2.5   Avoidance

Adolescence is a time of uncertainty and decision making. This can be difficult for some young people, particularly if they already have low self-esteem. Developing an eating disorder can be a way of avoiding the uncertainties and complexities of life. Maintaining dietary restriction gives the illusion of a secure and predictable lifestyle.

21.4.2.6   Starvation state

The effects of starvation can contribute to the maintenance of the disorder. Resulting low mood and lack of energy make it hard to make active efforts to change. Physical symptoms in starvation, such as loss of hunger and a feeling of fullness, make eating more difficult because of fear of loss of control. Narrowing of interests and social withdrawal lead to an identity that is centred around anorexia, making it increasingly difficult to give up. Rigidity of thought makes it hard to take a rational viewpoint of problems and make healthy changes.

21.4.2.7   Binge eating

In some young people, excessive dieting will trigger binge eating, followed by compensatory methods of weight control such as vomiting. Vicious cycles help to keep this process going (see Fairburn *et al.*, 1986a).

21.4.2.8   Rescue factors

In developing a maintenance model, it is important to be aware of the 'rescue factors', i.e. the strengths that help the young person to recover. These may be individual resources, or related to supportive family or peer relationships.

21.5   Assessment

A comprehensive assessment is an essential first step in the management of eating disorders. Table 21.1 summarizes the components of the initial assessment. An important goal is to engage the young person and the family in treatment. Teenagers with eating disorders, particularly anorexia nervosa, are frequently ambivalent about treatment, and it is important to spend time in the assessment checking out positive and negative aspects of having an eating disorder and how they feel about treatment. A collaborative approach, right from the start, is essential. (For useful ideas on how to motivate patients see Chapter 5; Schmidt and Treasure, 1993; Treasure and Schmidt, 1997; Treasure and Ward, 1997.)

Table 21.1 Assessment

- Current eating habits (including eating patterns, bingeing, vomiting, other methods of weight control)
- Associated problems (depression, anxiety, deliberate self-harm, drug and alcohol abuse)
- Clinical history (including weight history, menstrual history, previous psychiatric history)
- Early development (including history of childhood abuse)
- Family background (including history of eating problems)
- Physical assessment (including height and weight, cardiovascular state, muscle strength, blood screening)
- Standardized questionnaires (including EDE–Q, EAT, BDI, BAI)
- Family assessment (including level of family support, attitudes to daughters' problems, marital relationship)
- Individual assessment (including attitudes to eating problem, motivation, goals)

EDE–Q, Eating Disorder Examination – Questionnaire; EAT, Eating Attitudes Test; BDI, Beck Depression Inventory; BAI, Beck Anxiety Inventory.

21.6 CBT

21.6.1 The phases of treatment and the role of the family

The approach now described draws on existing research in the fields of both CBT and family approaches to adolescent eating disorders, and is based on the cognitive model described earlier.

Similar to the approach with adults, CBT for both anorexia nervosa and bulimia nervosa occurs in three phases. While there is considerable overlap between the phases, the major focus of each phase differs. The first phase is primarily concerned with establishing normal patterns of eating and, in the case of anorexia nervosa, restoring weight. Strategies will be primarily behavioural in this phase. The second phase focuses on addressing the maintaining factors of the disorder including the overconcern about weight and shape and other unhelpful cognitions, as well as the need for control. The young person is helped to develop a more realistic and positive view of herself and to take responsibility. The final phase is concerned with relapse prevention, helping the young person and their family to develop strategies to cope in the future.

In anorexia nervosa, it is considered essential to involve the family throughout treatment, particularly with younger adolescents. The treatment approach described follows the same pattern as the family treatment model developed by the Maudsley group (Dare *et al.*, 1995), while incorporating an individual cognitive approach. In the first phase, the treatment is largely family based, with a behavioural approach to treatment adapted from the first phase of the Maudsley family model. The second phase involves considerable work with the young person on her own, taking a cognitive approach in addition to continued behavioural work. Work with parents (and siblings, if appropriate) will continue alongside this, and the young person is encouraged to take increasing responsibility for her eating and to view parents as allies. Family work in the final phase may need to address broader issues of adolescence such as independence and separation, along with relapse prevention, similar to the final phase in the Maudsley model.

Evidence is lacking on a family approach with adolescents with bulimia; however, clinical experience suggests that a similar approach can be used with young people with this condition. A family-based CBT for adolescent bulimia nervosa has been described by Lock (2002). The young person may be older at presentation in bulimia nervosa and may be more motivated to make changes. Therefore, for some adolescents, it may be appropriate to work more individually from the start, with family members seen as allies to this work.

21.6.2 Anorexia nervosa

21.6.2.1 Phase 1

The first phase of treatment involves working with the family to enable the young person to re-establish normal eating patterns and regain weight. Commonly, the young person is reluctant to attend treatment at this stage, and may not even acknowledge that they have a problem. Thus, family support is a crucial factor in promoting change. The family work has a number of components which include educating the family regarding the worrying consequences of the disorder, separating the patient from the eating disorder and encouraging parents to take charge of their daughter's eating. The therapist aims to strengthen and support the parents in their task of helping their daughter eat. The focus is on current issues, rather than on the cause.

Parents, initially, may find it hard to achieve a balance between empathy and firmness, and need encouragement to find ways of relating to their daughter that enable her to improve. Taking a detailed behavioural approach to mealtimes and working out how best to supervise and support their daughter is an essential part of this phase. As time goes on, parents become more confident. Joining a parent group and discussing difficulties relating to this phase with other parents can also be reassuring and helpful. Monitoring of food intake is helpful at this stage, and the drawing up of a meal plan with collaboration from the parents and the young person provides a useful structure for the family to follow. Input from a dietician can be helpful.

Family work may either involve the whole family meeting together or, alternatively, for some families, meetings with parents primarily on their own with parallel supportive work for the young person. Research suggests that where there is high expressed emotion in the family, outcome may be better if the family work is separated into parental work and work with the young person (Eisler *et al.*, 2000). Whichever style is chosen, it is essential to take time to engage the young person.

This phase has similarities to the first phase of CBT of anorexia nervosa in adults, the essential difference being the prominent role that the family takes. The attention to monitoring of food intake and the establishment of a structured (and increasing) meal plan are carried out in collaboration with parents.

21.6.2.2   Phase 2

For some young people, cognitions begin to change in phase 1 with family work, and more specific cognitive work does not prove necessary. In this case, family work continues with increasing responsibility given back to the young person and with the focus on areas other than the eating disorder. However, for others, particularly older adolescents or those with a longer history, negative cognitions remain and more specific work is required. Although there is no empirical basis at present, clinical experience suggests that some young people benefit from an individual cognitive behavioural approach at this stage.

Timing is crucial for this phase. The young person needs to be ready and motivated to undertake individual CBT. Usually, the weight deficit will be 15% or less, although some young people will be ready for cognitive work at lower weights than this and some will not be accessible to working cognitively even at higher weights. In order to assess suitability, the following criteria are used:

- Is the young person motivated to change?
- Does she want active participation?
- Does she have the ability to take a 'meta' approach to her problems?
- Does she have some ability to distinguish thoughts from feelings?
- Does a cognitive behavioural understanding make sense to her?

Early in treatment, a maintenance formulation of the problems (based on Figure 21.2) can be produced together. In phase 1, the maintenance factors relating to starvation will have been addressed. Other maintaining factors may now be addressed in therapy.

Given the fluctuating motivation that young people often show, a motivational approach should be continued throughout the treatment. It is helpful to spend time with the young person early on in treatment working out the pros and cons of weight gain, or no weight gain, both in the short and long term. Other useful questions are:

- What values are important to you?
- How does thinness relate to achieving these values?
- Is the eating disorder working for you?

Writing letters to the anorexia as friend or enemy (Serpell *et al.*, 1999) can increase motivation. As treatment progresses, helping the young person reconnect to other aspects of their life can be highly motivating.

Goals for treatment are identified early on. Usually, the young person will suggest a mixture of goals relating to eating, weight and shape, as well as to wider issues, such as confidence and self-esteem. Having clarified the goals, a decision is made about which goals to tackle first. It is usually preferable to start with the more immediate goals – e.g. *I would like to feel OK about eating with others, I would like to finish my meals more quickly, I would like to feel happier about my weight*.

Throughout this phase, there is continued emphasis on weight gain and normalization of eating. Weighing patients regularly gives an opportunity to identify negative thoughts. A structured meal plan continues to be important, although as time goes on the young person can take more responsibility and be more flexible. It is helpful to continue monitoring food intake, although also including systematic self-monitoring of thoughts and feelings. With some young people, it works well to include parents in the detailed discussions of food intake; parents are seen as a resource to help support the meal plan. Behavioural strategies to help the young person get through mealtime, such as having company, listening to music, getting parents to continue supervising, etc., may be helpful. Triggers to food restriction may be discussed. As time goes on, the young person is encouraged to develop more normal patterns of eating. There is a systematic introduction of avoided foods, often with the help of parents, and a broadening of the contexts in which food is eaten.

Through self-monitoring, the young person will learn to identify 'anorexic' thoughts which help to maintain the disturbed eating pattern. Examples of these are:

- I may not be able to stop eating once I start.
- People will think I am greedy if they see me eating.
- I will feel better when I lose some more weight.
- If I eat one more biscuit, it will go straight to my stomach.

Understanding the nature of automatic thoughts – in particular, that they are interpretations rather than facts – is important. Identifying unhelpful thinking patterns can be helpful. Examples of unhelpful thinking patterns are given in Table 21.2.

The next stage is to help the young person develop more helpful thoughts. Having identified an 'anorexic' thought, the young person is encouraged to examine the evidence for and against the validity and usefulness of the thought. Having done this, she is encouraged to come to a reasoned conclusion, develop an alternative thought and make behavioural changes that are consistent with

Table 21.2   Unhelpful thinking patterns

Jumping to conclusions
I am special to people if I am thin
Magnification
Everyone must be able to see how unattractive I am
Overgeneralization
I enjoyed my food – therefore, I must be a greedy person
Black and white thinking
If I am not in complete control, I lose all control
Personalizing
People laugh at me when I eat
Magical thinking
If I eat one more biscuit, it will immediately turn into body fat

Table 21.3   Self-monitoring

Situation	Emotion	NAT	Alternatives	Feeling
Looking at a photo	Unhappy	I look awful Why do I need to put on weight? No one will want to be my friend	My friend also looked bad There are people more unattractive than me and they have friends People value me for my personality	Happier

NAT, negative automatic thought.

the conclusion. Using role play to challenge thoughts can be very useful with adolescents – e.g. the young person role plays a friend with the therapist acting as the patient. Table 21.3 shows a self-monitoring sheet with more realistic alternative thoughts added in.

During the therapy, it becomes evident that behaviour or events such as loss of weight or cutting down meals can initially lead to positive thoughts, such as:
- It's an achievement having skipped lunch.
- I am pleased that I lost 300 g today.
- It's good to be in control of my eating.

These positive thoughts can be challenged in the same way as negative automatic thoughts. It may be necessary at this stage to remind the young person of the decisional balance of pros and cons and their goals for therapy. Although she may initially feel proud of her achievement in losing weight, she realizes that it will not help achieve the goals formulated at the start of treatment.

Table 21.4 Behavioural experiments

Date	Situation	Prediction	Experiment	Outcome	What I learned

Many negative automatic thoughts in anorexia nervosa relate to concerns about shape and weight. Systematic work relating to these cognitions is essential. Young people with anorexia nervosa can have very strong feelings about their body, becoming convinced that the body actually looks as bad as it feels. Body image dissatisfaction may be maintained by focusing exclusively on negative aspects of the body, and disregarding the positive features. Perfectionism can contribute to body image dissatisfaction. Re-attribution of 'feeling fat' to other feelings, such as low mood, enables the young person to deal with these other feelings.

Behavioural experiments can be an excellent way of challenging negative cognitions. For example, frequent checking in the mirror or weighing is likely to increase concern about weight and shape. Setting up an experiment in which the checking behaviour is reduced can help the young person identify these links for themselves. Keeping track of behavioural experiments, with predictions and outcome, is helpful (see Table 21.4 for monitoring sheet).

As therapy proceeds, the young person may become more aware of wider cognitions unrelated to weight, shape and eating concerns, but linked to other anxieties about self or others. Examples of negative thoughts are:

- My friend did not ring me, therefore she does not like me.
- I only got 80% in my maths exam, therefore I am a failure.
- My parents are fed up with me.

These negative thoughts are examined in the same way, and alternative thoughts developed.

In some young people, as the eating disorder improves, self-esteem may improve and the young person becomes more confident and engaged in other aspects of life. However, in others, particularly those with a history of negative core beliefs that predate the eating disorder, the young person continues to hold negative beliefs about herself despite weight gain and normalization of eating; the therapy may then need to move to areas related to underlying assumptions and beliefs. The areas shown below typically arise at this stage of therapy; these areas may link to the original goals that the young person identified at the start of therapy or may be linked to problems that have emerged in therapy:

- **Perfectionism**
  Dysfunctional assumption: I must do everything perfectly otherwise people will not like me
- **Lack of confidence/assertiveness**
  Dysfunctional assumptions: no-one will listen to me, my views are useless
  If I say something wrong, people will laugh at me
- **Low self-esteem, underdeveloped identity**
  Core belief: I am worthless
- **Problems with relationships (family and peers)**
  Core belief: no-one likes me
  Dysfunctional assumptions: if I recover, no-one will care for me
  I need to be ill for people to take notice of me
- **Difficulty in expressing or dealing with feelings**
  Dysfunctional assumption: if I say what I feel, I must be out of control
- **Difficulties with sexuality/growing up**
  Dysfunctional assumptions: growing up is too difficult to cope with
  Being an adult means being unhappy
- **Difficulties with sexuality/growing up**
  Dysfunctional assumptions: growing up is too difficult to cope with
  Being an adult means being unhappy

Producing a formulation together, which includes early experience and development of core beliefs and assumptions, may be helpful at this stage. There are a number of ways in which these underlying beliefs or assumptions can be tackled.

It can be helpful to represent the beliefs on a continuum, e.g. I am worthless -----------------------------------I am of value. Work is done identifying the meaning at each end of the continuum – e.g. questioning what it really means to be of value. The young person is asked to place herself on the continuum but also to place herself where her best friend or parents would see her. In this way, it soon becomes apparent that the place on the continuum can be variable and may also depend on mood and context. It may be helpful to think of other people she knows and where she would place them on the continuum. How does she decide where to place them? It also emerges that the young person may have different standards for herself as compared with those for other people. It is useful, at this point, to discuss the prejudice model (Padesky, 1991). This model suggests that people with low self-esteem are prejudiced against themselves, viewing their negative aspects through maximizing glasses and their positive aspects through minimizing glasses. Work can be done on developing a more realistic view of self.

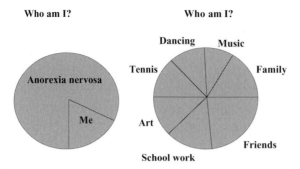

Figure 21.3   Work on identity.

Pie charts can be a useful way of tackling identity and core beliefs about self. Figure 21.3 shows firstly a typical pie chart for a young person with anorexia nervosa showing the importance that the anorexia has in their life. Work can be done identifying the aspects that they would like to add in (as in the second pie chart), encouraging them to develop specific ideas as to how they might do this. A key aspect to this part of the therapy is building up a positive sense of self. The young person may have focused on her eating disorder for a considerable time, neglecting other aspects of herself. The aim is to develop the belief that she is a person of value. The young person can be asked to keep a log of data that fits in with positive self-beliefs. Initially, it is apparent that the young person minimizes, distorts or does not notice the positive data. As she becomes aware of this, she can become more realistic about her achievements.

Using behavioural experiments to test out dysfunctional assumptions can be helpful. Some examples of assumptions which can be tested include:

- Being assertive will lead to being laughed at.
- Expressing feelings will lead to an out of control explosion.

Teaching assertiveness skills can be an important part of this process. Once the skill is learnt, then behavioural experiments can help to test out the validity of beliefs and strengthen more positive beliefs.

It is helpful for work with parents/family to proceed during the period of cognitive therapy, although the frequency may decrease. The family has to learn to step back from the intensive support/supervision that they may have provided initially and allow the young person to take responsibility. Parents can be anxious during this process, as they have become used to responding to their daughter as if she were much younger and more dependent. Other family relationship issues may emerge during this stage and the young person may learn to express feelings more assertively.

Table 21.5   Action plan

- How did my eating problem develop?
- What kept it going?
- What did I do that made a difference?
- How has my view of things changed?
- How can I build on changes I have made?
- What should I do if my eating problem starts to come back again?

21.6.2.3   Phase 3 – relapse prevention

By this time, the young person will have reached their target weight range and will be integrated into normal adolescent activities (school, socializing, etc.). The eating disorder will now have much less hold on them. Family work may need to deal with separation and independence as the young person grapples with growing up. It is helpful at this stage to consider the warning signs of relapse and to use relapses as a way of learning and progressing. Before discharge, it is useful to review with the young person what they have learnt throughout treatment and how they can build on that for the future. This can be in the form of an action plan, which the young person can keep in a folder to remind her of the work done during therapy (Table 21.5).

21.6.3   Bulimia nervosa

The CBT of bulimia nervosa in adolescents follows the same general pattern as described in Fairburn and Wilson (1993), although with much greater involvement of the family. The extent of the family involvement is variable depending on the developmental needs of the adolescent and the relationship the young person has with parents. Parents may often be seen as a helpful resource for the young person.

21.6.3.1   Phase 1

The first phase of treatment is focused on two major aims. The first aim is to collaborate with the young person to produce a cognitive behavioural formulation based on Fairburn's model (Fairburn *et al.*, 1986b, 1999b) and incorporating other relevant factors in the young persons life – in particular, family, peers, school, etc. – as described earlier in the maintenance model (it is important to take time to discuss this model thoroughly). The second aim is to introduce behavioural strategies to decrease bingeing and vomiting.

The young person is asked to self-monitor her eating (see Table 21.6 for an example of a self-monitoring sheet). The purpose of the self-monitoring is to

Table 21.6 Example of a self-monitoring sheet

Date	Time	Food eaten	Situation	B	V	L	Context

B, binge; V, vomiting; L, laxative abuse.

help the young person understand more clearly her eating habits and the context in which problems arise. Educating the young person is an important part of this phase of treatment. This will include healthy weight range, the physical consequences of binge eating, vomiting and laxative abuse, ineffectiveness of vomiting as a means of weight control and adverse effects of dieting. The focus is on helping the young person to normalize the eating pattern. The young person is encouraged to eat regular main meals three times a day, plus planned snacks in between. Gradually, the young person's day becomes structured by a pattern of regular eating. Self-monitoring helps the young person identify problem times when binge eating is more likely, and she is encouraged to develop alternative activities which make binge eating less likely. Other measures are introduced, such as limiting the supply of food. Finally, activities that can distract from vomiting after a meal are introduced.

It may be useful to enlist the help of parents and other members of the family during this phase, although, frequently, the young person wishes to tackle the problems herself. When enlisting family help, it works best to ask the young person first how her family can help. Occasionally, the young person wants active help with stopping bingeing and vomiting – e.g. support and supervision after meals, or even preventing access to food between meals. As therapy proceeds, involvement of parents becomes less as the young person develops strategies to stop bingeing and vomiting. Parents may need encouragement to stand back from the young person at this stage, giving her control again.

It is easier for family members to be supportive and helpful if they are provided with education about the nature of the disorder.

21.6.3.2 Phase 2

In the second phase, an emphasis on regular eating remains, but the focus broadens to address dieting, concerns about weight and shape and more general distorted cognitions. Later on, other problems such as low self-esteem, family and peer difficulties, anxiety and perfectionism may be addressed.

An important initial goal is to increase understanding of the relationship between binge eating and dieting, and to decrease dieting. Characteristically, young people follow a rigid set of dietary rules and when they inevitably break a rule they relax all control and binge eat. This is followed by re-establishment of a strict pattern of eating, or fasting, which in turn makes bingeing more likely. Over time, the young person is encouraged to add forbidden foods gradually to the meal plan and eat in a wider variety of situations. Self-monitoring will identify situations in which binge eating occurs, and she is encouraged to take a problem-solving approach to minimize the risk of bingeing.

A major focus of this phase of treatment is addressing concerns about shape and weight, which are a core feature of this disorder. Research indicates that if these are not addressed, relapse is more likely (Fairburn *et al.*, 1993b). The first step is to identify negative thoughts about weight, shape and eating through self-monitoring, and to increase awareness of how these thoughts relate to mood, behaviour and physical state. The next step is to help the young person challenge these thoughts and develop alternative, more realistic thoughts, using a process of cognitive restructuring (as described previously). Other cognitive distortions, unrelated to shape and weight, may also emerge and are addressed in this phase.

As therapy proceeds, problematic attitudes and beliefs emerge – e.g. the young person may judge her self-worth in terms of her shape or weight, or may believe that she has to be perfect in every way to be approved of. She may also demonstrate other wider problems, such as unassertiveness, anxiety or difficulties in peer or family relationships. As with anorexia nervosa, these may be addressed systematically, identifying the underlying beliefs or assumptions and working to establish more realistic and helpful attitudes and beliefs.

Patients with bulimia nervosa may have symptoms such as self-harm or drug misuse, which become a way of dealing with emotions that are too difficult to bear. Treatment may need specifically to address chaotic mood states. Strategies from DBT (dialectical behaviour therapy) can be useful here – e.g. learning to regulate moods, to cope with stress and to minimize self-harm (see Linehan, 1993).

Parents and other family members may continue to have an important role in helping their daughter to change her eating pattern and manage stressful situations.

21.6.3.3   Phase 3 – relapse prevention

As with anorexia nervosa, the young person is encouraged to consolidate changes and develop strategies for preventing relapse. Further family work may be necessary to address patterns in family relationships that have emerged during the process of recovery.

21.6.4   Number and frequency of sessions

CBT in bulimia nervosa is usually given in 16–20 treatment sessions. It is suggested that, early in treatment, the patient should be seen two or three times per week (Fairburn, 1981). Where there are additional areas to deal with – e.g. low self-esteem or interpersonal difficulties – treatment may need to be longer. In anorexia nervosa, the initial phase may continue for a number of months before the young person is ready for the individual cognitive phase. Phase 2 will require at least 20 sessions. In the relapse prevention phase, sessions may be spaced at longer intervals over a period of 2–3 months.

21.6.5   Case illustration

Jane, aged 15, was referred to the adolescent service because of weight loss along with low mood, decreased energy, poor motivation for school work, impaired concentration and mood swings. Menstruation had stopped 8 months previously. At the time of referral, she was avoiding sugary and fatty foods and exercising to lose weight. She disliked her body shape and size, feeling that she was fat and out of proportion, despite being underweight.

In her background, her older brother was successful with A levels and had obtained a place at university to study medicine. Jane had a younger sister who excelled at school. Both parents were academics with high expectations of her. She described putting on weight at puberty and feeling very uncomfortable with this. At the same time, she suffered losses at school, with two friends moving away. She became very unhappy with her appearance and started dieting. She began to lose weight and was pleased with the positive comments she got from new friends at school.

The initial phase of her treatment involved working closely with the family. Her parents were encouraged to supervise and support her at meal times; they found this very difficult, as they believed their children should be autonomous and independent. They were encouraged to view Jane's problems as serious and her mother took some time off to work at home so that she could support Jane with her meals. Jane herself was reluctant to make changes, so motivational work was done to help her identify the benefits of gaining weight. Gradually, her weight began to increase and her physical state improved. Her energy levels returned. However, she continued to feel dissatisfied about her shape and weight, with low self-esteem. She was assessed for individual CBT and found to be suitable. She had individual CBT over a period of 6 months.

Initially, this involved working with her on identifying goals; these involved eating-related goals, as well as more general goals relating to self-esteem and confidence. She decided to tackle the eating-related goals first. An example was to be able to eat in front of her friends. She was able to identify negative cognitions such as: *they will think I am greedy, they will laugh at me*. She tackled this goal by devising a behavioural experiment to eat a sandwich at break-time with her friends. She set up the experiment carefully and made predictions beforehand. When she did the experiment, she was surprised to find that her friends did not pay any attention to her. There was no evidence for the prediction that they would think she was greedy. Another goal was to feel better about herself and she tackled this first by noting negative automatic thoughts about herself. She started challenging these thoughts (see Table 21.3 for self-monitoring of thoughts and alternatives) and began to develop a more balanced view of herself. During therapy, it became apparent that her identity was bound up with anorexia nervosa with little else in her life. This fitted in with her core belief that she was of no value. Through therapy, she worked hard to identify other aspects of her life that she wanted to regain, and began to develop these aspects. An important goal was to feel more confident; with self-monitoring, she noticed that she paid far more attention to situations in which she was not confident. She found it helpful to log situations that demonstrated confidence and was able to build on these situations, growing further in confidence.

Towards the end of therapy, further family meetings proved useful. Her parents had become anxious about her desire for independence, having become used to close support. It was useful to discuss Jane's need for independence and her assertiveness.

In the final phase, Jane worked on identifying factors indicating relapse. Approaching exams she noticed that she focused more on her eating and became anxious about certain foods. She realized that this might lead to abnormal eating patterns and developed ways of coping with her anxiety other than by controlling her food. At the end of therapy, she devised an action plan, indicating the things she had learnt through therapy and what she could build on for the future.

21.7   Predictors of outcome

Research on outcome in bulimia nervosa indicates that poor prognostic signs are lower body mass index at start of treatment (Turnbull *et al.*, 1996), premorbid obesity (Fairburn *et al.*, 1995), low self-esteem (Fairburn *et al.*, 1993b) and comorbid personality disorders (Wonderlich *et al.*, 1994). There are no studies, to date, which indicate the predictors of outcome for CBT in anorexia nervosa.

21.8   Conclusion and implications for research

CBT is proving a promising treatment for adolescents with eating control problems, although the research basis for this patient group is lacking. The content and nature of distorted cognitions, as well as the impact of starvation on cognitions, needs further clarification. Clinical practice suggests that cognitive elements are best introduced in line with improvements in cognitive functioning.

Core belief work with this group is an area that needs exploration. Many young people with eating disorders have negative core beliefs, but it is not clear to what extent these need to be addressed directly. Family issues are very relevant in this patient group. Research has already established the need for involvement of the family. However, an area that needs further exploration is that of intergenerational transmission of beliefs and whether it is useful to address parental beliefs that may be activated by their daughter's illness.

There is a need to work jointly with practitioners in the adult field to develop and test theoretical models that span the age groups. Finally, there is an urgent need for randomized controlled trials of CBT in adolescents, comparing it with other individual approaches, alongside family therapy.

21.9   Acknowledgements

The author wishes to acknowledge the helpful comments of Zafra Cooper and Linette Whitehead on an earlier draft of this chapter.

21.10   REFERENCES

Agras, W. S., Rossiter, E. M., Arnow, B. *et al.* (1992). Pharmacologic and cognitive-behavioural treatment for bulimia nervosa: a controlled comparison. *American Journal of Psychiatry*, **149**, 82–7.

(1994). One-year follow-up of psychosocial and pharmacologic treatments for bulimia nervosa. *Journal of Clinical Psychiatry*, **55**, 179–83.

Agras, W. S., Schneider, J. A., Arnow, B., Raeburn, S. D. and Telch, C. F. (1989). Cognitive behavioural and response prevention treatments for bulimia nervosa. *Journal of Consulting and Clinical Psychology*, **57**, 215–21.

Beck, A. T. (1976). *Cognitive Therapy and the Emotional Disorders*. New York: International Universities Press.

Button, E. J., Sonuga-Barke, E. J. S., Davies, J. and Thompson, M. (1996). A prospective study of self-esteem in the prediction of eating problems in adolescent school girls: questionnaire findings. *British Journal of Clinical Psychology*, **35**, 193–203.

Carter, J. C. and Fairburn, C. G. (1998). Cognitive-behavioural self-help for binge eating disorder: a controlled effectiveness study. *Journal of Consulting and Clinical Psychology*, **66**, 616–23.

Channon, S., Da Silva, P., Hemsley, D. and Perkins, R. (1989). A controlled trial of cognitive-behavioural and behavioural treatment of anorexia nervosa. *Behaviour Research and Therapy*, **27**, 529–35.

Childress, A., Brewerton, T., Hodges, E. and Jarell, M. (1993). The kids eating disorder survey (KEDS). A study of middle school children. *Journal of the American Academy of Child and Adolescent Psychiatry*, **32**, 843–50.

Cooper, M. (1997). Cognitive theory in anorexia nervosa and bulimia nervosa: a review. *Behavioural and Cognitive Psychotherapy*, **25**, 113–45.

Cooper, P. (1995). *Bulimia Nervosa and Binge Eating: A Guide to Recovery*. London: Robinson Publishing.

Cooper, P. and Fairburn, C. G. (1984). Cognitive-behavioural treatment for anorexia nervosa: some preliminary findings. *Journal of Psychosomatic Research*, **28**, 493–9.

Cooper, P. J., Coker, S. and Fleming, C. (1996). An evaluation of the efficacy of supervised cognitive-behavioural self-help for bulimia nervosa. *Journal of Psychosomatic Research*, **28**, 493–9.

Dare, C., Eisler, I., Colahan, M., Crowther, C., Senior, R. and Asen, E. (1995). The listening heart and the chi square: clinical and empirical perceptions in the family therapy of anorexia nervosa. *Journal of Family Therapy*, **17**, 31–57.

Dodge, E., Hodes, M., Eisler, I. and Dare, C. (1995). Family therapy for bulimia nervosa in adolescents: an exploratory study. *Journal of Family Therapy*, **17**, 59–77.

Eisler, I., Dare, C., Hodes, M., Russell, G., Dodge, E. and Le Grange, D. (2000). Family therapy for adolescent anorexia nervosa: the results of a controlled comparison of two family interventions. *Journal of Child Psychology and Psychiatry*, **41**, 727–36.

Fairburn, C. G. (1981). A cognitive-behavioural approach to the management of bulimia nervosa, *Psychological Medicine*, **11**, 707–11.

(1995). *Overcoming Binge Eating*. New York: Guilford Press.

Fairburn, C. and Beglin, S. J. (1990). Studies of the epidemiology of bulimia nervosa. *American Journal of Psychiatry*, **147**, 401–8.

Fairburn, C. G. and Wilson, G. T. (1993). *Binge Eating: Nature, Assessment and Treatment*. New York: Guilford Press.

Fairburn, C. G., Agras, S. and Wilson, G. T. (1992). The research on the treatment of bulimia nervosa: practical and theoretical implications. In G. H. Anderson and S. N. Kennedy (eds.), *The Biology of Feast and Famine Relevance to Eating Disorders*. New York: Academic Press, pp. 318–40.

Fairburn, C. G., Cooper, Z. and Cooper, P. (1986a). The clinical features and maintenance of bulimia nervosa. In K. D. Brownell and J. P. Foreyt (eds.), *Handbook of Eating Disorders: Physiology, Psychology and Treatment of Obesity, Anorexia and Bulimia*. New York: Basic Books, pp. 389–404.

Fairburn, C. G. Cooper, Z., Doll, H. and Welch, S. (1999a). Risk factors for anorexia nervosa: a community based case-control study. *Archives of General Psychiatry*, **56**, 468–76.

Fairburn, C. G., Cooper, Z. and Shafran, R. (2003). Cognitive behaviour therapy for eating disorders: a transdiagnostic theory and treatment. *Behaviour, Research and Therapy*, **41**, 509–28.

Fairburn, C. G., Jones, R., Peveler, R. C. *et al.* (1991). Three psychological treatments for bulimia nervosa. *Archives of General Psychiatry*, **48**, 463–9.

Fairburn, C. G., Jones, R., Peveler, R. C., Hope, R. A. and O'Connor, M. (1993a). Psychotherapy and bulimia nervosa: the longer term effects of interpersonal psychotherapy, behavioural therapy and cognitive behavioural therapy. *Archives of General Psychiatry*, **50**, 419–28.

Fairburn, C. G., Kirk, J., O'Connor, M. and Cooper, P. J. (1986b). A comparison of two psychological treatments for bulimia nervosa. *Behaviour Research and Therapy*, **24**, 629–43.

Fairburn, C. G., Norman, P. A., Welch, S. L., O'Connor, M. E., Doll, H. A. and Peveler, R. C. (1995). A prospective study of outcome in bulimia nervosa and the long term effects of three psychological treatments. *Archives of General Psychiatry*, **52**, 304–12.

Fairburn, C. G., Peveler, R. C., Jones, R., Hope, R. A. and Doll, H. A. (1993b). Predictors of twelve-month outcome in bulimia nervosa and the influence of attitudes to shape and weight. *Journal of Consulting and Clinical Psychology*, **61**, 696–8.

Fairburn, C. G., Shafran, R. and Cooper, Z. (1999b). A cognitive behavioural theory of anorexia nervosa. *Behaviour, Research and Therapy*, **37**, 1–13.

Fairburn, C. G., Welch, S. L., Doll, H., Davies, B. and O'Connor, M. E. (1997). Risk factors for bulimia nervosa: a community based case-control study. *Archives of General Psychiatry*, **54**, 509–17.

Garner, D. M., Vitousek, K. M. and Pike, K. M. (1997). Cognitive-behavioural therapy for anorexia nervosa. In D. M. Garner and P. E. Garfinkel (eds.), *Handbook of Treatment for Eating Disorders*, 2nd edn. New York: Guilford Press, pp. 94–144.

Hill, A. J., Oliver, S. and Rogers, P. J. (1992). Eating in the adult world: the rise of dieting in childhood and adolescence. *British Journal of Clinical Psychology*, **31**, 95–105.

Killen, J., Taylor, C. and Hayward, C. (1994). The pursuit of thinness and the onset of eating disorder symptoms in a community sample of adolescent girls: a three-year prospective analysis. *International Journal of Eating Disorders*, **16**, 227–38.

Koff, E. and Rierdan, J. (1993). Advanced pubertal development and eating disturbances in early adolescent girls. *Journal of Adolescent Health*, **14**, 472–91.

Levine, M. P., Smolak, L. and Hayden, H. (1994). The relation of socio-cultural factors to eating attitudes and behaviours among middle school girls. *International Journal of Eating Disorders*, **15**, 11–20.

Linehan, M. M. (1993). *Skills Training Manual for Treating Borderline Personality Disorder.* New York: Guilford Press.

Lock, J. (2002). Treating adolescents with eating disorders within the family context: empirical and theoretical considerations. *Child and Adolescent Psychiatric Clinics*, **11**, 331–42.

Padesky, C. (1991). Schema as self-prejudice. *International Cognitive Therapy Network*, **6**, 16–17.

Patton, G., Johnson-Sabine, E., Wood, K., Mann, A. and Wakeling, A. (1990). Abnormal eating attitudes in London schoolgirls – a prospective epidemiological study: outcomes at twelve month follow-up. *Psychological Medicine*, **23**, 175–84.

Rathner, G. and Messner, K. (1993). Detection of eating disorders in a small rural town: an epidemiological study. *Psychological Medicine*, **23**, 175–84.

Robin, A. L., Siegel, P. T., Moye, A. W., Gilroy, M., Dennis, A. B. and Sikand, A. (1999). A controlled comparison of family versus individual therapy for adolescents with anorexia nervosa. *Journal of the American Academy of Child and Adolescent Psychiatry*, **38**, 1482–9.

Russell, G. F. M., Dare, C., Eisler, I. and Le Grange, P. D. F. (1992). Controlled trials of family treatments in anorexia nervosa. In K. A. Halmi (ed.), *Psychobiology and Treatment of Anorexia Nervosa and Bulimia Nervosa*. Washington, DC: American Psychiatric Press.

Serfaty, M. A., Turkington, D., Heap, M., Ledsham, L. and Jolley, E. (1999). Cognitive therapy versus dietary counselling in the outpatient treatment of anorexia nervosa: effects of the treatment phase. *European Eating Disorders Review*, 7, 334–50.

Serpell, L. T., Treasure, J., Teasdale, J. and Sullivan, V. (1999). Anorexia nervosa: friend or foe? *International Journal of Eating Disorders*, 25, 177–86.

Schmidt, U. and Treasure, J. (1993). *Getting Better Bit(e) by Bit(e)*. London: Lawrence Erlbaum Associates.

Shore, R. A. and Porter, J. E. (1990). Normative and reliability data for 11–18 year old on the Eating Disorder Inventory. *International Journal of Eating Disorders*, 9, 201–7.

Smolak, L. and Levine, M. P. (1994). Towards an empirical basis for primary prevention of eating problems with elementary school children. *Eating Disorders: The Journal of Treatment and Prevention*, 2, 293–307.

Thackwray, D. E., Smith, M. C., Bodfish, J. W. and Meyers, A. W. (1993). A comparison of behavioural and cognitive-behavioural interventions for bulimia nervosa. *Journal of Consulting and Clinical Psychology*, 61, 639–45.

Treasure, J. and Schmidt, U. (1997). *Clinicians' Guide to Getting Better Bit(e) by Bit(e)*. Hove: Lawrence Erlbaum Associates.

Treasure, J. and Ward, A. (1997). A practical guide to the use of motivational interviewing in anorexia nervosa. *European Eating Disorder Review*, 5, 102–14.

Treasure, J., Schmidt, U., Troop, N., Tiller, J. and Todd, G. (1994). First step in managing bulimia nervosa: a controlled trial of a therapeutic manual. *British Medical Journal*, **308**, 686–9.

Turnbull, S., Treasure, J., Schmidt, U., Troop, N., Tiller, J. and Todd, G. (1996). Predictors of short term and long term outcome of bulimia nervosa. *International Journal of Eating Disorders*, 21, 17–22.

Van Hoeken, D., Lucas, A. R. and Hoek, H. W. (1998). Epidemiology. In H. W. Hoek, J. L. Treasure and M. A. Katsman (eds.), *Neurobiology in the Treatment of Eating Disorders*. Chichester: John Wiley and Sons, pp. 97–126.

Vitousek, K. B. and Orimoto, L. (1993). Cognitive-behavioural models of anorexia nervosa, bulimia nervosa and obesity. In P. Kendall and K. Dobson (eds.), *Psychopathology and Cognition*. New York: Academic Press, pp. 191–243.

Walsh, B. T., Wilson, G. T., Loeb, K., Pike, K. and Devlin, M. J. (1997). Pharmacological and psychological treatment of bulimia nervosa. *Journal of Psychiatry*, **154**, 523–31.

Whitaker, A., Johnson, J., Shaffer, D. *et al.* (1990). Uncommon troubles in young people. Prevalence estimates of selected psychiatric disorders in a non-referred psychiatric population. *Archives of General Psychiatry*, 47, 487–96.

Wilson, G. T., Fairburn, C. G. and Agras, W. S. (1997). Cognitive-behavioural therapy for bulimia nervosa. In D. M. Garner and P. E. Garfinkel (eds.), *Handbook of Treatment for Eating Disorders*, 2nd edn. New York: Guilford Press, pp. 67–93.

Wolff, G. and Serpell, L. (1998). A cognitive model and treatment strategies for anorexia nervosa. In H. W. Hoek, J. Treasure and M. A. Katzman (eds.), *Neurobiology in the Treatment of Eating Disorders*. London: Wiley.

Wonderlich, S. A., Fullerton, D., Swift, W. J. and Klein, M. H. (1994). Five-year outcome from eating disorders: relevance of personality disorders. *International Journal of Eating Disorders*, **15**, 233–43.

22

Chronic fatigue syndrome

Trudie Chalder

Guy's, King's and St. Thomas' School of Medicine, London, UK

22.1 Introduction

Chronic fatigue syndrome (CFS), sometimes known as myalgic encephalomyelitis (ME), is a condition characterized by physical and mental fatigue which is made worse by exercise and is associated with profound disability (Sharpe *et al.*, 1991; Fukuda *et al.*, 1994). The consensus document issued by the three UK Royal Colleges considered the diagnostic criteria developed for adults were equally applicable to children, with the exception of the 6-month criterion, which is considered to be too long for children (Anon, 1996). Muscle pain, headache, sore throat and increased somnolence are typical in children (Marshall *et al.*, 1991; Smith *et al.*, 1991; Feder *et al.*, 1994; Carter *et al.*, 1995) and disability can be profound. Children referred to specialist centres often have had long periods of time away from school accompanied by impairment in social and leisure activities. Loss of peer relationships is frequent (Smith *et al.*, 1991; Feder *et al.*, 1994; Carter *et al.*, 1995). Despite the severity of the condition, a systematic review found that 54–94% of children made good recoveries (Joyce *et al.*, 1997). Good prognostic factors included specific physical triggers to the illness, start of illness in the autumn school term and higher socioeconomic status (Rangel *et al.*, 2000a), while poor prognosis was associated with somatic (de Jong *et al.*, 1997) or biological (Garralda and Rangel, 2001) attributions and illness enhancing cognitions and behaviours of parents as well as physical inactivity (de Jong *et al.*, 1997).

Like most disorders, evidence to date suggests that CFS is a heterogeneous condition which results from a complex interaction of physiological, cognitive, behavioural and affective factors in the child and the other family members.

Cognitive Behaviour Therapy for Children and Families, ed. Philip J. Graham.
Published by Cambridge University Press. © Cambridge University Press 2004.

The purpose of this chapter is to describe a family-orientated cognitive behavioural approach to CFS in adolescents, which is the approach the author and colleagues are currently evaluating at King's College Hospital, London. It is psychoeducational in that it is based on the idea that all illnesses are affected by physiological, cognitive, behavioural, affective, familial and social processes and much of the initial work with families involves information giving and explanation.

22.2   Epidemiology

Fatigue as a symptom is rarely reported by children prior to adolescence (Morrell, 1972; OPCS, 1985; Essen-Moller, 1956). However, after puberty, the prevalence of fatigue starts to rise (Eminson *et al.*, 1996). At one end of the spectrum, newspaper headlines such as 'Schools swept by M.E. plague' (Boseley, 1997) suggest that CFS or ME in children is of epidemic proportions, while, at the other end, the existence of the disorder is refuted (Plioplys, 1997). A recent population study suggests that the prevalence rate of CFS in children is comparable to some of the less common disorders found in childhood, such as eating disorders or severe tic disorders (Chalder *et al.*, 2003). In this study, 0.19% of children aged 11–15 years met criteria for CFS while only 0.04% of parents reported their child (5–15 year olds) had ME. There was no overlap between children's symptom reporting and parental labelling, indicating that parent and child may have different perceptions of symptomatic experience. Lack of concordance has been found previously in a community study examining bodily experiences and health concerns in adolescents (Taylor *et al.*, 1996), where there was virtually no agreement between parents and adolescents on the presence or absence of individual somatic symptoms.

22.3   Clinical description

Affected adolescents complain of feeling exhausted. They say that this subjective state is unfamiliar and unlike the sort of tiredness they used to feel when well. The fatigue is usually exacerbated by activity and even minor exertions can leave the patient feeling unwell for days. Many patients complain of additional symptoms such as headache, pain and 'flu-like' symptoms. Associated disability varies considerably. At the more severe end of the spectrum, an inability to go to school is common with some confined to a wheelchair or with some being bed bound. Most patients will complain of abnormal sleep patterns, particularly onset or sleep maintenance insomnia, hypersomnia and daytime sleepiness.

Of particular interest are patients' beliefs about the cause of their problem. Although some hold strong physical illness attributions, the majority do have a fairly sophisticated understanding of the factors associated with the onset. More importantly, most will not feel competent in managing the illness and will be confused about how to move forwards consistently.

22.4 Comorbidity

The overlap between psychiatric disorder and CFS in children has been investigated by a number of authors in secondary care, using questionnaires (Smith et al., 1991; Vereker, 1992; Walford et al., 1993; Carter et al., 1996). More recently, however, Garralda et al. (1999), in a carefully conducted, controlled study, used research psychiatric interviews as well as self-report scales to investigate psychiatric adjustment in affected youngsters, some of whom had recovered. Fifty per cent of adolescents with CFS had a psychiatric disorder (usually anxiety or depressive disorders) at assessment. Recovered CFS patients were more likely to have an anxiety disorder than those with active illness.

It has been argued that the psychiatric comorbidity found in patients with CFS is secondary to the experience of having a chronic physical disease. However, research from cross-sectional studies, using both questionnaires and standardized interviews, has indicated that adolescents with CFS display more psychological distress and depressive symptoms than those with debilitating chronic medical conditions such as cystic fibrosis, juvenile idiopathic arthritis and cancer (Walford et al., 1993; Pelcovitz et al., 1995; Brace et al., 2000; Rangel et al., 2003).

22.5 Medical management

In order to ensure patients do not have a comorbid disease or indeed a disease which would produce fatigue as a main symptom, a battery of screening tests may be carried out. This may include a full blood count, erythrocyte sedimentation rate or C-reactive protein, liver function tests, urea and electrolytes, thyroid-stimulating hormone and thyroid function tests and creatinine phosphokinase. However, usually a careful history and physical examination will be sufficient. This may be carried out by the general practitioner or paediatrician who may have been asked for an opinion. Generally, patients respond well to being given a diagnosis of CFS. Deale and Wessely (2001) reported on the perceptions of medical care that adult patients with CFS had received. Two-thirds of patients were dissatisfied, many with the dispute or confusion over the diagnosis. They perceived doctors as sceptical or not knowledgeable about CFS and felt the advice they were given was inadequate or conflicting. Confirming a diagnosis of CFS, if appropriate, can therefore pave the way for a more fruitful relationship, if it is then backed up by some specific advice about how to manage the problem.

22.6   A multi-factorial model of CFS

Cognitive behavioural therapy (CBT) is a pragmatic approach to managing and rehabilitating patients with CFS. It is based on a model of the condition that distinguishes between predisposing, precipitating and perpetuating factors.

22.6.1   Predisposing and precipitating factors

There are a number of factors both in the parents and child which may result in the child being vulnerable to developing CFS. In adults with CFS, there is some evidence from a small cross-sectional study that CFS patients, compared with controls, report their mothers as having been more overprotective (Fisher and Chalder, 2003). This certainly fits with this author's experience in the clinical setting, although the direction of causality is always difficult to ascertain. There are cases in the medical literature where illness in the child appears to be linked to beliefs and behaviours of the parents (Harris and Taitz, 1989; Marcovitch, 1997).

A possible reason for overprotectiveness in the mother may be related to her own level of distress. In a large cross-sectional study in the community, mother's psychological distress as assessed by the general health questionnaire (GHQ) was associated with fatigue in the child (Chalder et al., in press). In other psychiatric disorders, cross-sectional evidence suggests that mothers' distress may impact negatively on their child's health (Meltzer et al., 2000). It is possible that parents who are anxious themselves may be more focused on symptoms in their children, thereby influencing symptom reporting and help-seeking behaviour. This was borne out in a study using the national birth cohort where paternal 'nerves' were associated with unexplained hospital admissions and maternal neuroticism was associated with an increased risk of unexplained hospital admissions in males (Hotopf et al., 2000).

Although maternal or paternal behaviour will undoubtedly affect the child, the child's response to their parents will depend to some extent on their personality. Rangel et al. (2000b) recently reported impaired personality problems in one-half of the CFS adolescents, which is a replication of their early findings. The CFS adolescents were sensitive, vulnerable and conforming, with a tendency to depend on others. They were also anxiety prone, with a tendency to rigidity, conscientiousness and thoughtfulness. As Rangel points out, as desirable as these qualities are, they may compromise adaptation to common stresses such as infection and school pressures which are often associated with the onset of CFS.

Throughout childhood and adolescence, the types of stimuli which elicit concern and fear change. These changes parallel developments in cognitive and social competencies (Ollendick *et al.*, 1994). In late childhood, failure in academic and athletic performance at school becomes a source of fear as does fear about peer rejection. These issues are often salient topics for adolescents with CFS, particularly once activities have been increased and a return to school is being discussed. A recent, as yet unpublished study found that, although CFS adolescents and normal controls had similar IQs, parental and child expectations of IQ were higher in the CFS group (Coddington and Chalder, 2003). Thus, internal and external pressure to perform may have the paradoxical effect of lowering levels of performance. It also appears to be a general trait. Two other independently conducted studies have found similar results. In one study, CFS adolescents underestimated normative adolescent energy levels compared with healthy controls (Garralda and Rangel, 2001). In another study, adolescents with CFS and their parents underestimated the child's activity levels and furthermore the adolescent would have liked to have achieved higher levels of activity in the future than they expected to achieve. Parents also had this expectation (Fry and Martin, 1996). These findings do suggest that, if an individual's goals are out of proportion to what they may realistically achieve, the result may be avoidance of future attempts. These findings and observations in the clinical setting indicate a general tendency towards perfectionism, in many domains of life, which leads to all or nothing criteria for performance.

Two studies have noted a close connection between an exacerbation of symptoms and the start of a new term at school (Wilson *et al.*, 1989; Vereker, 1992). However, in the context of an individual who may be vulnerable for the aforementioned reasons, clinical experience suggests that a number of events such as stress, overactivity and a viral illness converge, resulting in the onset of severe acute fatigue.

22.6.2   Perpetuating factors

Once triggered, other influences, such as reducing activity due to concern about making symptoms worse and inappropriate advice from health professionals, may inadvertently perpetuate the fatigue and other symptoms, leading to substantial disability. In adults, fears about the nature of the illness, the meaning of symptoms, the consequences of activity and fear that activity or exercise will make symptoms worse are common (Deale *et al.*, 1998). Children have all these fears and more. They also worry about school performance and fear being rejected by friends.

Longitudinal studies have demonstrated that making physical illness attributions for fatigue predicts the degree of disability in adults with CFS (Sharpe et al., 1992; Chalder et al., 1996). In an effort to control and reduce symptoms, patients become hypervigilant and oversensitized to bodily sensations. This symptom focusing may serve to exacerbate unpleasant sensations and has been shown to be associated with fatigue in adult patients with CFS (Ray et al., 1995).

Prolonged rest and avoidance of activity is central in sustaining the cycle of symptoms and disability in CFS. Sharpe et al. (1992) found that avoiding exercise predicted disability, while Ray et al. (1995) found an association between functional impairment and accommodating to the illness in patients with CFS. For the majority of patients and their families, rest appears to be an effective coping strategy because it reduces symptoms in the short term. However, the long-term effects of decreased activity results in more symptoms at progressively lower levels of exertion. In reality, patients will often adopt a 'boom and bust' approach to activity, characterized by periods of prolonged rest interspersed with bursts of activity. This pattern is often driven by boredom, personal expectations or social pressures. In essence, activity has become symptom dependent and, as time goes on, the symptoms become more and more controlling.

The long-term physiological consequences of inactivity are deleterious. Very quickly, the individual becomes unfit and starting activity and exercise gets harder. Many adolescents with CFS will be engaged in very little exercise or activity and many will have developed a poor sleep routine, resulting in them sleeping during the day and being awake at night. The longer this persists, the more confidence is lost and returning to full-time education becomes all the more daunting. Despite the evidence, many families are advised to rest by ill-informed health professionals. The iatrogenic damage caused by this advice is profound. Many families feel very confused and upset by the contradictory advice they receive.

Cognitive behavioural interventions are based on the model described. In the first instance, the more obvious behavioural and cognitive responses, such as fear and avoidance, are addressed. Once a therapeutic alliance has been formed and trust developed, then more complex issues such as perfectionism and black and white thinking are approached.

22.7   A rehabilitation programme based on CBT

The main aim of treatment is to enable patients, with the help of their families, to carry out their own rehabilitation with some support and guidance from their therapist. Initially, treatment will involve the introduction of a consistent graded approach to activity and establishing a sleep routine (Chalder *et al.*, 2002). Cognitive strategies may be used but are sometimes unnecessary. It is important that parents are reassured about the safety of the approach and are given support in encouraging their child to engage in rehabilitation. Once the process of change has begun, the difficulties associated with being absent from school, such as loss of confidence, can be addressed. Given that the illness has occurred at a crucial stage of development, particularly in older teenagers, it is important to address issues of individuation and separation – just as it is to acknowledge how difficult it is for parents who have had to cope with the stress of caring for a child or children with a chronic illness, the difficulties of which are well recognized (Eiser, 1997). Throughout treatment, the therapist endeavours to focus on the end goal, i.e. enabling the child to return to school full time. Temptations to explore other issues within the family, i.e. difficulties within the parental relationship, are resisted, unless it is clear that progress will be facilitated by such a diversion.

Success with treatment seems to depend as much on the qualities of the therapist as on the activity scheduling itself. It is important that the therapist is positive and optimistic about the possibility of change while at the same time remaining mindful of how long change can sometimes take. It is not unusual for end of treatment goals to take up to 1 year to achieve, especially if the child is wheelchair or bed bound.

22.8   Assessment

The assessment should include not only a detailed description of symptoms but also, more importantly, a detailed behavioural analysis of what the adolescent is able to do in relation to school, home, private and social aspects of their lives. The quality and quantity of sleep should be enquired about. A detailed account of activity, rest and sleep patterns should be obtained by asking the patient to keep a diary for 2 weeks. This will be used as a guide for setting the initial behavioural goals and can be used throughout treatment to monitor progress. Specific fears about the consequences of activity and exercise should be elicited as should more general ideas about the nature of the illness. Circumstances surrounding the onset should be discussed as this information may be useful when giving the patient a rationale for treatment and lifestyle factors may need to be addressed during treatment. It is important at this stage to enquire about the presence of depression and/or anxiety. If severe, such disorders may require treatment in their own right, either before CBT or concurrently.

22.9   Engagement

Engaging the patient and family in treatment and forming a therapeutic alliance is a continual process. From the outset, the entire family is invited to attend, but the adolescent is the main focus of attention during treatment. This is done with a view to empowering them to take responsibility for their own progress and increasing the clarity of boundaries to facilitate the individuation of all family members.

During the assessment, various family members, who may be sensitive to being disbelieved, may be on the look out for evidence that the therapist thinks the problem is 'all in the mind'. During the early stage of treatment, it is helpful for the therapist to be explicit in conveying belief in the real and physical nature of the symptoms. Careful attention should be paid to the language that is used. The term 'psychological' is probably best avoided – first, because it is a broad term which means different things to different people and, secondly, because it may set the scene for unnecessary disagreement between the family and the therapist. The patient's symptoms are real and it helps to state and restate this. Rather than debating whether the problem is physical or psychological – a mind/body split which is unhelpful in any illness – it is far more useful to direct the discussion towards how the problem can best be managed, taking into account physiological, behavioural and cognitive factors.

22.10   Rationale for treatment

Once a thorough assessment has been carried out, the therapist should share with the family an initial formulation of the problem. While openly acknowledging that this is to some extent hypothetical, it should help the process of engagement and will form part of the rationale for treatment, which is a prerequisite to any intervention. It stands to reason that having an understanding of how and why treatment works will aid compliance.

The rationale will obviously vary depending on the individual's circumstances but essentially the patient should be told that the emphasis in treatment will be on perpetuating factors. Initially, diary keeping of activity and sleep patterns will highlight areas of inconsistency. These are used to set goals with a view to establishing a consistent level of activity every day regardless of symptoms. The amount of activity is then gradually increased and rest decreased as the patient becomes more confident. It can be helpful to point out that rest is useful in an acute illness but is rarely restorative in the longer term. A sleep routine should also be established as quickly as possible.

The rationale may be discussed several times throughout treatment. It can be useful to ask the patient to describe how they think the approach works in order to check out whether the potential benefits of treatment have been clearly understood and to discuss any concerns. Before commencing treatment, it is important that the entire family is clear about what it entails. The aims of treatment should be explicitly negotiated and agreed with the patient. These aims are best defined in terms of specific and realistic achievements or goals which are worked towards gradually and depend on the individual needs of the child.

22.11   Structure

Families are usually seen fortnightly for up to 15 sessions of face to face treatment. Follow-ups are carried out at 3 and 6 months and then at 1 year to monitor progress and tackle any residual problems. Written material and self-help books are offered (Chalder, 1995; Chalder and Hussain, 2002) to supplement verbal interactions. Questionnaires are given to assess fatigue and disability before and after treatment and at follow-up. At the beginning of treatment, long-term targets are negotiated with the patient to ensure therapist, patients and their families are working towards similar goals. At every subsequent session, short-term goals are agreed upon. Patients keep records of their activity and rest throughout treatment so that progress can be monitored and problems discussed.

At times, both the young person and other family members may be assigned homework. For example, a mother may agree to wake her son once at a certain time and make him a cup of tea once he's dressed and downstairs, while the adolescent person with CFS may take responsibility for setting an alarm and getting up at a pre-set time. Mothers may agree not to discuss their children's symptoms for more than 5 minutes per day.

Problems are anticipated and problem-solving strategies are used to elicit effective coping. Discussion during sessions often revolves around exploring issues in the family which may be preventing the patient from making changes. A variety of techniques are used to facilitate change. Socratic questions are used to explore specific concerns or difficulties. The therapist may need to slow down the expectation of success. Less pressure to succeed often results in quicker success, on the part of therapist and patient. Rewards for achieving goals can be helpful. Parents should be encouraged to praise their child or a specific reward can be negotiated during therapy for positive achievements.

22.12   Activity scheduling

Goals usually include a mixture of social, school and leisure-related activities. Short walks or tasks carried out in even chunks throughout the day are ideal and are interspersed with rests. The emphasis is on consistency and breaking the association between experiencing symptoms and stopping activity. The goals (for someone less disabled), e.g. walking for 10 minutes three times daily, are gradually built up as tolerance to symptoms increase, until the longer term targets are reached. Fatigue levels do not decrease very much initially but between discharge and follow-up marked reductions in fatigue would be expected. Tasks such as reading or school work, which require concentration, can be included but mental functioning does seem to improve in synchrony with physical functioning.

22.13   Establishing a sleep routine

Early on in treatment, patients are asked to keep a diary of bedtime, sleep time, wake up time and get up time. The total number of hours spent asleep is calculated and a variety of strategies can then be used both to improve quality and quantity of sleep. A routine of going to bed and getting up at a preplanned time, while simultaneously cutting out daytime catnaps, helps to improve both hypersomnia and insomnia. Change in sleep routine can be done slowly depending on the severity of the problem. For those who sleep too much, the amount of time they spend asleep can be reduced gradually. A detailed description of how to manage sleep problems is provided by Morin *et al.* (1994). It can be difficult for teenagers to establish a sleep routine, particularly when they are not at school but also because it is not uncommon for children of this age to sleep late into the morning. Some flexibility should be built into the negotiated programme.

22.14   Modifying negative and unhelpful thinking

The initial aim of this component is to prevent unhelpful thoughts from blocking progressive increases in activity. Information about the nature of CFS and the process of rehabilitation should be shared with the family throughout treatment as many patients will have been given incorrect or misleading information about their illness. Explanations regarding the physiological effects of inactivity can help patients understand the rationale for activity scheduling, while demonstrating the effect of attention on symptoms can also help patients use enjoyable activities as a form of distraction.

Information to assist self-help given at various stages of treatment can be helpful. In reality, unhelpful beliefs about the harmful effects of exercise will diminish as the patient becomes more active and confident. However, some will need more structured cognitive therapy using traditional methods (see Beck *et al.*, 1979). Specific negative thoughts such as 'My muscles will be damaged by exercising too much' should be recorded in a diary. Patients should be encouraged to elicit alternative, less catastrophic interpretations of events. These too should be recorded in a diary and discussed during consultations. In some patients, core beliefs and dysfunctional assumptions relating to perfectionism or self-worth can be tackled in the conventional way using Beck's cognitive therapy (Beck *et al.*, 1979). Excellent manuals for patient and therapist are now available (Greenberger and Padesky, 1996).

22.15 Treating comorbidity

Most adolescents will report symptoms of distress in one form or another throughout the process of therapy. Some with severe depression may benefit from antidepressants. A randomized controlled trial of fluoxetine in children and adolescents with non-psychotic depression provided some support for the use of this antidepressant with this age group (Emslie, 1997). Others will find their mood improves with activity scheduling and cognitive restructuring. For those with an anxiety disorder, discussion about the physiological aspects of the anxiety can be helpful. Many adolescents and their parents are unaware of how anxiety can show itself in physical symptoms. Giving information about the nature of autonomic arousal often helps explain the patient's experience of intrusive, frightening somatic sensations.

22.16 Tackling psychosocial problems

Related social or psychological difficulties will often emerge during treatment. It is important that these are tackled in a problem-solving way, otherwise they may prevent further progress. However, the focus needs to be on rehabilitation. Being distracted from the main task in hand may lead to treatment failure. Improvements in one particular area of a patient's life will usually generalize to other areas. A side effect of treatment, though, may be an increase in arguments within the family. Some of our adolescents who become more assertive and independent during the course of treatment become more confident in expressing their views which do not always concur with their parents. Merely acknowledging this change can be helpful.

22.17   Education

Negotiating a return to formal education can be difficult. Realistically, many adolescents present for treatment when they are only months off finishing school at age 16. Understandably, the patient may have reservations about returning to school towards the end of an academic year. There is no black and white rule about how to negotiate this aspect of care. From a therapeutic perspective, several factors need to be considered: the patient's level of fear; the degree of disability; the age of the patient; the time of year; plans for the future; and the school's view and their degree of support. The long-term goal usually involves a return to education or work, if age appropriate, outside the home. Some adolescents will be attending school part time, some will have home tuition, some will be working at home independently and liaising with the school, while others will not be receiving any education at all. All of these factors need to be carefully considered during the process. It is usually helpful to negotiate with the school and home tutor directly to ensure that all involved are being supportive and working towards similar goals. The child may need considerable encouragement, especially in the earlier stages of change.

Although a return to full-time education may take several months, it is important to consider the consequences of children not being at school, both educationally and socially. Clearly, the longer a child is away from school the more confidence that will be lost and the further behind with their work they will become, making a return even more daunting. It can be helpful to examine the possibility of reducing the number of GCSE or A level examinations undertaken. Examining perfectionism and all or nothing thinking can be particularly useful in relation to academic issues.

22.18   Facilitating change

Resistance to change is maintained by dissonance reduction. It can be recognized by the way in which patients and their families respond to situations or information which challenge or contradict their beliefs. A reluctance to accept an interpretation or advice is often a consequence of efforts to maintain a consistent interpersonal stance. Change has to occur slowly in order to maintain an adaptive and socially acceptable level of historical continuity. In the first instance, the therapist should support the patient's point of view, thus accepting the family and working with their attributions of cause and control. Therapeutic change can then occur slowly without arousing too much dissonance (Kirmayer, 1990). Minuchin discusses the use of mimesis, where the therapist adopts the family's tempo of communication – e.g. slowing pace in a family that is accustomed to long pauses and slow responses. In a jovial family, the therapist may become jocular and expansive; in a family with a restricted style, communications would be more sparse (Minuchin, 1974).

Contrary to popular belief, it is not necessary to challenge individuals' or families' beliefs about the aetiology of the illness directly (Deale *et al.*, 1998). Rather, specific cognitions about the danger of activity and exercise can be examined and, if appropriate, addressed. Joining and accommodating to the family's beliefs is far more advantageous to the process of change. All family members need to be supported throughout treatment and it can be helpful to discuss their different ways of coping with illness, thereby directing blame away from specific individuals.

22.19   Treatment evidence

A number of case studies and case reports suggest that an effective approach, which takes into account such factors, involves a combination of behavioural interventions often linked with a family therapy approach (Wachsmuth and MacMillan, 1991; Rikard-Bell and Waters, 1992; Vereker, 1992; Cox and Findley, 1994; Sidebotham *et al.*, 1994; Pipe and Wait, 1995; Chalder *et al.*, 2002). There are no randomized controlled trials demonstrating the effectiveness of a family-focused approach in children. However, this is not the case in adults. A number of studies have shown that, in the context of a supportive relationship, either CBT and/or graded exercise improves disability and symptoms in patients with CFS (Sharpe *et al.*, 1996; Deale *et al.*, 1997; Fulcher and White, 1997; Wearden *et al.*, 1998; Powell *et al.*, 2001; Prins *et al.*, 2001). We now await the results of two randomized controlled trials currently being conducted in adolescents with CFS.

22.20   REFERENCES

Anon (1996). *Chronic Fatigue Syndrome: Report of a Committee of the Royal Colleges of Physicians, Psychiatrists and General Practitioners.* London: Royal College of Physicians.

Beck, A., Rush, A. J., Shaw, B. F. and Emery, G. (1979). *Cognitive Therapy of Depression.* New York: Guilford Press.

Boseley, S. (1997). Schools swept by ME plague. London: *The Guardian.*

Brace, M., Scott Smith, M., McCauley, E. and Sherry, D. (2000). Family reinforcement of illness behaviour: a comparison of adolescents with chronic fatigue syndrome, juvenile arthritis and healthy controls. *Developmental and Behavioral Pediatrics,* **5**, 332–9.

Carter, B., Edwards, J., Kronenberger, W., Michalczyk, L. and Marshall, G. (1995). Case control study of chronic fatigue in pediatric patients. *Pediatrics*, **95**, 179–86.

Carter, B., Kronenberger, W., Edwards, F., Michalczyk, L. and Marshall, G. (1996). Differential diagnosis of chronic fatigue in children: behavioral and emotional dimensions. *Journal of Developmental and Behavioral Paediatrics*, **17**, 16–21.

Chalder, T. (1995). *Coping with Chronic Fatigue*. London: Sheldon Press.

Chalder, T. and Hussain, K. (2002). *Self Help for Chronic Fatigue Syndrome: A Guide for Young People*. Oxford: Blue Stallion Publications.

Chalder, T., Goodman, R., Wessely, S., Hotopf, M. and Meltzer, H. (in press). The epidemiology of chronic fatigue syndrome in 5–15 year olds: a cross sectional study. *British Medical Journal*.

Chalder, T., Power, M. and Wessely, S. (1996). Chronic fatigue in the community: 'a question of attribution'. *Psychological Medicine*, **26**, 791–800.

Chalder, T., Tong, J. and Deary, V. (2002). Family focused cognitive behaviour therapy for chronic fatigue syndrome. *Archives of Disease in Childhood*, **86**, 95–7.

Coddington, A. and Chalder, T. (2003). Do parents of children with CFS have higher expectations of them? Abstract, British Association of Behavioural and Cognitive Psychotherapists Annual Conference, York.

Cox, D. and Findley, L. (1994). Chronic fatigue syndrome in adolescence. *British Journal of Hospital Medicine*, **51**, 614.

Deale, A. and Wessely, S. (2001). Patients' perceptions of medical care in chronic fatigue syndrome. *Social Science and Medicine*, **52**, 1859–64.

Deale, A., Chalder, T., Marks, I. and Wessely, S. (1997). A randomised controlled trial of cognitive behaviour versus relaxation therapy for chronic fatigue syndrome. *American Journal of Psychiatry*, **154**, 408–14.

Deale, A., Chalder, T. and Wessely, S. (1998). Illness beliefs and outcome in chronic fatigue syndrome: is change in causal attribution necessary for clinical improvement? *Journal of Psychosomatic Research*, **45**, 77–83.

de Jong, L., Prins, J., Fiselier, T., Weemaes, C., Meijer-van den Burgh, E. and Bleijenberg, G. (1997). Chronic fatigue in young persons. *Nederlands Tijdschrift voor Geneeskunde*, **141**, 1513–16.

Eiser, C. (1997). Effects of chronic illness on children and their families. *Advances in Psychiatric Treatment*, **3**, 204–10.

Emison, M., Benjamin, S., Shantail, A., Woods, T. and Faragher, B. (1996). Physical symptoms and illness attitudes in adolescents: an epidemiological study. *Journal of Child Psychology and Psychiatry*, **37**, 519–28.

Emslie, G. (1997). A double blind, randomised, placebo controlled trial of fluoxetine in children and adolescents with depression. *Archives of General Psychiatry*, **54**, 1031–37.

Essen-Moller, E. (1956). Individual traits in a Swedish rural population. *Acta Psychologica*, **100** (suppl), 1–160.

Feder, H., Dworkin, P. and Orkin, C. (1994). Outcome of 48 pediatric patients with chronic fatigue; a clinical experience. *Archives of Family Medicine*, **3**, 1049–55.

Fry, A. and Martin, M. (1996). Cognitive idiosyncrasies among children with the chronic fatigue syndrome: anomalies in self-reported activity levels. *Journal of Psychosomatic Research*, **41**, 213–23.

Fulcher, K. and White, P. (1997). Randomised controlled trial of graded exercise in patients with chronic fatigue syndrome. *British Medical Journal*, **314**, 1647–52.

Fukuda, K., Straus, S., Hickie, I., Sharpe, M., Dobbins, J. and Komaroff, A. (1994). The chronic fatigue syndrome: a comprehensive approach to its definition and study. *Annals of Internal Medicine*, **121**, 953–9.

Garralda, E., Rangel, L., Levin, M., Roberts, H. and Ukoumunne, O. (1999). Psychiatric adjustment in adolescents with a history of chronic fatigue syndrome. *Journal of American Academy Child Adolescent Psychiatry*, **38**, 1515–21.

Garralda, M. and Rangel, L. (2001). Childhood chronic fatigue syndrome. *American Journal of Psychiatry*, **158**, 1161.

Greenburger, D. and Padesky, C. (1996). *Mind Over Mood*. New York: Guilford Press.

Harris, F. and Taitz, L. (1989). Damaging diagnosis of myalgic encephalomyelitis in children. *British Medical Journal*, **299**, 790.

Hotopf, M., Wilson-Jones, C., Mayou, R., Wadsworth, M. and Wessely, S. (2000). Childhood predictors of adult medically unexplained hospitalizations. *American Journal of Psychiatry*, **176**, 273–80.

Joyce, J., Hotopf, M. and Wessely, S. (1997). The prognosis of chronic fatigue and chronic fatigue syndrome: a systematic review. *Quarterly Journal of Medicine*, **90**, 223–33.

Kirmayer, L. J. (1990). Resistance, reactance and reluctance to change: a cognitive attributional approach to strategic interventions. *Journal of Cognitive Psychotherapy*, **4**, 83–104.

Marcovitch, H. (1997). Managing chronic fatigue syndrome in children. *British Medical Journal*, **314**, 1635–6.

Marshall, G., Gesser, R., Yamanishi, K. and Starr, S. (1991). Chronic fatigue in children: clinical features, Epstein–Barr virus and human herpes virus 6 serology and long term follow up. *Pediatric Infectious Diseases Journal*, **10**, 287–90.

Meltzer, H., Gatward, R., Goodman, R. and Ford, T. (2000). *Mental Health of Children and Adolescents in Great Britain*. London: The Stationery Office.

Minuchin, S. (1974). *Families and Family Therapy*. London: Tavistock Publications.

Morin, C. M., Culbert, J. P. and Schwartz, S. M. (1994). Nonpharmacological interventions for insomnia: a meta-analysis of treatment. *American Journal of Psychiatry*, **151**, 1172–80.

Morrell, D. (1972). Symptom interpretation in general practice. *Journal of the Royal College of General Practitioners*, **22**, 297–309.

Ollendick, T., King, N. and Yule, W. (1994). *International Handbook of Phobias and Anxiety Disorders in Children and Adolescents*. New York: Plenum.

OPCS (1985). *Morbidity Statistics from General Practice: The Third National Morbidity Survey*, 3rd edn. London: HMSO.

Pelcovitz, D., Septimus, A., Friedman, S., Krilov, L., Mandel, F. and Kaplan, S. (1995). Psychosocial correlates of chronic fatigue syndrome in adolescent girls. *Journal of Developmental and Behavioral Paediatrics*, **16**, 333–8.

Pipe, R. and Wait, M. (1995). Family therapy in the treatment of chronic fatigue syndrome in adolescence. *ACPP Review and Newsletter*, **17**, 9–16.

Plioplys, A. (1997). Chronic fatigue syndrome should not be diagnosed in children. *Pediatrics*, **100**, 270–1.

Powell, P., Bentall, P., Nye, F. and Edwards, T. (2001). Randomised controlled trial of patient education to encourage graded exercise in chronic fatigue syndrome. *British Medical Journal*, **322**, 387.

Prins, J., Bleijenberg, G., Bazelmans, E. *et al.* (2001). Cognitive behaviour therapy for chronic fatigue syndrome: a multi-centre randomised controlled trial. *Lancet*, **357**, 841–7.

Rangel, L., Garralda, M., Hall, A. and Woodham, S. (2003). Psychiatric adjustment in chronic fatigue syndrome of childhood and in juvenile idiopathic arthritis. *Psychological Medicine*, **33**, 289–97.

Rangel, L., Garralda, M., Levin, M. and Roberts, H. (2000a). The course of severe chronic fatigue syndrome in childhood. *Journal of Royal Society of Medicine*, **93**, 129–34.

  (2000b). Personality in adolescents with chronic fatigue syndrome. *European Child and Adolescent Psychiatry*, **9**, 39–45.

Ray, C., Jeffries, S. and Weir, W. (1995). Coping with chronic fatigue syndrome: illness responses and their relationship with fatigue, functional impairment and emotional status. *Psychological Medicine*, **25**, 937–45.

Rikard-Bell, C. and Waters, B. (1992). Psychosocial management of chronic fatigue syndrome in adolescence. *Australian and New Zealand Journal of Psychiatry*, **26**, 64–72.

Sharpe, M., Archard, L., Banatvala, J. *et al.* (1991). Chronic fatigue syndrome: guidelines for research. *Journal of the Royal Society of Medicine*, **84**, 118–21.

Sharpe, M., Hawton, K., Seagroatt, V. and Pasvol, G. (1992). Follow up of patients with fatigue presenting to an infectious diseases clinic. *British Medical Journal*, **302**, 347–52.

Sharpe, M., Hawton, K., Simkin, S. *et al.* (1996). Cognitive behaviour therapy for chronic fatigue syndrome; a randomized controlled trial. *British Medical Journal*, **312**, 22–6.

Sidebotham, P., Skeldon, I., Chambers, T., Clements, S. and Culling, J. (1994). Refractory chronic fatigue syndrome in adolescence. *British Journal of Hospital Medicine*, **51**, 110–12.

Smith, M., Mitchell, J., Corey, L., McCauley, E., Glover, D. and Tenover, F. (1991). Chronic fatigue in adolescents. *Pediatrics*, **88**, 195–201.

Taylor, D., Szatmari, P., Boyle, M. and Offord, D. (1996). Somatisation and the vocabulary of everyday bodily experiences and concerns: a community study of adolescents. *Journal of the American Academy Child Adolescent Psychiatry*, **35**, 491–9.

Vereker, M. (1992). Chronic fatigue syndrome: a joint paediatric-psychiatric approach. *Archives of Disease in Childhood*, **67**, 550–5.

Wachsmuth, J. and MacMillan, H. (1991). Effective treatment for an adolescent with chronic fatigue syndrome. *Clinical Pediatrics*, **30**, 488–90.

Walford, G., McCNelson, W. and McCluskey, D. (1993). Fatigue, depression and social adjustment in children with chronic fatigue syndrome. *Archives of Disease in Childhood*, **68**, 384–8.

Wearden, A., Morriss, R., Mullis, R. *et al.* (1998). Randomised, double-blind, placebo controlled treatment trial of fluoxetine and graded exercise for chronic fatigue syndrome. *British Journal of Psychiatry*, **172**, 485–90.

Wilson, P., Kusumaker, V., McCartney, R. and Bell, E. (1989). Features of Coxsackie B virus (CBV) infection in children with prolonged physical and psychological morbidity. *Journal of Psychosomatic Research*, **33**, 29–36.

23

Children's interpersonal problems

Caroline L. Donovan and Susan H. Spence

University of Queensland, Brisbane, Queensland, Australia

Children and adolescents present for therapy seeking assistance with a range of cognitive, behavioural and affective difficulties. Frequently, these difficulties are associated with, are the result of or at least contribute to difficulties in interpersonal relationships. Consequently, the improvement of social interaction is often a target of child and adolescent psychological interventions. Social competence is defined in this chapter as the ability to obtain successful outcomes from relationships with others. There are many reasons why a child may demonstrate deficiencies in social competence and, therefore, experience interpersonal problems. The initial section of this chapter outlines a number of these potential causal and maintaining factors and examines various approaches to the enhancement of children's social competence. The chapter then proceeds with an examination of the effectiveness of social skills training (SST) with children and its strengths and limitations. Finally, social skills assessment and the practical aspects of SST are discussed.

23.1 Factors that influence children's social competence

There are many reasons why a child may experience interpersonal problems and difficulties in social competence. The most proximal determinants of children's social competence relate to their actual behaviour within a social situation. This behaviour, however, is determined by many factors. In particular, the child's ability to engage in effective social–cognitive processes will strongly influence the way in which a child behaves. Thus, social perception and social problem-solving skills play a key role in determining how a child responds in a social situation. The child's attitudes, beliefs and thoughts also have a strong influence on the

Cognitive Behaviour Therapy for Children and Families, ed. Philip J. Graham.
Published by Cambridge University Press. © Cambridge University Press 2004.

way in which the child chooses to behave. However, we need to ask the question: 'what determines children's social cognition and in turn their social behaviour?' Some of the answers can be found in the child's learning environment.

The list in Table 23.1 is not exhaustive, but highlights some of the more common causal and maintaining factors associated with child social ineffectiveness.

23.2   What is SST?

Many people continue to assume that SST comprises training only in the more traditional areas of behavioural microskills and more complex behavioural skills. However, if the goal of SST is to improve the social interaction and social competence of children, then strategies aimed at the remediation of all possible causal and maintaining factors outlined above must be incorporated under the umbrella of SST. More contemporary SST conceptualizations and treatment packages therefore include techniques such as social problem-solving (SPS) training, cognitive therapy and contingency management, in addition to the more traditional procedures. The interventions aim to tackle the many factors that influence social competence as outlined above. Perhaps a more accurate term for contemporary approaches to SST should therefore be 'social competence training' or 'training in social interaction'. However, the term SST will be used throughout this chapter, while, at the same time, keeping in mind that it refers to the broader, rather than traditional, conceptualization.

Another distinction that appears to cause concern among researchers is that of social skill acquisition versus performance deficits (Gresham, 1997). A child is said to possess an acquisition skills deficit if he or she does not have the particular social skill in his or her behavioural repertoire. Alternatively, performance deficits refer to the situation where the young person possesses the skills to behave in a socially skilled manner, yet fails for some reason to demonstrate these skills in one or more social situations. It is the position of some that SST is appropriate only with children who demonstrate social skill acquisition deficits. However, this is not the authors' view. Take, for example, the child who actually possesses the requisite skills but who performs inadequately in a social situation due to negative cognitions and previous lack of reinforcement for appropriate skill demonstration. Cognitive therapy to reduce negative cognitions and contingency management to increase the likelihood that the child will use a socially skilled response are likely to form important components of intervention. Psychoeducation regarding the importance of appropriate social skill use, in addition to rehearsal of the appropriate social skills within the problem situation, is also likely to be required.

Table 23.1   Common causal and maintaining factors associated with child social ineffectiveness

Performance deficits

1. Behavioural microsocial skills such as inappropriate or deficient:
   - eye contact
   - posture
   - facial expression
   - social distance
   - tone, volume, clarity, rate and fluency of speech
   - latency of response
   - gestures
   - listening skills
2. Deficits in complex behavioural social skills such as:
   - asking questions
   - starting, maintaining and ending conversations
   - asking to join in
   - giving and receiving invitations
   - offering and asking for help
   - offering and accepting compliments
   - dealing with teasing and bullying
   - assertion

Deficits in cognitive processes or products

1. Difficulties associated with social perception skills including:
   - receiving information from others and the social environment
   - attention to relevant social cues
   - knowledge of social rules
   - knowledge of the meaning of social cues
   - correct interpretation of information received
   - ability to take the perspective of others
   - ability to monitor one's own behaviour and its outcome and alter it when necessary
2. Difficulties associated with social problem-solving skills such as:
   - identifying the nature and existence of a social problem
   - determining the goals for a situation
   - generating ideas for possible alternative responses
   - predicting the likely consequences of alternatives
   - deciding on a response likely to lead to a successful outcome
   - planning the chosen response
3. Maladaptive or distorted thoughts, attitudes and beliefs (i.e. cognitions)

The child's learning environment

1. Modelling of inappropriate behaviour by significant others (e.g. parents, peers, etc.)
2. Reinforcement for unskilled or inappropriate social behaviour
3. Punishment or lack of reinforcement for appropriate social behaviour
4. Lack of opportunity to acquire and practise social skills

Social performance deficits are frequently maintained by environmental contingencies and variables such as cognitive distortions and poor social problem-solving skills. However, the therapist should not assume that the presence of these factors rules out the possible existence of an acquisition deficit. Such factors may also serve to maintain and/or exacerbate acquisition skills deficits. For example, Spence *et al.* (1999) found evidence of cognitive distortions and social skill acquisition deficits in socially phobic children, suggesting that unhelpful cognitions were serving to maintain and/or exacerbate social skills acquisition deficits in these children. Thus, socially phobic children not only performed less well than their peers on social tasks, but also expected to perform poorly and evaluated themselves more negatively than was actually the case. The authors' position, therefore, is that various techniques subsumed under the more contemporary umbrella of SST are available to the therapist and may be used to enhance children's social relationships.

23.3   Is social skills training effective?

There have been a number of qualitative and quantitative reviews of the child social skills literature, the results and conclusions of which are varied, mixed and, in many cases, inconsistent. While earlier SST meta-analyses found moderate effect sizes of 0.40 (Schneider, 1992) and 0.47 (Beelman *et al.*, 1994), a more recent meta-analysis found only a minimal effect size of 0.199 (Kavale *et al.*, 1997). Similarly, a recent meta-analysis of SST effectiveness conducted with single-subject designs employing the mean percentage of non-overlapping data as the outcome measure indicated only a very modest intervention effect of 62% (Kavale *et al.*, 1997). To confuse the matter further, the various meta-analyses have suggested that the effectiveness of SST varies as a function of factors such as outcome measure, type of programme, age and presenting problem.

23.3.1   Outcome measure

The type of outcome measure employed appears to have differential effects on the results of SST efficacy studies. For example, Schneider (1992) found that studies employing role-play assessments demonstrated significantly higher effect sizes than studies employing peer- or child-report questionnaires, and that teacher measures demonstrated the lowest effect size. Beelman *et al.* (1994) found higher effect sizes for social–cognitive and behavioural observation outcome measures than for sociometrics or peer-, parent- or teacher-report measures. In contrast, Kavale *et al.* (1997) found that teacher-report measures produced larger effect sizes than peer or child ratings, which in turn produced larger effect sizes than experimenter and parental measures. For single-subject designs, SST appears to be most effective when interaction outcome measures are used and least effective when communication outcome measures are used (Kavale *et al.*, 1997). In summary, while the various meta-analyses suggest differential effects depending on the outcome measures employed, there is little consistency between their conclusions as to precisely what these effects are.

23.3.2   Type of programme

The effectiveness of SST has also been found to vary as a function of the type of programme employed. Schneider (1992) found that studies involving modelling and coaching demonstrated significantly higher effect sizes than social–cognitive or 'multiple technique' studies. Similarly, in an early qualitative review of cognitive behavioural SST studies, Gresham (1985) concluded that, while modelling and coaching were effective SST strategies, self-instruction and SPS strategies were less beneficial.

It would seem, however, that there is an interaction between outcome measure, programme content and the effectiveness of SST. Beelman *et al.* (1994) found that all multimodal SST programmes demonstrated at least moderate effect sizes in two outcome areas. Monomodal programmes, however, appeared to produce strong effects on their intended target variables, but evidenced few generalization effects. For example, SPS treatments produced large improvements on social–cognitive measures, but had little effect on social interaction skill measures. Similarly, Coleman *et al.* (1993) concluded that SPS strategies were effective in producing changes on SPS measures but not on behaviour ratings and observational measures. Conversely, Beelman *et al.* (1994) found that behavioural treatments produced large improvements on social interaction skill measures but produced lesser effects on SPS measures. In summary, it would appear that multimodal methods lead to greater generalization and a broader improvement of skills because individual components of the programmes are effective only in changing specific aspects of a child's social skill repertoire. The more components included within a particular programme, therefore, the greater the number of skills that are improved on.

23.3.3   Age

The conclusions of the various meta-analyses differ regarding the effect of child age on SST efficacy. Beelman *et al.* (1994) concluded that children under 6 years of age benefited most from SST, while children aged 12–15 years benefited moderately and children aged 6–11 years benefited least. In contrast, Kavale *et al.* (1997) found no effects for age in group-design SST studies and that preschool children benefited least from SST programmes incorporating a single-subject design.

23.3.4   Type of presenting problem(s)

The nature of the child's presenting problem(s) appears to affect the outcome of SST procedures. Schneider (1992) found that SST was more effective with withdrawn than with unpopular, aggressive, 'not atypical' or 'other' children. Similarly, Kavale *et al.* (1997) found that SST was most useful for anxious children and least effective for aggressive children. Beelman *et al.* (1994) found that at-risk children (i.e. those demonstrating social deprivation and/or confronted with critical life events) benefited most from SST, while children with externalizing and internalizing problems benefited moderately and 'normal' and intellectually disabled children benefited least. Similarly, Kavale *et al.* (1997) found that SST was most effective for delinquent participants, moderately effective for emotionally and behaviourally disordered children and relatively ineffective for autistic children.

Deficiencies and distortions of social skills are frequently present in all types of emotional and behavioural disorders, as well as learning difficulties. Interventions to improve social skills in other disorders, especially conduct, depressive and attention deficit disorders (and the strength of the evidence that exists to support their use) are discussed in the relevant chapters elsewhere in this volume. Here, detailed discussion is limited to the use of SST with rejected children and children with social phobia, conditions for which social deficits and distortions are central and may be unaccompanied by other disorders.

23.3.4.1   Rejected children

Children who are rejected by their peers have been found to demonstrate lower levels of social skill and a greater number of interfering problem behaviours compared with more popular children (Frentz *et al.*, 1991; Stuart *et al.*, 1991). It would seem logical, therefore, that training rejected children in social skills may improve their rejected status. An early study by Tiffen and Spence (1986) suggested that SST was ineffective in producing long-term beneficial effects with either isolated or rejected 7–11-year-old children. However, more recent studies appear to support the efficacy of SST with rejected children. For example, Gumpel and Frank (1999) found that a SST programme conducted with two sixth-grade and two kindergarten-grade rejected children increased the number of positive social interactions demonstrated by these children both following treatment and at 5-week follow-up. Similarly, a study conducted by Berner *et al.* (2001) with fifth- and sixth-grade girls with few friends found that, following

SST, the girls spent less time alone, more time initiating conversations and more time interacting with others than did the control group.

Not surprisingly, perhaps, children exhibiting externalizing behaviours are also frequently rejected. An interesting study by Lochman *et al.* (1993) attempted to distinguish between these two groups of children by investigating the relative effectiveness of a SST programme on both aggressive–rejected children and non-aggressive–rejected children. The results of the study suggested that SST improved prosocial behaviour and reduced both aggression level and rejected status in aggressive–rejected children, but failed to lead to improvements with non-aggressive–rejected children. While the findings of this study require replication, it may be important to screen for the presence/absence of aggression in rejected children before implementing SST. The non-aggressive–rejected youngsters may require an alternative approach to SST, highlighting the need for greater research into the causal factors of peer rejection.

23.3.4.2   Social phobia

By definition, social phobia comprises deficits in social functioning. However, a controversy continues to rage in both the adult and child literature as to whether the negative expectancies and evaluations regarding social performance reflect a history of poor performance (i.e. social skills deficits) and negative outcomes in social situations or whether they represent a focus on, and exaggeration of, features of their behaviour. In their review of the adult social anxiety literature, Rapee and Heimberg (1997) concluded that the findings were mixed as to whether adult social phobics indeed demonstrate social skills deficits. Very few studies, however, have investigated this question with socially phobic children.

Spence *et al.* (1999) provided evidence to support the supposition that social phobic children indeed demonstrate deficits in social skill. Compared with non-anxious children, children with social phobia were rated as being less socially skilled and competent by both self- and parent-report, and chose less assertive responses on a self-report measure. Even more convincing was the evidence from behavioural observations both in naturalistic and role-play settings. Specifically, compared with non-anxious children, children with social phobia were found to initiate and participate in fewer social interactions in a school setting, and demonstrated shorter response lengths on a role-play task. Furthermore, the naturalistic observations also suggested that social phobic children were significantly less likely than their non-anxious counterparts to receive positive outcomes from peers during social interactions.

The implications of the study for the treatment of social phobia in children are important. Exposure and cognitive challenging are frequently and effectively used for many types of anxiety in both children and adults. However, it will be of no therapeutic benefit to encourage children to participate in social situations (i.e. exposure) and challenge their cognitions regarding social ability if in fact they have social skills deficits as the Spence *et al.* (1999) study suggests. In fact, exposure and subsequent failure in social situations is likely to exacerbate the child's anxiety concerning interaction with others. It would, therefore, appear that SST is indicated as a component in the treatment of child social phobia.

Few investigations of SST with social phobic children have been undertaken to date. Beidel *et al.* (2000) compared the usefulness of Social Effectiveness Therapy for Children (SET-C) with an active non-specific intervention for 67 socially phobic children aged 8–12 years. SET-C comprised child and parent education, SST, peer generalization and *in vivo* exposure. Results indicated that compared with children in the non-specific intervention, children in the SET-C condition significantly improved in social skill and social interaction, and demonstrated reductions in social fear, anxiety and psychopathology. More importantly, perhaps, compared with 5% of the non-specific treatment group, 67% of participants in the SET-C condition no longer met criteria for social phobia following treatment.

Spence *et al.* (2000) also examined the benefits of SST in the treatment of 50 social phobic children aged 7–14 years, using the Spence (1995) SST programme outlined in detail below. Results indicated significant reductions in social anxiety and improvements in social skill. The reduction in social and general anxiety was statistically and clinically significant, with an average of 66% of children in the treatment condition being free from clinical diagnosis following the programme. Overall, the limited research to date suggests not only that social phobic children demonstrate social skills deficits, but that SST is effective in reducing social anxiety with many of these children.

23.3.5   Summary

In answer to the question 'is SST effective?', the research has produced very mixed results. Overall, the meta-analyses suggest small to moderate treatment effects that vary inconsistently as a function of outcome measure, type of programme and age. Yet another factor that has been shown to lead to variation in SST effectiveness is that of the child's presenting problem. Overall, it may be concluded that, while SST has been shown to be effective in many studies, there is a good deal of conflicting data. In particular, the evidence is weak when outcome is assessed in terms of long-term change on indicators of social effectiveness, such as improved social relationships. The following section examines some possible reasons why SST has not lived up to its expectations.

23.4   Why has SST failed to live up to expectations?

Several authors have proposed potential reasons to explain why SST has not produced the degree of improvement in social functioning that would be expected
from a theoretical perspective. These explanations can be subsumed into two
major categories pertaining to: (1) deficiencies in tailoring interventions to individual children and (2) failure to programme for generalization of behaviour
change.

23.4.1   Deficiencies in tailoring interventions

Researchers in the clinical area are in a bind. On the one hand, they must adhere
to 'good research practice' by providing all participants with identical training
to ensure treatment effects are due to the procedure implemented and not to
extraneous variables. On the other hand, they are attempting to emulate real
clinical settings where 'good clinical practice' dictates that treatment is tailor-
made to each client.

Hansen *et al.* (1998) suggested that, when interventions are not tailored to the
individual child, there is a reduced likelihood that:

* the goals selected are agreed on by the child, parents and teacher;
* achievement of the goals will lead to real improvement in the child's life;
* the treatment is fully explained and understood by all parties;
* all parties find the treatment agreeable; and
* the procedures are gender and culture sensitive.

It would appear, therefore, that attempts by clinical researchers to work within
the confines of experimental procedures through providing children with standard programmes that are not tailored to their individual needs has decreased
the apparent effectiveness of SST.

23.4.2   Deficiencies in programming for generalization

The limitation of SST to demonstrate generalization effects is certainly a major
problem in the literature. Gresham (1997, 1998) distinguished between topographical and functional generalization. Topographical generalization refers to
the occurrence of a particular behaviour under conditions other than the training condition and includes generalization across settings, responses and time.
Gresham (1997) suggested that conducting SST in less relevant contexts (e.g.
the clinic) is one of the main reasons why topographical generalization is not
evident in SST research. Emphasizing the importance of the context in which
social skills are learned, Gresham (1997) proposed that SST should take place
within the school setting for maximum benefit. This is not to say, however,

that initial training within the therapeutic environment is unnecessary or unimportant. Not only does initial clinic training allow the child to practise their new-found skills in a safe environment, it has the potential to begin the generalization process if procedures such as exposure to multiple models and settings and the use of multiple role plays with different situations and peers are programmed into therapy. However, once initial training is complete, teachers and parents should become involved in treatment so that modelling, prompting and reinforcing of acquired skills may continue in contextually relevant environments.

Functional approaches to generalization, however, are less frequently discussed and yet are of equal, if not greater, importance in determining the effectiveness of SST. A functional approach to generalization examines the reasons *why* a particular social skill is or is not demonstrated. Gresham (1997, 1998) and Hansen *et al.* (1998) suggested that, while training a child in a particular social skill may allow them to acquire the skill, competing stimuli in situations outside the therapeutic environment may lead to old, undesirable behaviours and subsequent suppression of newly acquired skills. Furthermore, the competing behaviours may be more effective or efficient in achieving a desired outcome. For example, a child may effectively learn appropriate social skills for conflict resolution in the clinic. However, it may be more appropriate within his or her 'deviant' peer group (or indeed more effective and easier in the short term) to attack physically rather than attempt to engage another person in conversation. Targeting contextual factors is, therefore, important for enhancing the generalization of prosocial behaviour change (Hansen *et al.*, 1998). Contextual factors such as peer group influences, major life stressors, family difficulties, time, money and competing responsibilities must be taken into consideration as they may contribute to problems with skill acquisition and performance in 'real world' settings.

23.5   Assessment of children's interpersonal functioning

It has been said so far that interpersonal problems may be the result of many factors, including difficulties with social perception, behavioural micro- or macroskills, cognitions, modelling, contingency management or SPS. It has also been suggested that these difficulties may be either acquisitional or performance in nature. The initial role of the therapist, therefore, is to conduct a thorough assessment investigating each of these areas in order to determine precisely where the child's difficulties lie. In this way, an accurate conceptualization and subsequent treatment plan tailored specifically to the individual child can be developed. Below is a summary of some useful assessment tools for investigating each of the potential deficit areas.

23.5.1   Social perception

Social perception skills are perhaps the most basic social skills on which the more complex social skills depend. For example, if a child is unaware of social cues and frequently misinterprets social information, they are unlikely to be able to begin, maintain and end a conversation appropriately. There are very few assessment tools developed specifically for social perception. Spence (1995) provides a number of photographs depicting a range of adult and child facial expressions and postures that are used to test the child on their interpretation of these social cues. The Child and Adolescent Social Perception Measure (CASP; Magill Evans *et al.*, 1995), the Social Perspective-Taking Task (Chandler, 1973), the Affective Situation Test for Empathy (Feshbach and Roe, 1968) and the Borke Test (Borke, 1971) may also be useful measures in the assessment of social perception.

23.5.2   Behavioural social skills

Behavioural social skills include microskills (e.g. posture, gaze or facial expression) and more complex social behavioural skills (e.g. asking questions, listening, asking for help and positive and negative assertion). A number of different assessment instruments have been designed for measuring behavioural social skills, the most useful of which are discussed below.

23.5.2.1   Behavioural observation

Naturalistic observation is one of the most valid forms of behavioural social skills assessment (Merrell, 2001). There are few published methods of behavioural observation, although the PLAY behavioural observational system (Farmer Dougan and Kaszuba, 1999), the Peer Social Behaviour Code (PSBC) of the Systematic Screening for Behaviour Disorders (SSBD; Walker and Severson, 1992) and the Furman and Masters (1980) system are examples the reader may wish to refer to. Spence *et al.* (1999) also reported a method for observing children within a naturalistic setting at school. For some of the systems mentioned above, the observations are coded 'live', whereas other systems have used videotaped recordings that are subsequently transcribed back in the clinic or laboratory.

From the authors' experience, while providing a wealth of important information, naturalistic observations are time consuming and extremely difficult to conduct. An alternative is to conduct observations of the child interacting with parents, peers or confederates within the clinic setting through use of video equipment or two-way mirror systems. Alternatively, a structured role-play task such as the Revised Behavioural Assertiveness Test for Children (BAT-CR; Ollendick, 1981), a role-play task adapted from the Behavioural Assertiveness Test for Children (BAT-C; Bornstein *et al.*, 1977), may be employed. While not as valid perhaps as naturalistic observation, clinic observations and structured role plays retain many of the benefits of naturalistic observations while removing many of the associated difficulties.

23.5.2.2 Behaviour rating scales

Behaviour rating scales are suggested to be the most valid, economical and useful methods of assessing child social skill (Merrell, 2001). Behaviour rating scales require a person close to the child (usually either a parent or teacher) or the young person himself/herself to rate the frequency with which the specific behaviours occur. Examples of behaviour rating scales include the School Social Behaviour Scales (Merrell, 1993), the Social Skills Rating System (Gresham and Elliott, 1990), the Walker–McConnell Scales of Social Competence and School Adjustment (Walker and McConnell, 1995; Walker *et al.*, 1995), the Waksman Social Skills Rating Scale (Waksman, 1985), the Matson Evaluation of Social Skills with Youngsters (MESSY; Matson *et al.*, 1983; Matson, 1990), the School Social Skills Rating Scale (S3; Brown and Greenspan, 1984), the Preschool and Kindergarten Behavior Scales (Merrell, 1996) and the parent-, teacher- and child-report versions of the Social Skills Questionnaire (Spence, 1995). While behaviour rating scales may be valid and useful indicators of a child's social skill, they are somewhat insensitive to small changes in behaviour and require relatively large changes in social skill before changes on the measures are evident (Elliott *et al.*, 2001).

23.5.2.3 Interviews

Interviewing should not be used in isolation to assess a child's social skill. However, this method allows the therapist to obtain important information from parent, child or teachers concerning various aspects of the child's social environment. When interviewing parents, clinicians should ask questions regarding the child's relationship with family members, the type of contact the child has with peers outside school, romantic relationships (in adolescents), the type of social life the parents and family members have, the child's relationship with peers and teachers at school and the child's general conversation skills. Interviews with the teacher should inform the therapist about relationships with classmates and teachers, general conversational skills and other school-related background information such as academic achievement and participation in school activities.

Finally, interviews with the child should centre around discussion of relationships with family, friends or romantic partner, contact with peers both within and outside school, relationships with teachers and other general issues such as loneliness, desire for more friends, etc. If a structured interview is required, the Social Adjustment Inventory for Children and Adolescents (SAICA; John *et al.*, 1987) may be a useful tool.

23.5.2.4   Sociometry

Sociometric techniques should only be used as an adjunct to observation or behaviour rating scales for the assessment of child social skill. There are two main forms of sociometry. The peer nomination method requires each child in a class to list a certain number of children who they particularly like or dislike, or with whom they would most prefer (or prefer not) to play or work with (e.g. Tiffen and Spence, 1986; Christopher *et al.*, 1991). In contrast, rating methods require each child in a class to rate each classmate on a scale of like–dislike or preference (e.g. La Greca and Santogrossi, 1980; Ladd, 1981). Such procedures do not actually measure social skills *per se*. However, sociometric techniques may inform the therapist about why a child is liked or disliked by peers and provide information pertaining to social standing and popularity.

23.5.3   Cognitions

Children's negative cognitions may hinder the appropriate performance of social skills, or may maintain/exacerbate an acquisition skills deficit. A number of questionnaires are available to assess child cognitions including the Children's Cognitive Error Questionnaire (Leitenbertg *et al.*, 1986), the Children's Negative Cognitive Error Questionnaire (CNCEQ; Messer *et al.*, 1994), the Cognitive Bias Questionnaire for Children (Haley *et al.*, 1985) and the Children's Attributional Style Questionnaire (Kaslow and Nolen-Hoeksema, 1991). Other procedures such as role play and/or recall of social events in conjunction with thought-listing procedures may also be useful. Similarly, requiring the child to fill in empty thought bubbles in response to cartoons and vignettes of social situations may also be a helpful technique.

23.5.4   Modelling and contingency management problems

Parents or significant others may contribute to a child's social deficits by modelling inappropriate social behaviour, reinforcing inappropriate social behaviour and/or providing little reinforcement or even punishment for appropriate behaviour. The parent interview will provide the therapist with some insight into the parents' level of social skill and, therefore, their modelling influence. If parental social skill deficits are evident, then additional probing or observation may reveal more information. Similarly, interviews with the child and parent may provide the therapist with information regarding the behaviour and potential modelling influences of significant peers.

Information regarding contingency management may also be obtained through observation and parental, teacher and child interviews. The therapist should question parents, teachers and the child themselves about the antecedents and consequences of the child's appropriate and inappropriate behaviour with parents, teachers and peers. Observation of child–parent and/or child–peer interactions may also provide the therapist with information pertaining to reinforcement contingencies.

Therapists must examine whether competing behaviours exist that are more efficient or effective in some way than socially appropriate behaviours. It is imperative that the therapist identify such competing behaviours, assess their efficiency and determine the stimuli with which they are associated. In some instances, an interview with the child is a valuable source of information regarding these difficulties, as the child may simply be asked the reasons *why* they engage in X behaviour rather than Y.

Finally, the therapist must assess for contextual difficulties that may prevent the child from performing in a socially appropriate manner. As noted above, there may be a variety of contextual issues such as peer group influences, time management, resources and life stressors that interfere with effective interpersonal functioning. Interviews with the child and parents are the most likely sources of information regarding these difficulties.

23.5.5   Social problem-solving

Children are unlikely to act appropriately in social situations if they are unable to detect that a social problem exists, to examine potential solutions to the problem and to choose the most appropriate response for enactment. A number of inventories and role-play measures have been developed specifically to assess child SPS ability. Examples include the Open Middle Inventory (OMI; Polifka *et al.*, 1981), the Means-Ends Problem-Solving Test (MEPS; Platt and Spivack, 1995), the Social Problem-Solving Inventory (D'Zurilla *et al.*, in press), the Interpersonal Problem-Solving Assessment Technique (IPSAT; Getter and Nowinski, 1981), the Adolescent Problems Inventory (API; Freedman *et al.*, 1978) and the Inventory of Decisions, Evaluations and Actions (IDEAs; Goddard and McFall, 1992).

23.5.6   Summary

In summary, the therapist must assess all factors that may potentially contribute to the child's difficulty with interpersonal relationships, including social perception, behavioural social skills, cognitions, modelling, contingency management and interpersonal problem-solving skills. Competing behaviours and contextual issues also need to be examined carefully. Only when these variables are thoroughly assessed will an accurate conceptualization of the child's case be possible.

23.6 Components of SST

As with all treatments, the content of the SST intervention must be driven by the conceptualization of the individual child's interpersonal difficulties. The specific procedures employed, therefore, will depend on the outcome of the assessment. Below is a brief description of various procedures that may be employed as components of SST.

23.6.1 Social perception skills training

Remediation of social perception deficits, if found, is a necessary first step as these skills provide the foundation for the other, more complex, social skills. Milne and Spence (1987) described a social perception skills training programme employing pictures, videotapes, audiotapes and role plays depicting a range of non-verbal cues. Children were taught to:

- recognize and discriminate their own emotions;
- recognize and discriminate other people's emotions from both verbal and non-verbal cues;
- identify characteristics of the social situation such as deciphering social rules and determining the aims of those involved in the social interaction;
- understand how others may interpret or view social situations; and
- be aware when a social problem exists.

23.6.2 Behavioural SST

Children may display deficits in any or all of the social behavioural skills outlined above. Behavioural microskills are typically targeted as an early component of SST as they provide a platform for the more complex social behavioural skills. The following steps are generally used in behavioural skills training.

23.6.2.1 Information and discussion

In order to motivate the child to engage in behavioural SST, he/she first must understand *why* a particular skill is important and how it should be performed. Pictures, role plays and videotapes may be used to illustrate the importance of each skill. Examples of interactions where the skill is absent or deficient, in addition to examples where the skill is performed effectively, can also be used to encourage discussion regarding social skill importance.

23.6.2.2   Modelling

Modelling may be conducted by the therapist, co-therapist, peers, videotapes or audiotapes. However, Bandura (1977) suggested that models who are of similar age to the child, who receive positive reinforcement for following performance of the target skill and who are seen to work through the steps competently but not perfectly are the most effective. Conducting therapy within a group situation of similarly aged peers is of enormous benefit in this regard, as group members may act as models for the various skills. Alternatively, skilled peers may be brought into individual or group therapy to demonstrate effective performance of a particular skill.

23.6.2.3   Behavioural rehearsal

Initially, behavioural rehearsal is conducted within the safe confines of the therapeutic environment. The use of group therapy is advantageous in this regard as children are able to role play various social situations with group members. A variety of scenarios and practise in 'real life' contexts should be included in order to facilitate skill generalization. Repetition is also necessary to ensure adequate skill acquisition.

Self-instructional training (Meichenbaum and Goodman, 1971) is frequently used to aid behavioural rehearsal. Once the therapist or peer has modelled the behaviour while vocalizing the procedure out loud, the child attempts the behaviour while the model vocalizes the steps. He/she then rehearses the behaviour, vocalizing the instructions out loud initially and then in a whisper. Finally, the child rehearses the behaviour using inner speech.

23.6.2.4   Reinforcement and feedback about performance

The SST procedure should be viewed as one of shaping the child's behaviour – that is, the therapist and group members should reinforce closer and closer approximations of the target behaviour. In order to provide the child with a safe environment for learning, feedback from the therapist and/or group members should first emphazise and reinforce the correct or effective aspects of the performance. Suggestions for improvement should then be provided constructively, in a non-critical manner.

23.6.2.5   Training outside the therapeutic environment

Adequate demonstration of the skill within the therapeutic environment in no way guarantees its performance in the child's natural environment. As discussed above, generalization is one of the major difficulties associated with SST, and lack of contextual training may be at the root of the problem. After training within the clinic setting has occurred, the young person must practise their new-found skills within their natural environment, i.e. in the school and home. To this end, homework tasks corresponding to the skills being taught should be set, and teachers, parents and even peers should be educated to model, prompt and reinforce performance of each particular skill.

Two approaches may be particularly helpful here. The first concerns using behaviour modification strategies to encourage the child to use their social skills in their natural environment. Many teachers are already trained in behaviour modification techniques and thus making the teacher aware of the particular social skills being targeted and encouraging them to model, prompt and reinforce these skills is likely to be beneficial. Parents are likely to require specific training in behaviour modification methods and must be provided with a strong rationale both for child skill acquisition and parental involvement in the programme. Parents can also assist by encouraging homework task completion and reinforcing their child for their social skill attempts.

The second approach involves using behaviour modification strategies to counteract competing behaviours, reinforcement of inappropriate behaviour and negative modelling influences. If negative parental modelling and reinforcement influences are found to exist, more intense parent training in both behaviour management and social skills will be necessary. If the competing behaviours are identified, the therapist must attempt to decrease the efficiency and frequency of these behaviours and increase the efficiency of the appropriate behaviours by enlisting the assistance of peers, teachers and parents (Hansen *et al.*, 1998).

23.6.2.6   Monitoring of child progress

As noted above, individual tailoring of interventions requires that the length and intensity of the programme be adjusted to the particular needs of the child. In order to ensure that the programme is neither too short nor too long for a particular child, frequent monitoring of the child's progress is necessary. To this end, Gresham (1997, 1998) highlights the necessity of employing meaningful outcome measures in order to ensure social validity – that is, the degree of change evident should not only be statistically significant, but should also make a difference in the child's life and be noticeable by parents, teachers and peers (Sechrest *et al.*, 1996). If such changes are not evident, the utility of the programme is questionable.

23.6.3   Changing maladaptive cognitions

As noted above, the presence of unhelpful cognitions may be a causal and/or maintaining factor for interpersonal problems with children. The actual content of the negative cognitions demonstrated by the child will vary depending on the child's presenting problem. For example, for some children, social responding may be disrupted by negative thoughts about a lack of ability to cope and anticipation of negative outcomes, leading to avoidance of the situation. For others, the maladaptive thoughts may relate to inaccurate attributions of threat from other people, thereby increasing the chance of an aggressive response. Whatever the nature of the maladaptive cognitions, the steps for remediation are similar. The basic steps are outlined below. The clinician may use stories, cartoons with thought bubbles and toys to illustrate the concepts in an interesting and child-friendly way. The complexity of the concepts to be taught will, of course, need to be adjusted to the developmental level of the child.

23.6.3.1   Step 1: explain the link between thoughts and feelings

A simple discussion of Ellis' (1958) ABC model using cartoons and stories about other children or fictional characters may be used to illustrate the important link between thoughts and feelings in children as young as 8 years. This stage begins with a focus on identification of different emotions and their situational triggers. Children are then taught to identify thoughts that occur in various situations and the different feelings that may be triggered in response to specific, hypothetical scenarios.

23.6.3.2   Step 2: assist the child to identify their own unhelpful thoughts

Children may be asked to recall the last time they felt scared (or sad, mad, etc.) and to explain the context in detail. The therapist may then prompt the child to vocalize their thoughts at various stages during the child's recital of the story regarding the event. Children may also be asked to write down their unhelpful thoughts for homework using a child version of the dysfunctional thoughts record. Unhelpful thoughts are described as those thoughts that, in a challenging situation, are likely to lead to a 'poor' outcome in terms of causing unwanted feelings or behaviours that lead to further problems. From the authors' experience, elementary school children appear able to understand this concept and quickly learn to identify and label their own 'unhelpful' thoughts.

23.6.3.3   Step 3: replace unhelpful thoughts with helpful thoughts

A simplified version of cognitive challenging may be employed for younger children. Using this technique, the child is simply asked to identify more constructive 'helpful' thoughts that may substitute for unhelpful thinking in a particular situation. Helpful thoughts in this context are defined as those thoughts that are likely to lead to a more positive outcome in terms of positive emotions for the child and behaviours that reduce the problem in a situation. Thus, children are taught to replace their unhelpful thoughts with more helpful ones that are likely to lead to a better outcome from a challenging situation. Older children are able to comprehend a more complex approach to cognitive restructuring in line with the work of Beck (1967). Examples may be provided of common forms of maladaptive thinking, such as catastrophizing, personalization and overgeneralization. Experiments may also be undertaken to illustrate the rationality and evidence relating to specific thoughts and attributions in a particular situation.

23.6.4   Social problem-solving difficulties

Some children act inappropriately because they have limited interpersonal problem-solving abilities. These children tend to respond impulsively or prefer to avoid attempts at dealing with a challenging social situation. The difficulty may lie in any one or all of the steps of SPS outlined above. Spence (1995) uses the analogy of the 'social detective' in her multimodal SST-based programme. The social detective model integrates many of the techniques described above into one model that children find easy to remember. The steps of the model are indicated below.

23.6.4.1   Step 1: detect

During the first step, children are taught to: (1) stop before acting further in order to reduce impulsive and emotionally cued responding and (2) identify the social problem.

23.6.4.2   Step 2: investigate

During the second step, children are taught to: (1) relax in order to reduce anxiety, anger, impulsivity, etc. that frequently prevents them from using their social skills; (2) brainstorm as many possible solutions to the problem as they can, regardless of usefulness or valence; (3) logically consider the positive and negative consequences of each solution; (4) choose the best solution based on consideration of the consequences; and (5) watch out for and replace unhelpful thoughts (adolescents only).

23.6.4.3   Step 3: solve

During step 3, children are taught to: (1) plan their approach to the social problem; (2) remember their social skills in order to increase their chances of a positive social outcome; (3) carry out the plan; and (4) evaluate their performance constructively and positively.

23.6.5 Summary

Once the assessment has been conducted, there are a number of useful procedures that may be used to address the child's presenting difficulties. Social perception deficits should be dealt with first as they constitute the most basic level of social skill acquisition. Difficulties with behavioural social skills, particularly microskill deficits, should be tackled next as they comprise the next step in the social skills acquisition ladder. To ensure optimal behavioural SST, techniques such as discussion of social skills, modelling, behavioural rehearsal, reinforcement, feedback, training outside the therapeutic environment and monitoring of child progress should be included within the programme. Problems with unhelpful cognitions may be rectified using cognitive restructuring approaches. Finally, a number of effective SPS skills training programmes exist that teach effective methods of approaching life challenges.

23.7 Conclusions

A number of causal and maintaining factors may contribute to a child's difficulty with social interaction. Deficits in social perception, behavioural social skills and social problem-solving and problems with unhelpful cognitions, inappropriate modelling influences and reinforcement contingencies may all contribute to interaction difficulties. Contemporary views of SST take a comprehensive approach, suggesting that intervention needs to integrate a range of strategies aimed at influencing a broad spectrum of causal and maintaining factors.

The various reviews investigating the efficacy of SST with children have indicated only minimal to moderate effect sizes. However, the reviews are frequently inconsistent in their conclusions and appear to vary as a function of the outcome measure employed, the type of programme implemented, the age of the child and the type of presenting problem. Prompted by the less than optimal results demonstrated by SST studies, various authors have theorized about the possible reasons behind the lack of efficacy. Deficiencies in tailoring interventions to the individual child in terms of programme content, length and intensity represent one potential reason for the observed ineffectiveness of SST with children. A second suggested reason is that SST studies frequently fail to programme for topographical and functional generalization.

A thorough assessment is the first step in combating these difficulties and improving the effectiveness of SST. The therapist should conduct a thorough assessment to determine the possible contribution of deficits in social perception, behavioural social skills and social problem-solving, in addition to unhelpful cognitions, modelling and contingency management effects. The content of intervention is then driven by the information derived from the assessment. A treatment strategy that is programmed for skill generalization and that is individually tailored to the needs of the child can then be devised from a variety of techniques available to the therapist.

23.8   REFERENCES

Bandura, A. (1977). *Social Learning Theory.* New York: Prentice-Hall.

Beck, A. T. (1967). *Depression.* New York: Harper and Row.

Beelman, A., Pfingsten, U. and Losel, F. (1994). Effects of training social competence in children: a meta-analysis of recent evaluation studies. *Journal of Clinical Child Psychology*, **23**, 260–71.

Beidel, D. C., Turner, S. M. and Morris, T. L. (2000). Behavioral treatment of childhood social phobia. *Journal of Consulting and Clinical Psychology*, **68**, 1072–80.

Berner, M. L., Fee, V. E. and Turner, A. D. (2001). A multi-component social skills training program for pre-adolescent girls with few friends. *Child and Family Behavior Therapy*, **23**, 1–18.

Borke, H. (1971). Interpersonal perception of young children: egocentrism or empathy? *Developmental Psychology*, **5**, 263–9.

Bornstein, M. R., Bellack, A. S. and Hersen, M. (1977). Social skills training for unassertive children: a multiple-baseline analysis. *Journal of Applied Behavior Analysis*, **10**, 183–95.

Brown, G. M. and Greenspan, S. (1984). Effect of social foresight training on the school adjustment of high-risk youth. *Child Study Journal*, **14**, 61–77.

Chandler, M. J. (1973). Egocentrism and antisocial behavior: the assessment and training of social perspective-taking skills. *Developmental Psychology*, **9**, 326–32.

Christopher, J. S., Hansen, D. J. and MacMillan, V. M. (1991). Effectiveness of a peer-helper intervention to increase children's social interactions: generalization, maintenance, and social validity. *Behavior Modification*, **15**, 22–50.

Coleman, M., Wheeler, L. and Webber, J. (1993). Research on interpersonal problem-solving training: a review. *RASE: Remedial and Special Education*, **14**, 25–37.

D'Zurilla, T. J. , Nezu, A. M. and Maydeu-Olivares, A. (in press). *Manual for the Social Problem Solving Inventory Revised (SPSI-R).* North Tonawanda, NY: Multi-Health Systems, Inc.

Elliott, S. N., Malecki, C. K. and Demaray, M. K. (2001). New directions in social skills assessment and intervention for elementary and middle school students. *Exceptionality*, **9**, 19–32.

Ellis, A. (1958). Rational psychotherapy. *Journal of General Psychology*, **59**, 35–49.

Farmer Dougan, V. and Kaszuba, T. (1999). Reliability and validity of play-based observations: relationship between the PLAY behaviour observation system and standardised measures of cognitive and social skills. *Educational Psychology*, **19**, 429–40.

Feshbach, N. D. and Roe, K. (1968). Empathy in six- and seven-year-olds. *Child Development*, **39**, 133–45.

Freedman, B. J., Rosenthal, R., Donahue, C. P., Schlundt, D. G. and McFall, R. M. (1978). A social behaviour analysis of skill deficits in delinquent and nondelinquent adolescent boys. *Journal of Consulting and Clinical Psychology*, **46**, 1445–62.

Frentz, C., Gresham, F. M. and Elliott, S. N. (1991). Popular, controversial, neglected, and rejected adolescents: contrasts of social competence and achievement differences. *Journal of School Psychology*, **29**, 109–20.

Furman, W. and Masters, J. C. (1980). *An Observational System for Measuring Reinforcing, Neutral and Punishing Interactions in Children*. Minneapolis, MN: University of Minnesota, Institute of Child Development.

Getter, H. and Nowinski, J. K. (1981). A free response test of interpersonal effectiveness. *Journal of Personality Assessment*, **45**, 301–8.

Goddard, P. and McFall, R. M. (1992). Decision-making skills and heterosocial competence in college women: an information-processing analysis. *Journal of Social and Clinical Psychology*, **11**, 401–25.

Gresham, F. M. (1985). Utility of cognitive-behavioral procedures for social skills training with children: a critical review. *Journal of Abnormal Child Psychology*, **13**, 411–23.

(1997). Social competence and students with behavior disorders: where we've been, where we are, and where we should go. *Education and Treatment of Children*, **20**, 233–49.

(1998). Social skills training: should we raze, remodel, or rebuild? *Behavioral Disorders*, **24**, 19–25.

Gresham, F. M. and Elliott, S. N. (1990). *Social Skills Rating System*. Circle Pines, MN: American Guidance Service.

Gumpel, T. P. and Frank, R. (1999). An expansion of the peer tutoring paradigm: cross-age peer tutoring of social skills among socially rejected boys. *Journal of Applied Behavior Analysis*, **32**, 115–18.

Haley, G. M., Fine, S., Maniage, K., Moretti, M. M. and Freeman, R. J. (1985). Cognitive bias and depression in psychiatrically disturbed children and adolescents. *Journal of Consulting and Clinical Psychology*, **53**, 535–7.

Hansen, D. J., Nangle, D. W. and Meyer, K. A. (1998). Enhancing the effectiveness of social skills interventions with adolescents. *Education and Treatment of Children*, **21**, 489–513.

John, K., Gammon, G. D., Prusoff, B. A. and Warner, V. (1987). The Social Adjustment Inventory for Children and Adolescents (SAICA): testing of a new semistructured interview. *Journal of the American Academy of Child and Adolescent Psychiatry*, **26**, 898–911.

Kaslow, N. J. and Nolen-Hoeksema, S. (1991). *Children's Attributional Style Questionnaire: Revised*. Atlanta, GA: Emory University.

Kavale, K. A., Mathur, S. R., Forness, S. R., Rutherford, R. B. Jr and Quinn, M. M. (1997). Effectiveness of social skills training for students with behavior disorders: A meta-analysis. In T. E. Scruggs and M. A. Matropieri (eds.), *Advances in Learning and Behavioral Disabilities*, Volume 11. Greenwich, CT: JAI Press, pp. 1–26.

Ladd, G. W. (1981). Effectiveness of a social learning method for enhancing children's social interaction and peer acceptance. *Child Development*, **52**, 171–8.

La Greca, A. M. and Santogrossi, D. A. (1980). Social skills training with elementary school students: a behavioral group approach. *Journal of Consulting and Clinical Psychology*, **48**, 220–7.

Leitenbertg, H., Yost, L. W. and Carroll-Wilson, M. (1986). Negative cognitive errors in children: questionnaire development, normative data, and comparisons between children with and without self-reported symptoms of depression, low self-esteem, and evaluation anxiety. *Consulting and Clinical Psychology*, **54**, 528–36.

Lochman, J. E., Coie, J. D., Underwood, M. K. and Terry, R. (1993). Effectiveness of a social relations intervention program for aggressive and nonaggressive, rejected children. *Journal of Consulting and Clinical Psychology*, **61**, 1053–8.

Magill Evans, J., Koning, C., Cameron Sadava, A. and Manyk, K. (1995). The child and adolescent social perception measure. *Journal of Nonverbal Behavior*, **19**, 151–69.

Matson, J. L. (1990). *Matson Evaluation of Social Skills with Youngsters: Manual*. Worthington, OH: International Diagnostic Systems.

Matson, J. L., Rotatori, A. F. and Helsel, W. J. (1983). Development of a rating scale to measure social skills in children: the Matson Evaluation of Social Skills with Youngsters (MESSY). *Behaviour Research and Therapy*, **21**, 335–40.

Meichenbaum, D. and Goodman, J. (1971). Training impulsive children to talk to themselves: a means of developing self-control. *Journal of Abnormal Psychology*, **77**, 115–26.

Merrell, K. W. (1993). Using behavioral rating scales to assess social skills and antisocial behavior in school settings: development of the School Social Behavior Scales. *School Psychology Review*, **22**, 115–33.

(1996). Social-emotional assessment in early childhood: the Preschool and Kindergarten Behavior Scales. *Journal of Early Intervention*, **20**, 132–45.

(2001). Assessment of children's social skills: recent developments, best practices, and new directions. *Exceptionality*, **9**, 3–18.

Messer, S. C., Kempton, T., Van Hasselt, V. B. *et al.* (1994). Cognitive distortions and adolescent affective disorder: validity of the CNCEQ in an inpatient sample. *Behavior Modification*, **18**, 339–51.

Milne, J. and Spence, S. H. (1987). Training social perception skills with primary school children: a cautionary note. *Behavioural Psychotherapy*, **15**, 144–57.

Ollendick, T. H. (1981). Assessment of social interaction skills in school children. *Behavioral Counseling Quarterly*, **1**, 227–43.

Platt, J. J. and Spivack, G. (1995). *Manual for the Means-Ends Problem-Solving Procedures (MEPS)*. Philadelphia: DHMS.

Polifka, J. A., Weissberg, R. P., Gesten, E. L., de Apodaca, R. F. and Picoli, L. (1981). *The Open-Middle Interview Manual*. New Haven, CT: Department of Psychology, Yale University.

Rapee, R. M. and Heimberg, R. G. (1997). A cognitive-behavioral model of anxiety in social phobia. *Behaviour Research and Therapy*, **35**, 741–56.

Schneider, B. H. (1992). Didactic methods for enhancing children's peer relations: a quantitative review. *Clinical Psychology Review*, **12**, 363–82.

Sechrest, L., McKnight, P. and McKnight, K. (1996). Calibration of measures for psychotherapy outcome studies. *American Psychologist*, **51**, 1065–71.

Spence, S. H. (1995). *Social Skills Training: Enhancing Social Competence in Children and Adolescents*. Windsor, UK: The NFER-NELSON Publishing Company Ltd.

Spence, S. H., Donovan, C. and Brechman Toussaint, M. (1999). Social skills, social outcomes, and cognitive features of childhood social phobia. *Journal of Abnormal Psychology*, **108**, 211–21.

(2000). The treatment of childhood social phobia: the effectiveness of a social skills training-based, cognitive-behavioural intervention, with and without parental involvement. *Journal of Child Psychology and Psychiatry and Allied Disciplines*, **41**, 713–26.

Stuart, D. L., Gresham, F. M. and Elliott, S. N. (1991). Teacher ratings of social skills in popular and rejected males and females. *School Psychology Quarterly*, **6**, 16–26.

Tiffen, K. and Spence, S. H. (1986). Responsiveness of isolated versus rejected children to social skills training. *Journal of Child Psychology and Psychiatry and Allied Disciplines*, **27**, 343–55.

Waksman, S. A. (1985). The development and psychometric properties of a rating scale for children's social skills. *Journal of Psychoeducational Assessment*, **3**, 111–21.

Walker, H. M. and McConnell, S. R. (1995). *The Walker-McConnell Scale of Social Competence and School Adjustment (SSCSA)*. San Diego, CA: Singular.

Walker, H. M. and Severson, H. H. (1992). *Systematic Screening for Behavior Disorders (SSBD)*, 2nd edn. Longmont, CO: Sopris West.

Walker, H. M., Colvin, G. and Ramsey, E. (1995). *Antisocial Behaviour in School: Strategies and Best Practices*. Pacific Grove, CA: Brooks/Cole.

24

Pain in childhood

Patrick McGrath
Dalhousie University, Halifax, Nova Scotia, Canada

Julie Goodman
Hotel Dieu Hospital, Kingston, Ontario, Canada

24.1 Introduction

The International Association for the Study of Pain has established a standard definition of pain as: 'an unpleasant sensory and emotional experience associated with actual or potential tissue damage or described in terms of such damage' (Merskey and Bogduk, 1994, p. 210). Cognitive behaviour therapy (CBT) has been used both to influence the presumed cause of pain (usually when the cause is related to 'stress') and to ameliorate the sensory and emotional aspects of pain. In this chapter, CBT will be examined in relation to both of these elements in specific pain problems.

There is a wide diversity of pain problems in children and adolescents that can be assisted by CBT. However, discussion will be focused on those problems that are common and for which there is most clinical experience and research. These include: pain from procedures, headache, recurrent abdominal pain and fibromyalgia. Similar strategies used to treat these problems can also be applied to neuropathic pain, pain from sickle cell disease, irritable bowel syndrome and pain from cancer. However, there is little research on disease-related pain interventions.

24.2 Why CBT works in pain relief

As will be discussed, there is solid evidence for the effectiveness of CBT in some areas of pain and promising evidence in others. In contrast, there is little or no evidence that simple counselling, psychodynamic or other psychotherapeutic approaches have any effectiveness in paediatric pain. A major problem

Cognitive Behaviour Therapy for Children and Families, ed. Philip J. Graham.
Published by Cambridge University Press. © Cambridge University Press 2004.

is that, because of the lack of clinical trials, there is no evidence to determine whether other approaches are not effective or merely that effectiveness has not been demonstrated. Unlike other psychotherapeutic approaches, CBT takes an evidence-based approach.

The mechanism for the effectiveness of CBT in paediatric pain appears to differ with different treatments. So, for example, distraction seems to work because it consumes attentional resources that are required for the processing of pain. In headache, the mechanism appears to be stress reduction. However, little work has examined mechanisms.

When we see a child in pain, we often do not have randomized trials to refer to in order to guide treatment. As a result, lesser forms of evidence must be used. For example, the Pediatric Pain List (http://www.dal.ca/~pedpain/ppml/ppmlist.html) is a listserv that has over 700 subscribers in 45 countries. Clinicians consult with each other on management of paediatric pain using the list. The evidence base is growing but there must be more research on paediatric pain. The authors believe that an evidence-based approach is ethically and scientifically the most legitimate strategy to use in helping the children suffering from pain.

24.3   Pain from procedures

Pain from procedures includes the pain from relatively common and minor procedures such as injection and venepuncture, as well as pain from more uncommon and major procedures such as bone marrow aspiration and lumbar puncture. The most predominant strategies used for reducing pain from procedures are distraction and hypnosis. In addition to giving control to the child, relaxation training, breathing exercises and positive reinforcement have been used to augment the positive effects of these strategies. Distraction has been commonly used for minor procedures such as finger pricks, immunization and venepuncture. Hypnosis has been used for minor procedures, as well as more invasive procedures such as bone marrow aspiration.

24.3.1   Distraction

The rationale underlying the use of distraction is that it divides or limits the child's attention to painful stimuli. Thus, there is limited attentional capacity available to feel pain: if attention is focused elsewhere, pain will be noticed less. It is important, however, to ensure that the distraction technique being used is captivating enough to be effective.

24.3.1.1   Case illustration

James is a 3-year-old child with diabetes who requires repeated finger pricks, up to four times daily, for blood tests to assess his blood sugar levels and gauge his insulin requirements. He has become quite resistant to and apprehensive of these tests. Whenever his mother approaches him with the test kit, he cries and tries to run away. As a strategy to prevent him from running from her, his mother had tried using the 'sneak attack' approach (trying to surprise him) and assumed that this approach would give him less time and opportunity to become upset. He subsequently became very suspicious of his mother, and avoided her whenever he suspected a surprise finger prick. As a result, each finger prick turns into a 1-hour battle. Unfortunately, his blood sugar levels are somewhat erratic and frequent testing is necessary to enhance good control. His mother consulted the psychologist from the diabetes clinic, who developed the following individualized programme for her:

(1)   Do not try to fool James about what is to happen.
(2)   Set up a bowl of his favourite 'diabetic' ice cream for him to eat immediately following the finger prick.
(3)   Allow him to watch his favourite video during the finger prick (reserve his favourites for this).
(4)   Let James choose the finger that will be pricked.
(5)   Hold his hand firmly, wait until he is involved in the video and then proceed with the prick.
(6)   Ignore any crying.
(7)   Give praise and the ice cream immediately when finished.

This programme was effective in reducing the turmoil surrounding the finger pricks, but it still took 10 minutes to complete a finger prick. Gradually, over the following 2 weeks, finger pricks became more routine and much more predictable for James. He no longer feared 'sneak attacks' and the process became less onerous. James' mother sometimes omitted the ice cream reward or the video distraction. However, 2 months later, the problem recurred and the full programme was reinstated for 2 weeks.

As described in this vignette, distraction is usually embedded in the context of other behavioural methods. For example, being forthcoming with James about exactly what was going to happen and when it would happen probably reduced excessive anticipatory anxiety. Furthermore, the videotape distraction was combined with an immediate positive tangible reward (ice cream) as well as positive, verbal feedback, regardless of James' crying behaviour. Crying behaviour was ignored, so that he was not scolded for crying nor was he given excessive sympathy for crying. Cohen *et al.* (1999) found that coaches using distraction were more effective and less costly than was no treatment or EMLA for a series of three injections for vaccination over a 6-month period. For longer and more invasive procedures, distraction can be combined with EMLA, a topical analgesic containing lidocaine and prilocaine (Halperin *et al.*, 1989).

Research examining the use of distraction has shown variable treatment effect size. For example, Fowler-Kerry and Lander (1987) found a small effect ($d = 0.39$) when using music distraction to reduce self-reported pain in 200 4.5–6.5-year-old children undergoing intramuscular immunization. Other studies have evaluated the use of distraction during venepuncture. Vessey *et al.* (1994) found a medium effect ($d = 0.65$) of kaleidoscope distraction in reducing pain in 100 3–11-year-old children undergoing venepuncture. Arts *et al.* (1994) found no significant effect of music distraction in reducing pain in 180 4–16-year-olds undergoing routine venepuncture.

Teaching 3–7-year-old children coping skills without an adult to coach them appears to be insufficient to reduce distress (Cohen *et al.*, 2002). It may be more effective to combine teaching coping skills and coaching.

Tips to ensure good distraction include:

(1)   Allow enough time for the child's attention to be as fully engaged as possible by the method of distraction being used. Clinical judgement and the age and developmental level of the child should be used to gauge how long the preprocedure distraction time should be.

(2)   Choose a method of distraction that is interesting and appropriate to the age and developmental level of the child. Potential distractors include: blowing bubbles or other blowing games, listening to music, singing, watching videos or mobiles, reading aloud to the child or playing with toys. For example, watching videotapes of cartoons during a finger prick may be appropriate for preschool or younger, school-aged children, whereas listening to a favourite CD might be more appropriate for adolescents.

(3)   Allow the child to have some choice in selecting the method of distraction to give the child a sense of control over the procedure but do not allow them to avoid the procedure.

(4)   Do *not* deceive or criticize the child.

24.3.2 Hypnosis

There is considerable controversy in the literature on hypnosis. Some believe it is an altered state of consciousness (e.g. Hilgard and LeBaron, 1984), whereas others (e.g. Spanos, 1986a,b) regard the hypnotic state simply as one of heightened suggestibility. Both sides to the argument agree that hypnosis involves a focusing of attention with suggestions. As such, attention is diverted away from pain and pain-inducing stimuli. The focusing of attention has included the use of 'favourite stories' in young children (Kuttner, 1988) and the more conventional techniques of visual or cognitive focusing that are widely used with adults. Although many believe it is clinically useful to assess hypnotic suggestibility prior to using hypnosis as a form of intervention, no clear relationship has been identified between hypnotic suggestibility and the effectiveness of hypnosis in children. Some families may have religious objections to the use of hypnosis and, therefore, the family's view of hypnosis should be known before recommending its use.

24.3.2.1   Case illustration

Marie, aged 5 years, has acute lymphoblastic leukaemia and is required to have numerous and frequent finger pricks and other invasive procedures. Pain from bone marrow aspirations and lumbar punctures is prevented by using conscious sedation, an anaesthetic procedure whereby the child is given a very brief anaesthesia in the treatment room. Generally, Marie does not show excessive anticipatory anxiety to these procedures. However, she often becomes distressed for up to an hour prior to each finger prick. In collaboration with the unit psychologist, Marie's mother developed a form of hypnosis that incorporated guided imagery to help Marie dissociate from the pain of the finger prick. The story described a medieval knight, whose suit of armour protected her from a dragon's fiery breath. In a variation on this story, Marie's mother suggested that Marie was the knight, whose suit of armour would protect her from the pain from the finger prick. Although this strategy did not eliminate the pain from the needle pricks, Marie reported that they felt less painful when she was 'wearing' her suit of armour.

Hypnosis can be combined with other medical and psychological therapies. Hypnosis is often conceptualized in other terms such as distraction, relaxation or guided imagery. Moreover, pharmacotherapeutic procedures can be used, in addition, if they are warranted.

There is good evidence that hypnosis can reduce pain from medical procedures. For example, in a randomized trial, Kuttner (1988) found that hypnosis in the form of favourite stories was superior both to a distraction treatment and to standard care in reducing behavioural distress in response to bone marrow aspirations.

24.4   Headaches

The two most common types of headaches that children and adolescents experience are tension-type headache and migraine. Tension-type headaches are typically associated with dull or pressing pain, often bilateral, not aggravated by physical activity, not accompanied by vomiting or severe nausea and generally less severe than migraine (Olesen *et al.*, 1988). Migraine headaches are of several types, but the most frequent are migraine with aura, previously known as classic migraine, and migraine without aura, previously known as common migraine. Migraine headaches are usually well-defined attacks of severe throbbing pain and are commonly unilateral. Significant nausea and vomiting are common and the pain is made worse by physical activity. The aura of migraine is usually visual and occurs about half an hour prior to the headache itself.

The reported prevalence of headaches in schoolchildren occurring once a month or more has varied from 23% to 51% (Egermark-Eriksson, 1982; Sillanpaa, 1983; Kristjansdottir and Wahlberg, 1993). More frequent unspecified headaches occurring once a week or more have been reported among 7–22% of schoolchildren (Egermark-Eriksson, 1982; Sillanpaa, 1983; Larsson, 1988; Kristjansdottir and Wahlberg, 1993). A smaller proportion of schoolchildren experience almost daily headaches (2.5–6%) and about 0.3–1.2% of the children report daily headaches (Egermark-Eriksson, 1982; Sillanpaa, 1983). A very marked increase in the prevalence of headache with age has been noted. In children below 10 years of age, headache is approximately equally distributed in both sexes. However, during adolescence, the prevalence of headache increases in both males and females, but generally increases more in females until there is a marked preponderance of female headache sufferers. This trend is maintained in adulthood. Clinical impressions suggest that there is a secular trend of increasing prevalence of headache. This has been confirmed by Sillanpaa and Anttila, who did a 20-year follow-up survey in which they examined children in the same schools using the same instrument (Sillanpaa and Anttila, 1996). They found a striking increase in the prevalence of migraine as well as unspecified headaches over a 20-year time period. The greatest increase in prevalence was observed in areas with high school instability. The authors suggested that changes in the psychosocial environment might explain the increase in prevalence.

The rationale for using CBT for children who have recurrent headaches is to reduce psychosocial stress that often triggers migraine, to reduce perceived pain intensity and severity and to reduce or prevent disability from headache. Three major techniques have been used: hypnosis, progressive muscle relaxation and cognitive restructuring. However, although headaches from pathological causes are rare, a careful history and physical examination by a physician should be completed prior to beginning CBT. Bilateral headaches and headaches that wake the child in the night require especially careful assessment for organic causes.

24.4.1   Hypnosis

There are many different forms of hypnosis. All of them involve the focusing of attention and usually also suggest relaxation and reduction of pain. Hypnosis is sometimes indistinguishable from forms of relaxation training.

24.4.2   Progressive muscle relaxation

Relaxation typically consists of a combination of relaxation with tension, relaxation without tension and abbreviated relaxation using breathing exercises. Although relaxation training has been shown to reduce the frequency of migraine and overall headache activity in children effectively (e.g. Richter *et al.*, 1986), relaxation training alone, in the absence of additional, concurrent cognitive behavioural strategies such as cognitive restructuring or coping-skills training, may not constitute a consistently effective therapy (McGrath *et al.*, 1988). Audio-taped instructions of relaxation exercises may also be used between sessions to facilitate training (e.g. McGrath *et al.*, 1990).

Cognitive behavioural approaches to headaches often include a psycho-educational component to teach children about the relationship between their headaches and psychosocial stress. Most programmes incorporate a series of steps and should include the following elements:

(1)   rationale of the relationship between headache and psychosocial stress;

(2)   prospective recording of pain and coping strategies prior to treatment, during treatment and following treatment;

(3)   learning to identify negative thoughts and to replace them with more positive thoughts;

(4)   examining unrealistic beliefs;

(5)   distraction strategies;

(6)   imagery, behaviour rehearsal and mental activities; and

(7)   problem-solving.

The major form of assessment needed prior to the implementation of CBT for headaches is the determination of whether the patient has the cognitive ability and the motivation to complete the programme. For example, it is unlikely that children under 9 or 10 years of age have the meta-cognitive ability to use cognitive restructuring (but see Chapter 2). Hypnosis and relaxation may be used with children over the age of 7 or 8 years, but a younger child would probably require considerable parental involvement and assistance with the exercises. Further, children with only occasional headaches are unlikely to be motivated enough to undertake such a demanding programme.

Relaxation and cognitive restructuring are often combined. Both of these methods have been delivered in a reduced therapist contact model in which the adolescent moves through the treatment programme by means of telephone contact and a manual. The programme is introduced to the adolescent in one or two introductory sessions, and compliance is encouraged and maintained through regular follow-up telephone calls. The reduced therapist contact approach is about three times more cost-efficient and equally effective to the therapist-directed approach (McGrath *et al.*, 1992).

24.4.3   Case illustration

Kerry is 15 years old and has had recurrent headaches that occur about twice a week for 2 years. They began just after she started to menstruate. She has two types of headaches: 'regular' headaches and 'killer' headaches. Her 'regular' headaches, which occur about 80% of the time, are tension-type headaches, while her 'killer' headaches are migraine headaches without an aura. Kerry usually does not miss school from her tension-type headaches but often must go home when she has a migraine. The tension-type headaches usually make it difficult for her to concentrate. She tries to keep up in school but feels she could work better if she had fewer headaches. Her mother also has had chronic tension-type and migraine headaches since about the same age. Kerry uses paracetamol sparingly because she is afraid of becoming addicted. When her doctor suggested a referral to the psychologist at the local hospital for treatment of her headaches, both she and her family were reluctant because they did not feel it was a psychological problem. However, Kerry decided to try it for a few sessions.

The treatment was a combination of psychoeducation, relaxation training, hypnosis and cognitive restructuring. Kerry found that the best part of the treatment was meeting five other girls who had the same problem. They learned all about headaches and were very supportive in encouraging each other to do the exercises and manage their headaches. Kerry learned to recognize the stressors that were most likely to trigger her headaches. These were skipping meals (i.e. not eating) and being worried about her school work. She really enjoyed the relaxation exercises and found the hypnosis and imagery exercises, as directed by the audiotape, to be very helpful. She also learned to use a full dose of paracetamol or ibuprofen as soon as her headache began, rather than waiting until the pain became unbearable. Over the 12 weeks of the programme, Kerry's migraines declined by about one-half in severity and about one-half in frequency. She almost eliminated the occurrence of her tension-type headaches. She attended booster sessions every 3 months for 1 year. On her own, she kept in contact with three of the other headache group members. She described the treatment group as a positive and helpful experience.

CBT should be combined with education about headache and, when indicated, appropriate use of over-the-counter analgesics (usually paracetamol/acetaminophen). Many parents are wary of the use of paracetamol for pain in children, with about 15% fearing drug abuse or addiction and about 30% fearing the development of tolerance (Forward *et al.*, 1996). As a result, parents frequently delay the administration of medication for over an hour after the headache begins (Forward *et al.*, 1996). Early aggressive use of over-the-counter analgesics may reduce the pain of significant headache.

Several randomized, controlled trials have been conducted to evaluate the effect of CBT of migraine and tension-type headache. For example, Larsson and colleagues (e.g. Larsson and Melin, 1986; Larsson *et al.*, 1987a,b; Larsson and Melin, 1988, 1989; Larsson *et al.*, 1990) have demonstrated that relaxation delivered in a school-based programme to children with tension-type headache was significantly more effective than a control condition. Similarly, Richter *et al.* (1986) demonstrated that a therapist-reduced treatment, in which the adolescents used a manual and tape in combination with two appointments and telephone calls from the therapist, was at least as effective as the same treatment delivered by a therapist.

The addition of a brief parent-training module that focuses on teaching parents to reward coping behaviour and ignore sick role behaviour may increase the effectiveness of CBT that is directed towards the child with headache (Allen and Shriver, 1998).

24.5   Recurrent abdominal pain

Recurrent abdominal pain refers to pain in the abdomen that occurs on at least three occasions over a period of greater than 3 months and that interferes with normal activities and for which no organic cause can be found (Apley, 1975). The rationale for the use of CBT in treating recurrent abdominal pain is that stress may be important in triggering attacks in susceptible children. Moreover, children may have secondary gain, most notably school avoidance and increased parental attention from having recurrent abdominal pain. The techniques used have included stress management and operant approaches. Sanders and his colleagues (Sanders *et al.*, 1994) have demonstrated the effectiveness of these strategies in well-designed trials.

The assessment should include a thorough history and physical examination conducted by a physician to rule out significant pathology causing recurrent abdominal pain. Approximately 10% of children who present with recurrent abdominal pain have an underlying organic pathology which explains the pain (e.g. lactose intolerance, appendicitis, parasites, etc.; Rappaport and Leichtner,

1993). In addition, the relationship between stressful life events and pain, and between secondary gain and pain, should be determined. The developmental capacity of the child to learn and use cognitive behavioural methods must be ascertained. Finally, the ability of the parents to function as effective agents of change must be assessed.

24.5.1   Case illustration

Mona, a 12-year-old child, has experienced bouts of abdominal pain since she was 7 years old. The pain has waxed and waned over the years, and there has been no apparent relationship with obvious stressors. Her parents are concerned because she has started to miss a significant amount of school. Until this year, she had reported pain once every week or so, and had been absent from school about 1 day per month. This year, she had been absent from school about 25% of the time. Her teacher reported that she was a quiet student who works hard. However, she was falling behind this year. Assessment revealed that she was very afraid of being embarrassed in school by vomiting (although she rarely vomited with her pain) and there was some concern expressed by her parents that she was 'enjoying' the time she spent at home watching television.

She was cooperative and compliant with CBT, and able to learn to relax well. Her fear of vomiting was directly attacked and her parents were encouraged to make sick time at home boring, with no access to television and to reward every 2 weeks of perfect school attendance with a movie for her and her friend. She was coached to increase her activity as she had a very sedentary lifestyle and was also helped to increase her consumption of dietary fibre (she especially liked popcorn). Her bouts of pain gradually decreased and her attendance at school increased dramatically.

The only other validated treatment for recurrent abdominal pain is supplementary dietary fibre (Feldman *et al.*, 1985). CBT can be combined with an increase of dietary fibre (about 10 g per day), but no empirical studies have been done to determine whether this combined approach improves long-term outcome.

The evidence for the effectiveness of CBT for recurrent abdominal pain is a series of randomized trials by Sanders and colleagues (1989, 1994) that have shown excellent outcome.

24.6   Fibromyalgia

Fibromyalgia is a non-inflammatory, soft tissue, rheumatic disorder of unknown aetiology, characterized by widespread aches, pains and stiffness. The presence of an excessive number of tender points, identified by pressure dolorimeter or thumb palpation, is typically noted. Fibromyalgia occurs both on its own and in conjunction with other rheumatic disorders. It is also often exacerbated by fatigue, stress, inactivity and cold, damp weather. Those affected have also reported experiencing sleep disturbances, headaches, irritable bowel syndrome, feelings of numbness and subjective feelings of swelling. Standard diagnostic criteria for fibromyalgia have been developed by the American College of Rheumatology (Report of the Multicenter Criteria Committee, 1990) and by the International Association for the Study of Pain (Merskey and Bogduk, 1994). Fibromyalgia is a chronic pain disorder and most adults seen in rheumatology clinics with fibromyalgia are significantly disabled.

Very little research on the prevalence, natural course and treatment of fibromyalgia in children and adolescents has been conducted. Malleson *et al.* (1992) reported a retrospective chart review of children with idiopathic, musculoskeletal pain presenting at a tertiary care children's rheumatology clinic. Most of the children (35/40) with diffuse pain fulfilled Yunus and Masi's (1985) diagnostic criteria for fibromyalgia. They found that these children had frequent recurrences and many had significant psychological morbidity. A recent epidemiological study (Buskila *et al.*, 1993) studied 338 healthy Israeli school children, aged 9–15 years, from a single school and found 6.2% to have fibromyalgia using the American College of Rheumatology's criteria (Report of the Multicenter Criteria Committee, 1990). There were no age or gender differences noted. Children with fibromyalgia had lower thresholds for tenderness than children without fibromyalgia at both tender point and control sites. There were seven children who had low pressure–pain thresholds at tender points who did not report widespread pain, and thus were not diagnosed as having fibromyalgia. A 30-month follow-up (Buskila *et al.*, 1995) found that 73% of the children originally diagnosed with fibromyalgia no longer fulfilled its diagnostic criteria. None of the children with low pain thresholds had developed fibromyalgia. The authors concluded the prevalence of fibromyalgia in a community sample of adolescents to be 1.7%.

The underlying cause of fibromyalgia is still unknown. A very wide variety of causes has been suggested, but none has been firmly established. Depression and sleep problems are common, but it is unclear if they are the cause or result of the disorder. Case control studies of clinical samples have found mixed results regarding the psychological concomitants of fibromyalgia in adolescents. Yunus and Masi (1985) compared 33 fibromyalgia patients and controls and found that the children with fibromyalgia had higher rates of sleep problems, fatigue, depression, anxiety, chronic headaches, numbness and irritable bowel symptoms compared with the controls. However, they used psychometrically weak measurements of anxiety, depression and sleep problems. Reid *et al.* (1996) found no differences between adolescents and their families with fibromyalgia, juvenile rheumatoid arthritis and pain-free controls on a variety of well-validated instruments measuring clinical psychopathology.

The one treatment trial of CBT for fibromyalgia in adolescents is a clinical series with seven patients (Walco and Illowite, 1992). The authors found that four of the five patients who completed more than four sessions of treatment were pain free, and the remaining patient who completed treatment had sharply reduced pain. Their treatment programme consisted of four to nine sessions of instruction, focusing on progressive muscle relaxation and guided imagery, or self-regulatory techniques directed at reducing pain and improving sleep and mood. They concluded that a cognitive behavioural approach may be useful in treatment of the pain and other symptoms, such as sleep and/or mood distur-bances, associated with fibromyalgia in children.

CBT might be effective in fibromyalgia by increasing restorative sleep, by decreasing pain sensitivity and by increasing physical fitness. The CBT strategies used with fibromyalgia have included cognitive restructuring, improving sleep hygiene and increasing activity.

24.6.1   Case illustration

Jill was a 14-year-old girl who has had widespread pain, fatigue and difficulty sleeping for 2 years. She had gradually become less physically active, quitting the swimming team, and was more socially withdrawn, sharply limiting her contact with her peer group. Her family doctor had thought that her symptoms would remit or significantly improve because she could find no physical basis for Jill's complaints. In addition, although Jill was a bit unhappy, she was not depressed. After a year without improvement, Jill's parents asked that she be referred to a specialist. Her doctor gave her parents the choice of seeing either a psychiatrist or a rheumatologist. Jill's parents chose to see a rheumatologist. A thorough physical examination showed that Jill's pressure–pain tolerance was lower than normal, and that she had 12 of 18 tender points. A series of blood tests revealed nothing abnormal. Jill was diagnosed with fibromyalgia and referred to a psychologist for treatment.

The treatment package consisted of a 10-week, time-limited treatment that included:

(1) An explanation of fibromyalgia as a non-articular rheumatic disorder that is negatively influenced by poor sleep, lack of exercise and increased psychosocial stress.

(2) Daily recording of pain, mood and fatigue using a detailed diary.

(3)   Relaxation training using diaphragmatic breathing.
(4)   Identification of negative thoughts.
(5)   Assistance in changing negative, self-defeating thoughts to more realistic and positive thoughts.
(6)   Instruction in appropriate sleep hygiene.
(7)   Assistance in gradually increasing activity level and developing a programme of mild exercise and activity to enhance physical fitness, endurance and tolerance.
(8)   Training in guided imagery, and distraction from pain.

Jill had individual sessions with a psychologist, who also had three sessions with her parents. Jill made good progress with her sessions and was able to decrease her pain and fatigue. She began a programme of mild exercise and increased her number and frequency of social contacts. She still had a sufficient number of tender points necessary for a diagnosis of fibromyalgia but had much less widespread pain and fatigue. She was followed for 1 year by telephone calls and remained relatively well.

When she was 16 years old, she was in a car accident and sustained a whiplash injury. Her doctor said the pain would just go away with time. When it did not, Jill became more withdrawn and depressed. Her sleep deteriorated and her pain returned. She declined further treatment, saying that it would not help her. Her family moved and she was lost to follow-up.

CBT for fibromyalgia is often combined with low-dose amitriptyline and physiotherapy. There are no data to determine the effectiveness of these combinations in children and adolescents.

24.7   Evidence for effectiveness

Cognitive behavioural approaches have contributed to major advances in the treatment of both acute and chronic pain in infants, children and youths. *The Journal of Pediatric Psychology* has published a series of papers on empirically supported treatments or 'treatments that work' in paediatric psychology. Four of the initial reviews focused on pain. In his review, Powers (1999) concluded that cognitive behavioural strategies were 'well established' for acute pain from procedures. Holden *et al.* (1999) reported that cognitive behavioural treatments were effective in treating both tension headaches and migraine headaches. Walco *et al.* (1999) reviewed the data on pain in chronic disease. Although they found that cognitive behavioural treatments held promise, they concluded that insufficient research had been done to determine if pain in chronic illness is effectively treated using cognitive behavioural interventions. Similarly, because of the lack of sufficient research, Janicke and Finney (1999) found that cognitive behavioural treatments were only 'probably efficacious' for recurrent abdominal pain.

24.8 Conclusions

CBT has been applied to many areas of children's health. Pain management provides an excellent model of the application of CBT with medical problems. A major challenge for the future is to integrate CBT into medical practice. Although cognitive behavioural approaches are widely accepted by mental health practitioners, there are still significant barriers to their implementation in medical settings. These barriers include, first, the fact that physicians and nurses are often unaware of cognitive behavioural approaches and are therefore unlikely to refer for them. Secondly, because it is commonly believed by professionals and the lay public that psychological interventions such as CBT are appropriate only for disorders that are psychologically based, most medical disorders are thought not to benefit from these approaches. Thirdly, many psychologists are not familiar enough with medical conditions to develop treatment strategies for them. Finally, in some countries, funding for the use of CBT for medical conditions or symptoms is either difficult to obtain or unavailable.

The reduced therapist contact methods that have proven extremely effective in headache may have applications to other disorders and have the advantage of being cost-effective. Furthermore, reduced therapist contact methods can be delivered to children who, because of distance from major centres, do not have ready access to specialist care. Elgar and McGrath (2003) have reviewed the evidence for reduced therapist contact methods across all child disorders and conclude that there is ample evidence to use these methods more broadly. In particular, use of information technologies to make treatments more available should be investigated. These might include telephone-enabled and web-enabled systems delivering care to families in their home or computer kiosks delivering care in doctors' offices. There is also a need for a great deal more systematic clinical research work applying cognitive behavioural treatments to pain from children's medical conditions. As wider experience is gained, single-subject studies, clinical series and well-designed clinical trials need to be developed to ensure an evidence-based approach to treatment.

24.9   REFERENCES

Allen, K. D. and Shriver, M. D. (1998). Role of parent-mediated pain behavior management strategies in biofeedback treatment of childhood migraines. *Behavior Therapy*, **29**, 477–90.

Apley, J. (1975). *The Child with Abdominal Pains*, 2nd edn. London: Blackwell.

Arts, S. E., Abu Saad, H. H., Champion, G. D. *et al.* (1994). Age-related response to lidocaine-prilocaine (EMLA) emulsion and effect of music distraction on the pain of intravenous cannulation. *Pediatrics*, **93**, 797–801.

Buskila, D., Neumann, L., Hershman, E., Gedalia, A., Press, J. and Sukenik, S. (1995). Fibromyalgia syndrome in children: an outcome study. *Journal of Rheumatology*, **22**, 525–8.

Buskila, D., Press, J., Gedalia, A. *et al.* (1993). Assessment of nonarticular tenderness and prevalence of fibromyalgia in children. *Journal of Rheumatology*, **20**, 368–70.

Cohen, L., Bernard, R. S., Greco, L. A. and McClellan, C. B. (2002). A child-focused intervention for coping with procedural pain: are parent and nurse coaches necessary? *Journal of Pediatric Psychology*, **27**, 749–57.

Cohen, L. L., Blount, R. L., Cohen, R. J., Schaen, E. R. and Zaff, J. F. (1999). Comparative study of distraction versus topical anesthesia for pediatric pain management during immunizations. *Health Psychology*, **18**, 591–8.

Egermark-Eriksson, I. (1982). Prevalence of headache in Swedish school children: a questionnaire survey. *Acta Paediatrica Scandinavica*, **71**, 135–40.

Elgar, F. and McGrath, P. (2003). Self-administered psychosocial treatments for children and adolescents. *Journal of Child Psychology*, **59**, 1–19.

Feldman, W., McGrath, P. J., Hodgon, C., Ritter, H. and Shipman, R. T. (1985). The use of dietary fiber in the management of simple, childhood, idiopathic, recurrent, abdominal pain. Results of a prospective, double-blind, randomized, controlled trial. *American Journal of Diseases of Children*, **139**, 1216–18.

Forward, S. P., McGrath, P. J. and Brown, T. L. (1996). Mothers' attitudes and behaviour towards medicating children's pain. *Pain*, **67**, 469–75.

Fowler-Kerry, S. and Lander, J. R. (1987). Management of injection pain in children. *Pain*, **30**, 169–75.

Halperin, D. L., Koren, G., Attias, D., Pellegrini, E., Greenberg, M. L. and Wyss, M. (1989). Topical skin anesthesia for venous, subcutaneous drug reservoir and lumbar punctures in children. *Pediatrics*, **84**, 281–4.

Hilgard, J. R. and LeBaron, S. (1984). *Hypnotherapy of Pain in Children with Cancer*. Los Altos, CA: Kaufmann.

Holden, E. W., Deichmann, M. M. and Levy, J. D. (1999). Empirically supported treatments in pediatric psychology: recurrent pediatric headache. *Journal of Pediatric Psychology*, **24**, 91–109.

Janicke, D. M. and Finney, J. W. (1999). Empirically supported treatments in pediatric psychology: recurrent abdominal pain. *Journal of Pediatric Psychology*, **24**, 115–27.

Kristjansdottir, G. and Wahlberg, V. (1993). Sociodemographic differences in the prevalence of self-reported headache in Icelandic school-children. *Headache*, **33**, 376–80.

Kuttner, L. (1988). Favorite stories: a hypnotic pain-reduction technique for children in acute pain. *American Journal of Clinical Hypnosis*, **30**, 289–95.

Larsson, B. S. (1988). The role of psychological, health behaviour and medical factors in adolescent headache. *Developmental Medicine and Child Neurology*, **30**, 616–25.

Larsson, B. S. and Melin, L. (1986). Chronic headaches in adolescents: treatment in a school setting with relaxation training as compared with information-contact and self-registration. *Pain*, **25**, 325–36.

  (1988). The psychological treatment of recurrent headache in adolescents – short-term outcome and its prediction. *Headache*, **28**, 187–95.

(1989). Follow-up on behavioural treatment of recurrent headache in adolescents. *Headache*, **29**, 249–53.

Larsson, B. S., Daleflod, B., Hakansson, L. and Melin, L. (1987a). Therapist-assisted versus self-help relaxation treatment of chronic headaches in adolescents: a school-based intervention. *Journal of Child Psychology and Psychiatry*, **28**, 127–36.

Larsson, B. S., Melin, L. and Doberl, A. (1990). Recurrent tension headache in adolescents: treatment with self-help relaxation training and a muscle relaxant drug. *Headache*, **30**, 665–71.

Larsson, B. S., Melin, L., Lamminen, M. and Ullstedt, F. (1987b). A school-based treatment of chronic headaches in adolescents. *Journal of Pediatric Psychology*, **12**, 553–66.

Malleson, P. N., Al-Matar, M. and Petty, R. E. (1992). Idiopathic muculoskeletal pain syndromes in children. *Journal of Rheumatology*, **19**, 1786–9.

McGrath, P. J., Cunningham, S. J., Lascelles, M. A. and Humphreys, P. (1990). *Help Yourself: A Treatment for Migraine Headaches, Professional Handbook*. Ottawa: University of Ottawa Press.

McGrath, P. J., Humphreys, P., Goodman, J. T. *et al.* (1988). Relaxation prophylaxis for childhood migraine: a randomized placebo-controlled trial. *Developmental Medicine and Child Neurology*, **30**, 626–31.

McGrath, P. J., Humphreys, P., Keene, D. *et al.* (1992). The efficacy and efficiency of a self-administered treatment for adolescent migraine. *Pain*, **49**, 321–4.

Merskey, H. and Bogduk, N. (eds.) (1994). *Classification of Chronic Pain: Descriptions of Chronic Pain Syndromes and Definitions of Pain Terms*, 2nd edn. Seattle: IASP Press.

Olesen, J., Bes, A., Kunkel, R. *et al.* (1988). Classification and diagnostic criteria for headache disorders, cranial neuralgias and facial pain. *Cephalgia*, **8** (suppl 7), 1–96.

Rappaport, L. and Leichtner, A. M. (1993). Recurrent abdominal pain. In N. L. Schecter, C. B. Berde and M. Yaster (eds.) *Pain in Infants, Children, and Adolescents*. Baltimore: Williams and Wilkins, pp. 561–70.

Reid, G. J., Lang, B. A. and McGrath, P. J. (1996). Primary juvenile fibromyalgia: psychological adjustment, family functioning, coping and functional disability. *Arthritis and Rheumatism*, **40** 752–60.

Report of the Multicenter Criteria Committee (1990). The American College of Rheumatology 1990 criteria for the classification of fibromyalgia. *Arthritis and Rheumatism*, **33**, 16–72.

Richter, I. L., McGrath, P. J., Humphreys, J., Goodman, J. T., Firestone, P. and Keene, D. (1986). Cognitive and relaxation treatment of paediatric migraine. *Pain*, **25**, 195–203.

Sanders, M. R., Rebgetz, M., Morrison, M. and Bor, W. (1989). Cognitive-behavioural treatment of recurrent nonspecific abdominal pain in children: an analysis of generalization, maintenance and side effects. *Journal of Consulting and Clinical Psychology*, **57**, 294–300.

Sanders, M. R., Shepherd, R. W., Cleghorn, G. and Woolford, H. (1994). The treatment of recurrent abdominal pain in children: a controlled comparison of cognitive-behavioural family intervention and standard pediatric care. *Journal of Consulting and Clinical Psychology*, **62**, 306–14.

Sillanpaa, M. (1983). Prevalence of headache in pre-puberty. *Headache*, **23**, 10–14.

Sillanpaa, M. and Anttila, P. (1996). Increasing prevalence of headache in 7-year-old school children. *Headache*, **36**, 466–70.

Spanos, N. P. (1986a). Hypnotic behavior: a social-psychological interpretation of amnesia, analgesia and 'trance logic'. *Behavioral and Brain Sciences*, **9**, 449–67.

   (1986b). More on the social psychology of hypnotic responding. *Behavioral and Brain Sciences*, **9**, 489–502.

Vessey, J. A., Carlson, K. L. and McGill, J., (1994). Use of distraction with children during an acute pain experience. *Nursing Research*, **43**, 369–72.

Walco, G. A. and Illowite, N. T. (1992). Cognitive-behavioral intervention for juvenile primary fibromyalgia syndrome. *Journal of Rheumatology*, **19**, 1617–19.

Walco, G. A., Sterling, C. M., Conte, P. M. and Engel, R. G. (1999). Empirically supported treatments in pediatric psychology: disease-related pain. *Journal of Pediatric Psychology*, **24**, 155–67.

Yunus, M. B. and Masi, A. T. (1985). Juvenile primary fibromyalgia syndrome. A clinical study of thirty-three patients and matched normal controls. *Arthritis and Rheumatism*, **28**, 138–45.

25

Conduct disorders in adolescence

John E. Lochman, Nancy C. Phillips and Heather K. McElroy
University of Alabama, Tuscaloosa, Alabama, USA

Dustin A. Pardini
University of Pittsburgh Medical Center, Pittsburgh, Pennsylvania, USA

In this chapter, the nature of conduct disorder and its symptoms will be reviewed briefly, and then an overview of a set of child, family, peer and community risk factors that can predict the emergence of serious antisocial behaviour in youth will be provided. Based on the contextual social–cognitive risk factors that have been implicated in the development of antisocial behaviour, a set of empirically supported cognitive behavioural interventions have been developed for youths from pre-adolescence through to the adolescent age periods. These programmes will be discussed, along with the research indicating their effectiveness.

25.1 Conduct disorder

The fourth edition of the *Diagnostic and Statistical Manual of Mental Disorders* (DSM-IV; American Psychiatric Association, 1994) defines conduct disorder (CD) as symptoms consisting of aggressive conduct that threatens physical harm to other people or animals or non-aggressive conduct that causes property loss or damage, deceitfulness and theft and serious violations of rules. CD is a repetitive and persistent pattern of behaviour which violates societal norms or the basic rights of others. These serious conduct problems are differentiated from oppositional defiant disorder which represents a recurrent pattern of defiant and disobedient behaviour (see Chapter 13). In the USA, rates of CD are estimated to be in the range of 6–16% for boys and 2–9% for girls (American Psychiatric Association, 1994), and to be more prevalent in boys than girls at a rate of about 3:1 (Kazdin, 1998).

Cognitive Behaviour Therapy for Children and Families, ed. Philip J. Graham.
Published by Cambridge University Press. © Cambridge University Press 2004.

The DSM-IV (American Psychological Association, 1994) distinguishes between children who begin showing conduct problems in early childhood from those who begin showing conduct problems closer to adolescence. If any symptoms are present prior to the age of 10 years, with the child meeting criteria for CD, he or she is classified as being of childhood-onset type. However, if criteria are met for CD and no symptoms are present prior to age 10, the child is classified as being of adolescent-onset type. Children classified as childhood-onset type are typically more aggressive with more behaviour problems than children classified as adolescent-onset type. Childhood-onset CD is also associated with prolonged aggressive and antisocial behaviour into adulthood. This subset typically has more difficulty with peer relationships than children diagnosed with adolescent-onset CD. Conversely, children classified as adolescent-onset type typically display disruptive behaviours, particularly in the company of peers, but do not usually exhibit severe behaviour problems or continued conduct problems into adulthood. This distinction between childhood-onset and adolescent-onset CD is consistent with Moffitt's (1993) identification of youths with life-course persistent antisocial behaviour, in contrast to other delinquent youths who have adolescent limited antisocial behaviour. The youths with life-course persistent antisocial behaviour are at early risk because of combined biological and family factors.

Longitudinal research has indicated that CD is often a precursor of antisocial personality disorder (APD) in adulthood (Myers *et al.*, 1998). It is estimated that approximately one-half of children with CD develop significant APD symptomatology. Two factors that predict the development of APD are the number of CD symptoms the child exhibits and early age of onset of symptoms (American Psychiatric Association, 1994). In addition, CD children who show pervasive symptoms in a variety of settings (e.g. home, school and community) and who develop 'versatile' forms of antisocial behaviour, including both overt (assaults or direct threats) and covert (theft) behaviours by early to mid-adolescence, are at risk for a wide range of negative outcomes in adolescence including truancy, substance use, early teenage parenthood and delinquency (Lochman and Wayland, 1994).

25.2 Comorbidity

Between 65% and 90% of children with CD have a comorbid diagnosis of attention deficit hyperactivity disorder (ADHD) (Frick, 1998), with symptoms of hyperactivity/impulsivity showing a stronger relationship to CD than symptoms of inattention. Children with significant conduct problems and symptoms of ADHD are at an increased risk for a severe and chronic form of antisocial behaviour than children with either ADHD or conduct problems alone. Given that stimulant medications have been shown to reduce behaviours specific to CD in youths with comorbid ADHD and CD, clinical interventions for children with conduct problems should assess for the presence of ADHD.

Internalizing problems are also common among children with CD (Angold and Costello, 2001). Research suggests that children with CD and significant depressive symptoms may be at particular risk for developing substance use problems, and exhibit a severe form of depression that often includes suicidal behaviours. Depressive symptoms may also increase the likelihood that adolescent boys with CD will exhibit antisocial personality disorder in adulthood (Loeber *et al.*, 2002). As a result, integrated treatment models designed to address the special needs of children with comorbid CD and depression have been proposed. In contrast, the presence of anxiety disorders in children with CD has been related to a less severe form of antisocial behaviour and low levels of fearfulness have been associated with higher levels of the callous and unemotional traits in delinquent adolescents (Pardini *et al.*, 2003).

Symptoms associated with CD in childhood, especially aggression, have consistently been associated with later substance-using behaviours (Angold and Costello, 2001). Adolescents with CD who use substances are also at increased risk for developing APD (Loeber *et al.*, 2002), even after receiving intensive treatment for their substance abuse problems (Myers *et al.*, 1998).

25.3 Aetiology

A number of specific factors and pathways that place youths at risk for CD and associated antisocial behaviour have been identified, including child factors, family factors and broader factors in the youths' peer and community contexts (Lochman *et al.*, 2001; see also Chapter 27). Adolescent CD, substance abuse and delinquent behaviour can be conceptualized in a developmental framework to be the result of a set of familial and personal factors, with children's aggressive behaviour often being part of that developmental course. This developmental course is set within the child's social ecology, and an ecological framework is needed to guide preventive and treatment efforts (Lochman and Wells, 2002a).

25.3.1 Child factors

Evidence indicates that children with conduct problems do exhibit social–cognitive distortions and deficits at different stages of information processing (Dodge *et al.*, 1986). Children and adolescents exhibiting antisocial behaviour are more likely than normal children to attend to and recall hostile and irrelevant cues, and to make hostile attributions about others' intentions, they are more action-orientated and they are less verbally assertive and compromising when thinking about solutions to social problems (Dunn *et al.*, 1997) and expect aggressive behaviour to have positive consequences. In addition, youths with conduct problems are less socially skilled at enacting positive interpersonal behaviours than children without conduct problems (Dodge *et al.*, 1986). Aggressive adolescents have social goals that place high value on dominance and revenge and relatively little value on affiliation, and these distinctive social goals have been found to have a direct effect on adolescents' delinquent behaviour and on their selection of solutions to social problems (Lochman *et al*, 1993).

Anger can play a particularly important role in the relationship between problematic information processing and aggressive behaviour (Lochman *et al.*, 1997). Anger has been shown to affect information processing in at least three different ways. First, the initial perception of threat can trigger anger and a physiological response. In addition to these physiological responses, anger can then activate schemas which lead to the aggressive child attributing more hostile intent towards others' actions. Finally, prior feelings of anger, left over from conflicts even hours earlier, can alter subsequent cue-encoding and thus the aggressive child's cognitive processing of the stimulus (Lochman *et al.*, 1997).

25.3.2 Family factors

There is a wide array of factors in the family that can affect child aggression, ranging from parenting practices to more general stress and discord within the family. Starting as early as the preschool years, marital conflict is likely to cause disruptions in parenting and these disruptions contribute to children's high levels of stress and consequent aggression (Dadds and Powell, 1992). Both boys and girls from homes in which marital conflict is high are especially vulnerable to externalizing problems like aggression and CD even after controlling for age and family socioeconomic status (Dadds and Powell, 1992).

Parental physical aggression, such as spanking and more punitive discipline styles, have been associated with oppositional and aggressive children in both boys and girls. Low parental warmth and involvement contribute to parents' use of physically aggressive punishment practices. Weiss *et al.* (1992) found that ratings of the severity of parental discipline were positively correlated with teacher ratings of aggression and behaviour problems. In addition to higher aggression ratings, children experiencing harsh discipline practices exhibited poorer social information processing even when controlling for the possible effects of socioeconomic status, marital discord and child temperament. It is important to note that, although such parenting factors are associated with childhood aggression, child temperament and behaviour also affect parenting behaviour. Such evidence indicates the bidirectional relationship between child and parent behaviour.

Poor parental supervision has also been associated with child aggression. Haapasalo and Tremblay (1994) found that boys who fought more often with their peers reported having less supervision and more punishment than boys who did not fight. Interestingly, the boys who fought reported having more rules than the boys who did not fight, suggesting the possibility that parents of aggressive boys may have numerous strict rules that are difficult to follow.

Parents' attributional styles, or the way they think about the causes of their children's behaviour, and the effectiveness of various parenting techniques are related to childhood aggression (Baden and Howe, 1992). For example, mothers of conduct-disordered children are more likely to see the children's misbehaviour as intentional and to attribute the causes to stable factors within the child that are outside of the mothers' control. Research also suggests that poor parental problem-solving skills in interactions with their children are linked with their children's aggression and behaviour problems (Pakasiahti *et al.*, 1996).

25.3.3 Peer and community factors

Children with disruptive behaviours are at risk for being rejected by their peers. Childhood aggressive behaviour and peer rejection independently predict delinquency and conduct problems in adolescence (Lochman and Wayland, 1994). Aggressive children who are also socially rejected tend to exhibit more severe behaviour problems than children who are either aggressive only or rejected only. Despite the compelling nature of these findings, race and gender may moderate the relationship between peer rejection and negative adolescent outcomes. For example, Lochman and Wayland (1994) found that peer rejection ratings of African-American children within a mixed-race classroom did not predict subsequent externalizing problems in adolescence, whereas peer rejection ratings of Caucasian children were associated with future disruptive behaviours. Similarly, while peer rejection can predict serious delinquency in boys, it can fail to do so with girls (Miller-Johnson *et al.*, 1999).

As children with conduct problems enter adolescence, they tend to associate with deviant peers. It is believed that many of these teens have been continually rejected from more prosocial peer groups because they lack appropriate social skills and, as a result, they turn to antisocial cliques as their only means for social support (Miller-Johnson *et al.*, 1999). The relationship between childhood conduct problems and adolescent delinquency is at least partially mediated by deviant peer group affiliation (Vitaro *et al.*, 1999).

In addition to family interaction problems, peer rejection and involvement in deviant peer groups, neighbourhood and school environments and low socio-economic status (SES) have also been found to be risk factors for aggression and delinquency over and above the variance accounted for by family characteristics (Kupersmidt *et al.*, 1995). For example, early onset of aggression and violence has been associated with neighbourhood disorganization and poverty partly because children who live in lower SES and disorganized neighbourhoods are not well supervised and engage in more risk-taking behaviours. Low SES assessed as early as preschool has predicted teacher- and peer-rated behaviour problems at school. Schools can further exacerbate children's conduct problems through the frustration from academic demands and from peer influences. The density of aggressive children in classroom settings can increase the amount of aggressive behaviour emitted by individual students (Kellam *et al.*, 1998).

25.4   Cognitive behavioural intervention

Based on these risk factors, typically conceptualized in contextual social–cognitive models (e.g. Lochman and Wells, 2002a), cognitive behavioural interventions have emerged as the approaches with the most promise and clearest evidence for efficacy for children with CD (Brestan and Eyberg, 1998). These interventions usually involve behavioural parent training, but can also include social problem-solving skills training, anger-management training and social skills training with the children (Lochman *et al.*, 2001). The nature of the intervention programmes varies to some degree across the pre-adolescent to adolescent age periods, and produces effect sizes on outcome analyses in the moderate to large range (from 0.3 to over 1.0).

25.4.1   Preadolescence to early adolescence
25.4.1.1   Problem-solving skills training (PSST)
This programme is targeted for school-age antisocial children between 7 and 13 years of age. Children attend 25 weekly sessions lasting approximately 50 minutes each (Kazdin *et al.*, 1992). PSST emphasizes the daily interpersonal situations that children face and specifically focuses on individual interpersonal deficits. Leaders teach problem-solving skills such as generating multiple solutions to a problem and thinking about the consequences. In addition, problem-solving skills are applied to interpersonal situations with teachers, peers, siblings and parents. Techniques such as role playing, reinforcement, modelling and feedback are all utilized to teach and reward effective problem-solving skills. Children are also given tasks called super-solvers which allow them to practise techniques

from the sessions outside of the group with other people. Parent participation is also a big component of the training and parents watch the sessions and serve as co-leaders in addition to supervising the use of the new skills at home (Kazdin *et al.*, 1992).

Outcome studies suggest that PSST significantly reduces antisocial behaviour during 1-year follow-up periods. In addition, the combination of PSST with an increased parent-focused intervention was found to have the greatest improvements in statistical and clinical significance, as compared with PSST or parent-focused interventions alone (Kazdin *et al.*, 1992).

25.4.1.2   Anger Coping and Coping Power Programmes

The Coping Power Programme is an extended version of an earlier Anger Coping Programme (Lochman, 1992), and includes 33 sessions in the Coping Power Programme Child Component. The Coping Power Programme is a school-based prevention programme designed to be delivered to children at the time of transition to middle school, as they approach the upcoming increases in anti-social behaviours during adolescence, and to last for 15–18 months. The group sessions focus on emotional awareness, anger management training, attribution retraining and perspective-taking, social problem-solving and social skills training, behavioural and personal goal-setting and handling peer pressure. Children also attend individual sessions every 4–6 weeks to ensure that the social–cognitive skills in the intervention are individualized for each child. A Coping Power Parent Component is designed to cover the same period of time as the Child Component. The parents meet for 16 sessions which address parental use of reinforcement and positive attention, establishment of clear rules and expectations, correct and effective use of punishment, family communication, positive school experience for the child and stress management. Parents are instructed on what their child is learning in each session so that they can help facilitate and reward the practise of these new skills at home.

Initially, research on the Anger Coping programme, which is an 18-session child intervention, indicated that the intervention produces reductions in independent observers' ratings of children's aggressive–disruptive off-task behaviour in the classroom and in parent-rated aggressive behaviour, in comparison with randomly assigned control children (e.g. Lochman *et al.*, 1984), and produced reduced substance use at a 3-year follow-up (Lochman, 1992). Subsequently, two studies have indicated the preventive effects of the multi-component Coping Power Programme, which was designed to enhance the Anger Coping Programme's effects on externalizing behaviours. Lochman and Wells (2002a) randomly assigned 183 teacher-rated aggressive boys to the Coping Power Child

Component only, the full Coping Power Programme including both the Child and Parent Components or to an untreated control group, and found that the Coping Power intervention had produced reductions in self-reported delinquency, parent-reported substance use and teacher-rated behavioural improvement for children at a 1-year follow-up, in comparison with a randomly assigned control group. In path analyses, these outcome effects at follow-up were found to be mediated by improvements in: intervention children's hostile attributional biases, expectations that aggressive behaviour leads to negative consequences, internal locus of control, person perception and parents' consistency of discipline (Lochman and Wells, 2002a).

In a second study, with 243 moderate to high aggressive fifth-grade boys and girls, the Coping Power Programme produced lower substance use rates and improved social competence, self-regulation and parental involvement at post-intervention (Lochman and Wells, 2002b), and replicated the prior study's results at a 1-year follow-up by finding lower rates of self-reported delinquency, self-reported substance use and teacher-rated physical aggression at school for Coping Power children in comparison with control children. In a dissemination study, CD and oppositional defiant disorder children had reduced levels of overtly aggressive behaviour following the Coping Power intervention in a Dutch outpatient clinic (Matthys *et al.*, 2001). Across this set of studies, the Coping Power cognitive behavioural interventions with pre-adolescent children and their parents have been found to have preventive effects on the children's subsequent serious conduct problems involving delinquency and substance use.

25.4.2   Middle to late adolescence

25.4.2.1   Multisystemic therapy

Multisystemic therapy (MST) is an individualized intervention that focuses on the interaction between adolescents and the multiple environmental systems that influence their antisocial behaviour, including their peers, family, school and community (Henggeler *et al.*, 1992). Strategies for changing the adolescent's behaviour are developed in close collaboration with family members by identifying the major environmental drivers that help maintain the adolescent's deviant behaviour. Services are delivered in the family's natural environment and can include a variety of treatment approaches including parent training, family therapy, school consultation, marital therapy and individual therapy. Although the techniques used within these treatment strategies can vary, many of them are either behavioural or cognitive behavioural in nature (e.g. contingency management and behavioural contracting). Clinicians are guided by a set of nine MST principles which include concepts like focusing on systems' strengths, delivering developmentally appropriate treatment and improving effective family functioning. Throughout the intervention, clinician adherence to these treatment principles is closely monitored through weekly consultation with MST experts.

Evaluations of the effectiveness of MST with chronic and violent juvenile offenders have produced promising results. Several investigations have shown that families who receive MST report lower levels of adolescent behaviour problems and improvements in family functioning post-treatment in comparison with alternative treatment conditions (Henggeler *et al.*, 1992; Borduin *et al.*, 1995). In the first randomized clinical trial, MST was compared with treatment as usual with a sample of 84 serious juvenile offenders. Juveniles in the MST condition had significantly fewer arrests (mean of 0.87 versus 1.52) and weeks of incarceration (mean of 5.8 versus 16.2) at a 59-week follow-up (Henggeler *et al.*, 1992), and showed reduced recidivism at a 2-year follow-up in comparison with youths receiving treatment as usual. Results from the most extensive evaluation of MST to date found lower recidivism rates in juvenile offenders assigned to MST in comparison with youths who completed individual counselling at 4-year follow-up (Borduin *et al.*, 1995). Among those offenders who continued to offend, those assigned to MST had a lower number of total arrests and were charged with less serious offences in comparison with youths assigned to individual counselling.

25.4.2.2 Functional Family Therapy

Functional Family Therapy (FFT) combines principles from both family systems theory and cognitive behavioural approaches to intervene with antisocial adolescents and their families. The clinical practice of FFT has evolved over the past 30 years, and the most recent version of FFT consists of three intervention phases: (1) engagement and motivation, (2) behaviour change and (3) generalization. During the engagement and motivation phase, the therapist addresses maladaptive beliefs within the family system in order to increase expectations for change, reduce negativity and blaming, build respect for individual differences and develop a strong alliance between the family and therapist. The behaviour change phase is then used to implement concrete behavioural interventions designed to improve family functioning by building relational skills, enhancing positive parenting, improving conflict management skills and reducing maladaptive interaction patterns. These behavioural interventions are individualized to fit the characteristics of each family member and the family relational system as a whole. Finally, the generalization phase of the intervention is used to improve the family's ability to influence competently the systems in which it is embedded (e.g. school, community and juvenile justice system) to help maintain positive change.

An early version of the FFT programme was evaluated using a sample of 86 adolescents charged with status offences and their families. Families were randomly assigned to FFT treatment, client-centred therapy, psychodynamic therapy or no treatment. Following treatment, families who received FFT exhibited better communication patterns than families in the other three conditions. Moreover, court records indicated that adolescents assigned FFT had lower rates of recidivism 6–18 months following treatment, while their siblings had fewer court contacts at 2.5–3.5 years post-treatment, in comparison with all other groups (Klein *et al.*, 1977). A subsequent investigation with repeat adolescent offenders found that youths who participated in FFT showed reduced recidivism and a lower number of new offences during a 15-month follow-up period in comparison with youths assigned to a group home condition (Barton *et al.*, 1985). Other studies have shown that repeat juvenile offenders who received FFT had lower levels of recidivism up to 5.5 years later (Gordon *et al.*, 1995) in comparison with a probation-only group consisting of lower risk delinquents.

25.4.2.3 Adolescent Transitions Programme

The Adolescents Transitions Programme (ATP) was designed as a preventive intervention for middle school youths exhibiting risk factors for the escalation of problem behaviour (Dishion and Andrews, 1995). The programme initially consisted of 12 weekly 90-minute parent and teen group sessions. The parent groups consisted of eight to 16 caregivers and were designed to teach family management skills such as monitoring, positive reinforcement, limit setting and problem-solving. Skills taught within the session were reinforced through the use of exercises, role plays and discussions about how the skills can be employed within the home. In addition to these group sessions, families received three individual consultation sessions. The teen groups consisted of seven to eight teenagers and were designed to enhance self-regulation by addressing self-monitoring and tracking skills, goal setting, developing prosocial peer relationships, limit setting with peers, problem-solving strategies and interpersonal communication skills. Groups begin with a discussion of events occurring during the previous week, including opportunities to practise the skills learned. Group leaders then introduce a new topic for the week, lead role plays and discussions and assign home practice work to be completed before the next session. Incentives are offered to group members for appropriate participation and reaching individual goals.

The initial evaluation of the ATP included 119 at-risk adolescents assigned to one of four conditions: parent groups, teen groups, parent and teen groups and self-directed change (Dishion and Andrews, 1995). Families that were involved in either of the three group interventions showed reduction in coercive parent–child interactions, while families in the self-directed intervention showed no change in coercive interactions over time. While evidence suggested that parent group-only intervention reduced teacher-rated behaviour problems immediately following treatment, these beneficial effects faded within 1 year. Surprisingly, both intervention conditions involving teen groups showed higher levels of tobacco use and teacher-rated behaviour problems in comparison with other conditions at a 1-year follow-up, suggesting that aggregating high-risk adolescents into groups may have iatrogenic effects. A recent, 3-year follow-up suggested that these iatrogenic effects endured over time (Dishion *et al.*, 1999). As a result, a recent version of ATP has eliminated peer groups and moved to a tiered intervention strategy that includes universal, selected and indicated family components.

25.4.2.4   Multidimensional Treatment Foster Care

Multidimensional Treatment Foster Care (MTFC) is an alternative to traditional group care settings for antisocial youths who are removed from the care of their parents or guardians. MTFC temporarily places antisocial youths with a community-based foster family where contingencies governing the youths' behaviour are systematically modified through consultation with a comprehensive treatment team (Fisher and Chamberlain, 2000). As the youths' behaviour improves, a gradual transition is made from the MTFC setting back to their parents' or guardians' home. Each foster family is assigned a behavioural support specialist, youth therapist, family therapist, consulting psychiatrist, parent daily report caller and case manager/clinical team manager to assist with programme implementation. Foster parents, who are informally screened for programme participation, engage in a 20-hour pre-service training which provides an overview of the treatment model and teaches techniques for monitoring and modifying adolescent behaviour. Adolescents are able to earn privileges within the foster home by following a daily programme of scheduled activities and fulfilling behavioural expectations. The youth's biological parents or guardians assist in the treatment planning, engage in family therapy to learn effective parenting skills and begin applying newly learned skills during short home visits. As the family's functioning improves, the visits are extended until complete reunification occurs. Family therapists continue to follow the case for 1–3 months following reunification to assist in the successful resolution of problems that arise.

Initial research on the effectiveness of MTFC has provided some encouraging results. An early version of MTFC was compared with placement in community-based group care (GC) facilities for adjudicated delinquent adolescents using a matched control design. Results from this investigation indicated that juveniles in MTFC condition were more likely than GC youths to complete their placement and had fewer days of incarceration 2 years following treatment. Another matched control design involving younger abused boys in the juvenile justice system revealed that youths in MTFC had significantly fewer arrests, less self-report criminal activities and fewer days incarcerated 1 year following treatment in comparison with GC controls (Fisher and Chamberlain, 2000). At 2-year post-discharge, MTFC boys reported using drugs less often than GC controls. A subsequent randomized clinical trial compared MTFC with placement in GC facilities in 79 adolescent boys, many of whom had been previously charged with several serious criminal offences and had a history of running away from previous placements (Eddy and Chamberlain, 2000). In comparison with GC, boys in the MTFC condition were more likely to complete their programme and spent 60% fewer days incarcerated a year following their referral to the programme. MTFC boys also had a fewer number of criminal referrals and reported lower levels of serious and violent crimes in comparison with boys in GC 1 year following programme completion.

25.5   Summary and implications

It is evident that, even though CD represents a chronic problem for youths and can be difficult to alter, certain forms of cognitive behavioural interventions have had very promising results in preventing and treating the behaviours associated with CD. These empirically supported interventions address an array of mutable risk factors within youths, their families and their peer and community contexts. It is notable that most of these interventions are targeting multiple risk factors and using multiple component programmes. This set of effective interventions for children at risk for, or with, CD are characterized by a strong focus on the contextual factors within the youths' family and peer groups which provide modelling and reinforcement of antisocial behaviours. Developmental factors may influence which components to include in an intervention. With pre-adolescents and early adolescent youths, effective interventions address both deficient parenting processes and distorted and deficient social–cognitive processes. However, when intervening with severely antisocial youths during the later adolescent years, the focus is more strongly on behavioural training approaches with parents and other adult caregivers. By mid-adolescence, there is increasing evidence that child-orientated group interventions may have deleterious effects, although, in the pre-adolescent to early adolescent period, group and individual interventions with children can have significant preventive and treatment effects in reducing children's antisocial behaviour, delinquency and substance use.

Future research on cognitive behavioural interventions with antisocial youths can usefully address four primary issues. First, although there is an increasing understanding of the important changes in outcome behaviours that can be evident at the end of intervention and during follow-up periods, research has generally not examined mediational processes. Thus, it is not clear if the positive outcome effects are occurring because of the intervention's focus on key mediating processes, which would support the development models underlying the intervention, or for other reasons. Secondly, intervention research should include attention to factors which moderate and predict intervention responsivity. These moderator variables can include characteristics of the children as well as characteristics of the children's family and neighbourhood. Despite evidence that an intervention can impact heterogeneous groups of antisocial youths, it is essential that we understand more clearly which types of youths benefit the most and which types benefit the least from the intervention. Thirdly, because aggressive behaviour in children and adolescents is highly stable over time, intervention research needs to examine the effects of booster interventions and intervention components which are specifically designed to promote relapse prevention can be empirically investigated. Fourthly, even though certain cognitive behavioural interventions have been found to be efficacious in controlled intervention trials, these empirically supported interventions may not be as effective in some real-life settings and they have had relatively little impact on clinical and prevention work in many communities. Agencies will need to allocate resources to implement these empirically supported interventions and to provide adequate opportunities for training. Although these programmes are based on well-established behavioural and cognitive behavioural strategies (e.g. focusing on antecedents and consequences, emphasizing social reinforcement, training in social problem-solving and perspective-taking skills) and mental health professionals who do not have access to the resources to implement the programmes formally must rely on their general training in these areas, the optimal use of the programmes will require specific training and supervision. Intervention research needs to examine factors in the training process and in the host systems (community agencies and schools) which affect dissemination.

25.6   Acknowledgements

The completion of this chapter has been supported by grants to the first author from the National Institute for Drug Abuse (DA 08453; DA 16135), the Center for Substance Abuse Prevention (UR6 5907956; KD1 SP08633), the Centers for Disease Control and Prevention (R49/CCR 418569) and the US Department of Justice (2000CKWX0091), as well as a National Research Service Award from the National Institute of Drug Abuse to the second author. Correspondence about this paper can be directed to John E. Lochman.

25.7   REFERENCES

American Psychiatric Association. (1994). *The Diagnostic and Statistical Manual of Mental Disorders*, 4th edn. Washington, DC: American Psychiatric Association.

Angold, A. and Costello, E. J. (2001). The epidemiology of disorders of conduct: nosological issues and comorbidity. In J. Hill and B. Maughan (eds.), *Conduct Disorders in Childhood and Adolescence*. New York: Cambridge University Press, pp. 126–68.

Baden, A. D. and Howe, G. W. (1992). Mothers' attributions and expectancies regarding their conduct-disordered children. *Journal of Abnormal Child Psychology*, **20**, 467–85.

Barton, C., Alexander, J. F., Waldron, H., Turner, C. W. and Warburton, J. (1985). Generalizing treatment effects of Functional Family Therapy: three replications. *American Journal of Family Therapy*, **13**, 16–26.

Borduin, C. M., Mann, B. J., Cone, L. T. *et al.* (1995). Multisystemic treatment of serious juvenile offenders: long-term prevention of criminality and violence. *Journal of Consulting and Clinical Psychology*, **63**, 569–78.

Brestan, E. V. and Eyberg, S. M. (1998). Effective psychosocial treatment of conduct-disordered children and adolescents: 29 years, 82 studies, and 5,272 kids. *Journal of Clinical Child Psychology*, **27**, 180–9.

Dadds, M. R. and Powell, M. B. (1992). The relationship of interparental conflict and global marital adjustment to aggression, anxiety, and immaturity in aggressive and nonclinic children. *Journal of Abnormal Child Psychology*, **19**, 553–67.

Dishion, T. J. and Andrews, D. W. (1995). Preventing escalation in problem behavior with high-risk adolescents: immediate and 1-year outcomes. *Journal of Consulting and Clinical Psychology*, **63**, 538–48.

Dishion, T. J., McCord, J. and Poulin, F. (1999). When interventions harm: peer groups and problem behavior. *American Psychologist*, **54**, 755–64.

Dodge, K. A., Pettit, G. S., McClaskey, C. L. and Brown, M. M. (1986). Social competence in children. *Monographs of the Society for Research in Child Development*, **51**, No. 213.

Dunn, S. E., Lochman, J. E. and Colder, C. R. (1997). Social problem-solving skills in boys with conduct and oppositional disorders. *Aggressive Behavior*, **23**, 457–69.

Eddy, J. M. and Chamberlain, P. (2000). Family management and deviant peer association as mediators of the impact of treatment condition on youth antisocial behavior. *Journal of Consulting and Clinical Psychology*, **68**, 857–63.

Fisher, P. A. and Chamberlain, P. (2000). Multidimensional Treatment Foster Care: a program for intensive parenting, family support, and skill building. *Journal of Emotional and Behavioral Disorders*, **8**, 155–64.

Frick, P. J. (1998). Conduct disorders. In T. H. Ollendick and M. Hersen (eds.), *Handbook of Child Psychopathology*, 3rd edn. New York: Plenum Press, pp. 213–37.

Gordon, D. A., Graves, K. and Arbuthnot, J. (1995). The effect of functional family therapy for delinquents on adult criminal behavior. *Criminal Justice and Behavior*, **22**, 60–73.

Haapasalo, J. and Tremblay, R. (1994). Physically aggressive boys from ages 6 to 12: family background, parenting behavior, and prediction of delinquency. *Journal of Consulting and Clinical Psychology*, **62**, 1044–52.

Henggeler, S. W., Melton, G. B. and Smith, L. A. (1992). Family preservation using multisystemic therapy: an effective alternative to incarcerating serious juvenile offenders. *Journal of Consulting and Clinical Psychology*, **60**, 953–61.

Kazdin, A. E. (1998). Conduct disorder. In R. J. Morris and T. R. Kratochwill (eds.), *The Practice of Child Therapy*, 3rd edn. Boston: Allyn and Bacon, pp. 199–230.

Kazdin, A. E., Siegal, T. C. and Bass, D. (1992). Cognitive problem-solving skills training and parent management training in the treatment of antisocial behavior in children. *Journal of Consulting and Clinical Psychology*, **60**, 733–47.

Kellam, S. G., Xiange, L., Mersica, R., Brown, C. H. and Ialongo, N. (1998). The effect of the level of aggression in the first grade classroom on the course and malleability of aggressive behavior into middle school. *Development and Psychopathology*, **10**, 165–85.

Klein, N. C., Alexander, J. F. and Parsons, B. V. (1977). Impact of family systems intervention on recidivism and sibling delinquency: a model of primary prevention and program evaluation. *Journal of Consulting and Clinical Psychology*, **45**, 469–74.

Kupersmidt, J. B., Griesler, P. C., DeRosier, M. E., Patterson, C. J. and Davis, P. W. (1995). Childhood aggression and peer relations in the context of family and neighborhood factors. *Child Development*, **66**, 360–75.

Lochman, J. E. (1992). Cognitive-behavioral interventions with aggressive boys: three-year follow-up and preventive effects. *Journal of Consulting and Clinical Psychology*, **60**, 426–32.

Lochman, J. E. and Wayland, K. K. (1994). Aggression, social acceptance, and race as predictors of negative adolescent outcomes. *Journal of the American Academy of Child and Adolescent Psychiatry*, **33**, 1026–35.

Lochman, J. E. and Wells, K. C. (2002a). Contextual social-cognitive mediators and child outcome: a test of the theoretical model in the Coping Power Program. *Development and Psychopathology*, **14**, 971–93.

(2002b). The Coping Power Program at the middle school transition: universal and indicated prevention effects. *Psychology of Addictive Behaviors*, **16**, S40–54.

Lochman, J. E., Burch, P. R., Curry, J. F. and Lampon, L. B. (1984). Treatment and generalization effects of cognitive behavioural and goal setting interventions with aggressive boys. *Journal of Consulting and Clinical Psychology*, **52**, 915–16.

Lochman, J. E., Dane, H. E., Magee, T. N., Ellis, M., Pardini, D. A. and Clanton, N. R. (2001). Disruptive behavior disorders: assessment and intervention. In H. B. Vance and A. J. Pumareiega (eds.), *Clinical Assessment of Child and Adolescent Behaviour*. New York: John Wiley and Sons, Inc, pp. 231–62.

Lochman, J. E., Dunn, S. E. and Wagner, E. E. (1997). Anger. In G. Bear, K. Minke and A. Thomas (eds.), *Children's Needs II*. Washington, DC: National Association of School Psychology, pp. 149–60.

Lochman, J. E., Wayland, K. K. and White, K. K. (1993). Social goals: relationship to adolescent adjustment and to social problem solving. *Journal of Abnormal Child Psychology*, **21**, 135–51.

Loeber, R., Burke, J. D. and Lahey, B. (2002). What are adolescent antecedents to antisocial personality disorder? *Criminal Behaviour and Mental Health*, **12**, 24–36.

Matthys, W., Van de Wiel, N., Maassen, G. and Van Engeland, H. (2001). *The Effect of Manualized Parent Training and Cognitive Behavioral Therapy with Referred Conduct Disordered Children*. Paper presented at the 10th Scientific Meeting of the International Society for Research in Child and Adolescent Psychopathology, Vancouver, British Columbia, Canada.

Miller-Johnson, S., Coie, J. D., Maumary-Gremaud, A., Lochman, J. E. and Terry, R. (1999). Relationship between childhood peer rejection and aggression and adolescent delinquency severity and type among African American youth. *Journal of Emotional and Behavioral Disorders*, **7**, 137–46.

Moffitt, T. E. (1993). Adolescence-limited and life-course persistent antisocial behavior: a developmental taxonomy. *Psychology Review*, **100**, 674–701.

Myers, M. G., Stewart, D. G. and Brown, S. A. (1998). Progression from conduct disorder to antisocial personality disorder following treatment for adolescent substance abuse. *American Journal of Psychiatry*, **155**, 479–85.

Pakasiahti, L., Asplund-Peltola, R. and Keltlkangas-Jarvinen, L. (1996). Parents' social problem solving strategies in families with aggressive and nonaggressive boys. *Aggressive Behavior*, **22**, 345–56.

Pardini, D. A., Lochman, J. E. and Frick, P. J. (2003). Callous/unemotional traits and social cognitive processes in adjudicated youth. *Journal of the American Academy of Child and Adolescent Psychiatry*, **42**, 364–71.

Vitaro, F., Brendgen, M., Pagani, L., Tremblay, R. E. and McDuff, P. (1999). Disruptive behavior, peer association, and conduct disorder: testing the developmental links through early intervention. *Development and Psychopathology*, **11**, 287–304.

Weiss, B., Dodge, K. A., Bates, J. E. and Petit, G. S. (1992). Some consequences of early harsh discipline: child aggression and maladaptive social information processing style. *Child Development*, **63**, 1321–35.

26

Drug and alcohol abuse

Renuka Arjundas

Newcastle Cognitive and Behavioural Therapies Centre, Newcastle upon Tyne, UK

Eilish Gilvarry

Centre for Alcohol and Drug Studies, Newcastle upon Tyne, UK

26.1 Introduction

There has been increasing interest in the problem of adolescent substance use and abuse over the last decade. This arises from the changing patterns of use, greater recognition of the problem, the complexity and heterogeneity of these young populations, the increased risk of later comorbid problems and the associated impairments in many domains of functioning. Significant substance use/abuse is associated with increased accidents, suicide and violence, mental health and behavioural problems, academic failure and school drop-outs, juvenile delinquency, impaired driving, sexual promiscuity and family difficulties (Gilvarry, 2000). Children and adolescents present not only with drug problems but often with multiple and complex problems, both antecedent and co-occurring mental health, educational and social problems. Often, these may date from preschool years, may occur in those with developmental vulnerabilities and may be deeply entrenched. Consequently, any successful treatment service must be capable of recognizing and adequately addressing a potentially wide range of predicaments and vulnerabilities. It is, therefore, important that drug and alcohol services for adolescents are integrated into children's systems to allow for multi-component responses (Gilvarry *et al.*, 2001).

The definitions applied to adolescent substance use have been intensely debated, reflecting different cultures and beliefs, society's tolerance of drug use, the application of adult classifications and illegality. Commonly used terms such as experimentation, regular or chaotic use are used to express individual opinion but are not necessarily backed by accepted definitions. Some clinicians, concerned about the stigmatization if terms such as abuse are used for all adolescents,

Cognitive Behaviour Therapy for Children and Families, ed. Philip J. Graham.
Published by Cambridge University Press. © Cambridge University Press 2004.

regard experimentation and/or use as a normative developmental trend. Although classifications such as the *Diagnostic and Statistical Manual* (DSM-IV) (American Psychiatric Association, 1994) and the International Classification of Diseases (ICD-10) are widely accepted, their use in adolescence remains controversial, as they have been largely derived from adult clinical work. In this chapter, the authors will refer to 'use' and terms appearing in DSM-IV – i.e. abuse/dependence and substance use disorder.

The age of a young person is important in considering interventions, particularly in terms of developmental issues, abstract thinking and speech and language development. The authors refer to adolescents as those less than 18 years of age; in fact, clinical referrals are usually aged between 12 and 18 years. It is unusual for children under 10 to be referred for drug use, although, by this age, they may have already initiated tobacco use. All services should assess substance use and abuse in an age-appropriate manner.

There is evidence of improved outcome following treatment for substance use disorders in adolescent groups (Hser *et al.*, 2001). Generally, these treatments are of packages of multiple components of care in various settings. Cognitive behavioural therapy (CBT) is one of the approaches used in the treatment of addiction, although there has been little specific research in this age group. Motivation to engage with services might be required prior to commencement of this intervention. For those adolescents who live chaotic lives, lack basic care and have not engaged with services, the initial priority of treatment is one of child protection and care, with CBT part of a management care plan when engaged.

26.2   Principles of CBT in substance use disorders

The basic principles of CBT are discussed elsewhere in this book. When applying these principles to the management of substance abuse, the assumption is that substance abuse, like any behaviour, is linked with thoughts and feelings and that these associations occur through learning. These associations can then act as triggers or cues (i.e. antecedents) for substance use.

Substance abuse is seen as a maladaptive form of coping with problems in the individual's life. Enhancing the individual's adaptive coping skills reduces the need for substance use as a coping mechanism and forms the rationale for cognitive behavioural interventions. Thus, teaching coping skills is the focus of most cognitive behavioural approaches in adolescent substance use disorders.

Interventions are targeted at high-risk situations that in the past have led to substance use, at recognizing those situations and at learning alternative, more effective ways of coping with them. The strategies used are both behavioural and cognitive, although most CBT interventions in substance abuse focus more on behavioural strategies. Teaching and practise of overt adaptive behaviours are important components of cognitive behavioural interventions for substance abuse. Maladaptive cognitions or thinking patterns and beliefs associated with substance abuse are also identified and modified to enhance coping skills.

There are several cognitive behavioural models that attempt to conceptualize the process and maintenance of addiction (Marlatt and Gordon, 1985; Abrams and Niaura, 1987; Beck *et al.*, 1993). The cognitive behavioural model of alcohol or drug relapse developed by Marlatt and Gordon (1985) has been important for its profound effect on the knowledge of substance use behaviours and influential in the evolution of thinking related to concepts of substance abuse.

26.3   Rationale for CBT in adolescent substance use disorders

Among adults with substance use disorders, cognitive behavioural interventions are one of the most frequently evaluated psychosocial treatment approaches and they have strong empirical support (American Psychiatric Association, 1995). For example, CBT has been effectively used in the treatment of adults with alcohol and cocaine dependence (Project Match Research Group, 1997; National Institute on Drug Abuse, 1998). Could this evidence be extrapolated to adolescents with similar problems?

There is evidence in children and adolescents that CBT is an effective intervention in treating various psychological disorders. These include childhood and adolescent depressive disorders (Lewinsohn and Clarke, 1999), generalized anxiety disorders and phobias (Silverman *et al.*, 1999). Evidence is emerging of CBT's positive effects in post-traumatic stress disorder (March *et al.*, 1998) and obsessive compulsive disorder (March, 1995).

The CBT models and techniques employed in these childhood and adolescent disorders are adapted from those used in adults. Hence, it would seem rational that CBT, with its proven effectiveness in treating adults with substance use disorders, might suit the treatment of young people with substance use disorders as well. Indeed, the evidence is now starting to emerge to support this assumption.

Azrin *et al.* (1994), investigating the effects of behavioural interventions such as Stimulus Control Response Training, Behavioural Contracting and Imaginal Rehearsal of Drug Use Consequences in reducing drug use in adolescents and adults, showed that behavioural therapy resulted in less frequent drug use and fewer positive urine drug screens compared with supportive group intervention.

Kaminer *et al.* (1998) similarly showed significant reduction in the severity of substance use in those who underwent group CBT therapy over those in an interactional therapy group (IT) in their study of adolescents (13–18-years old) with dual diagnosis of substance use disorder and a psychiatric disorder. However, this was a pilot study with a small sample size and the urine drug screens had not shown significant differences between the two treatment groups. In their 15-month follow up of the study population, Kaminer and Burleson (1999) reported long-term gains in both treatment groups with respect to substance abuse, family function and psychiatric status, with no significant difference between the two groups.

However, there is evidence that suggests that the positive effects of individual CBT in treating adolescent substance use disorders are not maintained in the long term. Waldron *et al.* (2001), studying reduction of marijuana use in adolescents (13–17 years), compared the efficacy of 12-week individual CBT with that of family therapy, combined individual and family therapy and psycho-educational peer-group intervention of similar duration. They found that each intervention, including CBT, had demonstrable efficacy at 4 months after treatment initiation in reducing substance use. However, at 7 months' follow-up, the interventions that involved family therapy and group therapy, learnt in the social context of the adolescents, were superior to individual CBT in maintaining this effect.

Preliminary results at 6 months' follow-up of the Cannabis Youth Treatment study (Dennis *et al.*, 2000) are encouraging in their support of CBT in treating adolescents with marijuana use disorders. This was a large multicentre randomized study comparing five different treatment models in managing this group of patients. The five approaches were: (1) three sessions CBT with two sessions Motivational Enhancement Therapy (MET); (2) ten sessions CBT with two sessions MET; (3) ten sessions CBT with two sessions MET combined with family support network; (4) Adolescent Community Reinforcement Approach; and (5) multidimensional family therapy (MDFT).

It was found that all interventions involving CBT were effective in significantly reducing marijuana use in those adolescents with low severity of abuse prior to entry into the study. However, those who entered the study with a high severity of marijuana abuse fared significantly better when CBT/MET was combined with family support network rather than with CBT/MET on its own.

Even though evidence is still emerging for the efficacy of CBT in substance abuse disorders, there are features about CBT that make it particularly useful in adolescents. During their development, adolescents go through a stage where they develop separate identities from their parents or significant caregivers (developmental task of individuation; Nowinski, 1990) and value their individuality. The CBT approach that focuses on individual responsibility for behavioural change could, therefore, be attractive to clients in this age group.

CBT is a flexible and individualized treatment that can be tailored to an adolescent's needs. It can be used in a wide variety of settings, is compatible with a range of other treatments such as pharmacotherapy, is a brief intervention that is affordable and is perhaps more suited to the resources of most substance abuse services.

CBT skills can be disseminated to healthcare professionals delivering treatments for substance use disorders. Manual-driven therapies are now available that facilitate this and the application of CBT, particularly in group settings.

26.4   Assessment

The American Academy of Child and Adolescent Psychiatrists (Bukstein *et al.*, 1997) has outlined the key domains of assessment of the adolescent with substance use disorders that include the nature and pattern of drug use, the presence of abuse/dependence, comorbid mental and physical problems, educational attainment, social functioning, peer relations, family conflict and parental substance misuse. The presence of comorbidity is important in the overall assessment and preparation of a care plan. Other problems that require assessment are the ability of the child to consent to the interventions, the competence of the young person, the developmental context, parental involvement and issues of confidentiality. To assess motivation, the Stage of Change model is used (Prochaska and DiClemente, 1984) to help assess and guide the therapist in matching appropriate interventions (see Chapter 5 for further discussion of motivational issues).

There are large numbers of assessment instruments used to assess criteria for classification of substance use disorders. Some have been adapted for adolescents – e.g. the Structured Clinical Interview for the DSM (SCID; Martin *et al.*, 2000).

There is no specific valid screening instrument available to assess an adolescent for suitability for CBT. In the cognitive behavioural treatment of substance use disorders in adolescents, assessment involves a detailed analysis of the substance use behaviour with emphasis on the antecedents to substance use and the consequences of use – i.e. functional analysis. Functional analysis leads to formulation of the problems unique to the particular client on the basis of which appropriate interventions can be applied.

Antecedents to adolescent substance use are environmental and individual factors. Among the environmental factors, parental attitude and behaviour and peer-related factors such as peer substance use behaviours and attitudes are strong predictors of adolescent substance use (Kandel *et al.*, 1978). Parental role modelling, quality of communication and parent behaviour management should be assessed as family factors which may predict an adolescent's response to treatment and maintenance of any gains from treatment (Kaminer and Burkstein, 1992). Similarly, assessment of peer relationships and their influence on adolescent substance use/abuse is important for treatment planning.

More specific to CBT assessment are individual factors such as beliefs and attitudes about substance use and the adolescent's anticipation of the effects of substance use (outcome expectancies). Positive expectancy could predict future use and must be a treatment target. For example, adolescent problem drinkers when compared with those who were not problem drinkers expected that alcohol would improve their cognitive and motor functioning (Kaminer and Burkstein, 1992). The Alcohol Expectancy Questionnaire (Brown *et al.*, 1987), a self-report instrument, measures the adolescents' expectancies, positive and negative, about alcohol consumption. A comparison of pretreatment and post-treatment scores would indicate if CBT was effective in changing the cognitions around substance use.

It is important to assess the current frequency of intoxication episodes, previous periods of abstinence and the coping skills and resources the adolescent used during these periods. If the client is frequently intoxicated, he/she will not be able to engage with CBT and will be, therefore, not suitable for CBT.

The therapist must be aware of potential problems that could exist in this group of clients such as a lower ability for abstract thinking, cognitive deficits and subtle language and speech problems. In such clients, the therapy could be tailored to the specific needs of the clients. Cognitive behavioural assessment is comprehensive and continues into treatment.

26.5 Cognitive behavioural interventions

26.5.1 Theoretical model

Marlatt's Cognitive Behavioural Relapse Prevention Model (Marlatt and Gordon, 1985) focuses clinical attention on the identification of high-risk situations or antecedents to substance use and on interventions that help patients to avoid or cope with these situations, thus interrupting the relapse process. This model is shown in Figure 26.1.

In this model, high-risk situations are thought to be precipitants of relapse. Three broad classes of high-risk situations are identified as precursors to relapse (Marlatt and Gordon, 1980):

(1) negative emotional states (e.g. anxiety, anger, depression and boredom);
(2) conflicts in interpersonal relationships; and
(3) social pressure (e.g. societal pressure to engage in the proscribed behaviour).

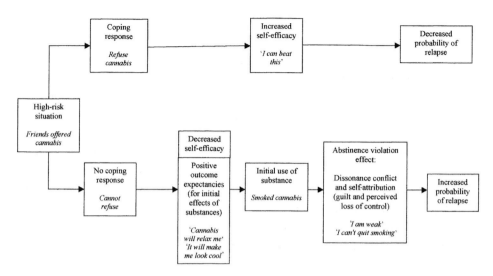

Figure 26.1   Cognitive behavioural model of the relapse process (Marlatt and Gordon, 1985).

The model further postulates that high-risk situations will act as precipitants of relapse only if the individuals lack an adaptive response for coping with that situation. These individuals are then thought to experience decreased confidence in their ability to cope with an impending high-risk situation (i.e. decreased self-efficacy; Bandura, 1977).

Outcome expectancy or individuals' anticipation of the effects of engaging in substance use is another important component of the model. Positive outcome expectations of using a substance (e.g. 'using will help me relax') are expected to interact with lowered self-efficacy to increase the chance of using the substance. The processes leading to discrete episodes of substance use following abstinence or lapse are illustrated with a case example below.

26.5.1.1   Case example

Seventeen-year-old Michael was referred for management of cannabis abuse. He had been smoking cannabis from the age of 14 with a group of friends. As a result of excessive cannabis use, he had been attending school irregularly and was unable to sit for his exams. He left school at the age of 15 and suffered from a brief psychotic episode 6 months before his referral. He recovered from his psychotic episode with pharmacological treatment and was advised to abstain from cannabis. Michael had been quite shocked by his psychotic episode and feared a recurrence. He had briefly abstained, but, despite his best attempts at abstinence, he lapsed frequently.

On assessment, it was found that common high-risk situations for Michael were peer pressure and boredom. Michael's group of friends smoked cannabis and since Michael spent a lot of time with them he found it difficult to refuse. He feared he would lose his only friends if he did not smoke with them. Michael did not know how to cope with the situation other than smoking cannabis (no adaptive coping response). He lacked confidence in his ability to deal with the situation (low self-efficacy) and also believed that smoking cannabis made him look 'cool' (positive outcome expectancy). This perpetuated his use of cannabis, which served to decrease his self-efficacy further.

The progress from lapse to further continued use to pre-abstinent levels – that is, relapse – is dependent on what the individuals attribute the cause of the lapse to and how they cope with the resultant affective and cognitive responses. A lapse is expected to be more likely to lead to a relapse if the individual attributes the lapse to an internal (supposedly stable) cause such as a personal weakness or failure and experiences negative affective states such as guilt. Marlatt and Gordon (1985) called the above cognitive affective components the 'abstinence violation effect'. Helping individuals to reattribute the cause for lapse to external, changeable factors can reduce this effect.

When Michael lapsed during his attempts at abstinence, he thought, 'I will never be able to stop smoking cannabis because I am weak'. As a result, he felt guilty and distressed and this led to more cannabis abuse which resulted in further erosion of his confidence in his ability to abstain. He therefore relapsed to using cannabis at pre-abstinent levels.

Marlatt's model for relapse prevention is usually targeted at individuals who have voluntarily ceased the use of substances and made a commitment to abstinence. Its principles can be applied to individuals yet to abstain from substance use but seeking help to do so, in the absence of more specific and comprehensive empirically validated treatment models.

26.5.2   Interventions

The aim of most cognitive behavioural interventions used in substance use disorder is abstinence. However, it may not be possible to achieve abstinence in all clients and reduced use and harm limitation should be considered as the goal in these clients. In the authors' experience, the goals of therapy are negotiated with the client and may change during the course of therapy. For example, clients who started therapy with a goal of achieving reduced use may go on to become abstinent and those whose initial aim was abstinence may change their goal during therapy to reduced use.

The initial treatment sessions focus on helping adolescents understand why they use substances. This can be done by involving the client in a functional analysis of his or her own use. The rationale behind the analysis is to help clients understand that substance abuse is a function of antecedents and consequences. To illustrate the concept, an example from the client's experiences, such as a recent episode of substance use, is used.

Table 26.1 Example of Michael's worksheet

Trigger/ situation	Thoughts	Feelings	Behaviour	Positive results	Negative results
In what situations am I more likely to use cannabis?	What was I telling myself at that time? What was going through my mind?	What was I feeling then?	What did I do?	What good things happened?	What bad things happened?
When I am with friends	*If I smoke 'pot', my friends will think I am cool*				
When I have nothing else to do	*'Pot' will help me pass time*	*Feeling bored*	*Smoked 'pot' with friends*	*Getting 'high' Feel like being part of the gang*	*Felt guilty about smoking 'pot' again Worried the psychosis will come back*

Adapted from Sampl and Kadden, 2001.

The client is helped to identify various events, thoughts and feelings that were associated with that episode. Analysis of the function of each of these identified components using the process of guided discovery enables the individual to understand what motivates their substance abuse. Further analysis helps them derive the positive and negative consequences of substance use. The client can record these on a worksheet, initially with help from the therapist before doing this independently as a means of self-monitoring. This is akin to the thought record diaries that are used during cognitive therapy of other psychological problems. An example of this is laid out in Table 26.1.

It is also important to ask the client to record situations where he/she had managed to avoid using the substance despite urges and cravings. This would help in determining the skills and strengths he/she already possesses. In CBT of substance use disorders, there are some critical tasks that are essential for effective treatment (Rounsaville and Carroll, 1992). These are:

(1) enhancing motivation for abstinence;
(2) developing coping skills;
(3) enhancing social support;
(4) increasing drug-free pleasant activities;
(5) managing negative affective states and cravings; and
(6) maintenance of abstinence or relapse prevention.

26.5.2.1   Enhancing motivation for abstinence

Marlatt proposed a technique called decisional balance exercise to help clients build their motivation to maintain changes in their behaviour (Marlatt and Gordon, 1985). This is an analysis of the negative and positive consequences of substance use. During therapy sessions, the client is guided through a decision-making process. It is important for the client to do the analysis and come to conclusions him/herself. At the end of the process, the client, coming to the conclusion that the negative consequences far outweigh the positive consequences, could be motivated to abstain.

This technique has some similarities to MET. MET (Miller and Rollnick, 1992) is an approach based on the premise that clients can achieve change in their substance abuse if motivation is internally generated rather than generated from external sources. MET and CBT can be complementary to each other, particularly in clients with low motivation and poor coping skills.

26.5.2.2   Developing coping skills

Once high-risk situations or triggers are identified, the client is guided to develop self-management and interpersonal skills to cope with them adaptively.

Development of refusal skills is an important part of coping skills training. Since clients tend to socialize with substance users and avoid friends who do not use substances, their social circle tends to narrow as substance use increases. The ideal for the client would be to avoid people who put them at high risk of using substances. However, this is not always possible; hence, learning to refuse when pressured to use substances is essential.

Techniques such as modelling by the therapist and role play may be used in therapy sessions to demonstrate how to refuse substance use. Real-life practice exercises that are repeated will help the client to generalize the skill to various situations. The practise of these techniques in a group therapy setting may offer advantages over individual therapy, as it involves behavioural change strategies in the usual social context of the adolescent. Active participation by the clients is essential, placing responsibility on them to use the new skills. This gives them a sense of self-control.

26.5.2.3   Enhancing social support

Increasing social support can help the client to abstain or reduce substance use. It also may increase the client's confidence in his or her ability to cope. This rationale is discussed with the client.

The therapist can help by guiding the client to identify existing social supports, and potential sources of support, including family, friends or acquaintances.

Substance use in young people may impair the development of effective social skills. This may need addressing by means of social skills training which involves improving interpersonal communication and coping with problematic social situations.

Adolescents can use substances to facilitate social interaction. Anxiety in social situations can act as an antecedent to substance use. Adolescents with social anxiety may need therapy to improve social functioning.

26.5.2.4   Increasing pleasant drug-free activities

Adolescents with substance use disorders tend to narrow their range of activities, limiting themselves to substance use and missing out on activities normally engaged in by adolescents. They also tend to hold beliefs that they can only have pleasure under the influence of substances.

Increasing pleasant drug-free activities could serve to help clients cope with common triggers for substance use such as boredom and challenge their beliefs that they can have 'fun' only under the influence of substances. One way of achieving this is the use of behavioural assignments. This could consist of collaboratively making a list of activities other than substance use that the client may consider to be fun. The client then engages in these activities without substance use and evaluates pleasure he / she derives from these activities. Activity scheduling, a technique used in the treatment of depression, can be used to increase drug-free pleasurable activities.

26.5.2.4.1   Example
Peer influence and lack of recreational activities and the resulting boredom appeared to maintain Michael's substance use problem. Its continuance was further influenced by his belief that his friends would accept him only if he shared their practice.

Reducing peer influence-related drug use was an important component of Michael's treatment. This involved teaching him refusal skills that he could use to refuse cannabis when this was offered. However, it was important to begin by enhancing Michael's social support and evaluating how realistic his assumptions were about his friends not accepting him should he refuse to smoke with them.

Without these interventions, teaching Michael refusal skills alone would not be effective in facilitating abstinence.

Establishing support from others who did not use drugs could enable Michael to spend more time away from his cannabis-smoking friends and risk potentially losing them. Towards this end, potential sources of support were identified such as his family – i.e his mother and older brother and old friends. However, there were difficulties in his relationship with his family that needed addressing. His mother found it difficult to deal with his substance use and criticized him often. His brother did not approve of it and kept away from him. Michael thought his immediate family did not understand or care for him.

During therapy, Michael's belief about his family was evaluated and modified. Socratic questioning was used to explore evidence and counter evidence for his belief. This led Michael to modify his belief that his mother and brother did not understand or care for him to a belief where his mother and brother did care for him but did not understand his drug use and found dealing with it difficult. Michael's mother and brother were involved in therapy at this stage with the aim of improving communication between them and Michael. This was done by educating them about the nature of Michael's substance use and ways to deal with it. Their involvement supported Michael's modified belief that they cared for him.

Avenues of other support such as Michael's old friends were considered. Michael had lost contact with them since he began to spend more time with his cannabis-smoking friends. He was encouraged to make links with them again after exploring the advantages and disadvantages of doing so. The advantages generated by Michael were that he could engage in drug-free activities with his old friends and he could spend less time with his substance-using friends, thus reducing the risks of using cannabis and increasing his ability to refuse it. This led to him re-establishing contact with a friend who did not use drugs. Michael began to go bowling with this friend, which he enjoyed. He gradually engaged in more drug-free activities and spent less time with friends who used substances.

The validity of his assumption that his drug-using friends would not accept him if he quit cannabis was explored. Evidence from the past such as his friends laughing at him when he tried to abstain strongly reinforced this belief. Michael also admitted that he did enjoy smoking cannabis with them. Hence, he found it difficult to refuse. An advantage–disadvantage analysis of both continuing smoking cannabis and quitting led to Michael recognizing that the long-term negative consequences of cannabis use outweighed the positive.

As Michael began to spend more time away from his cannabis-using friends, he was willing to consider refusing cannabis when he was with them and to cope with the consequences. He did manage to refuse on more occasions than he had done before therapy. He gradually reduced his cannabis use.

26.5.2.5 Management of negative affective states, urges or craving

Substances can act as powerful mood regulators. Adolescents may use them to modify negative affective states such as depression and anxiety. Thus, these negative states can act as triggers or high-risk situations for substance use. Hence, their management is essential to prevent relapse. Furthermore, these moods can be the direct effects of drugs. The management of negative affective states in people with substance use disorders by cognitive techniques is similar to those used in emotional disorders such as depression and is described elsewhere (see Chapter 16).

The management of craving is another important component of treatment. Individuals with problematic substance use commonly experience cravings or urges. Craving increases during withdrawals from substances, especially during the early phase of abstinence, although it can occur several months after abstinence. It is important to educate clients about the nature of craving: that it is common after abstinence and not a sign of weakness. Using their own experiences, they can be helped to become aware of the manifestations of craving, both physical and psychological. Helping them to recognize the triggers of craving will enable them to deal with it.

Since craving is often associated with memories and thoughts about positive effects of substance use, such as being high (positive outcome expectancy), cognitive techniques can play a role by the application of the decisional balance exercise discussed earlier. Recognizing that the positive outcomes of substance are transient and followed by negative outcomes that are more enduring can help in reducing craving and change behaviour. Clients can carry reminder sheets listing positive and negative consequences of substance use that they can refer to when experiencing craving.

However, in the initial stages of therapy, clients may need to use behavioural strategies to deal with craving, including the avoidance of situations that lead to craving, distraction, talking to a supportive person and self-reminding that craving is normal and will pass away.

26.5.2.6   Relapse prevention

Interventions based on Marlatt's cognitive behavioural model of relapse prevention described earlier fall into two categories:

(1)   intervention before a lapse (i.e. prevention of a lapse) – aimed at increasing coping skills to prevent a lapse; and

(2)   intervention after a lapse (i.e. prevention of progression into full-blown relapse). Once a lapse has occurred, interventions are used with the intention of altering the individual's maladaptive attributions and attitudes about their lapse.

Marlatt and Gordon (1985), drawing on techniques developed to modify cognitive errors and maladaptive assumptions associated with depression by Beck *et al.* (1979), formulated general strategies to counter faulty assumptions and cognitive errors associated with initial lapse.

These strategies help clients to see their lapse as a mistake rather than a failure and that their lapse was a unique event that could be attributed to factors other than their weakness. Common cognitive distortions associated with lapse such as black or white thinking, catastrophizing and overgeneralization are modified. Lapses are reframed as valuable opportunities for correction rather than as failures.

26.5.2.6.1 Example

As mentioned earlier, Michael tended to attribute his lapses after a period of abstinence to his inability to quit and personal weakness. He also tended to catastrophize lapses, for example, by saying to himself: 'I will never be able to stop smoking cannabis and end up a junkie'. These attributions and cognitive distortions were explored and guided discovery led Michael to reframe lapse as an opportunity to learn from rather than a failure. Increasing his skills to replace cannabis use with other activities helped him recognize that he did have control over his substance use and a lapse did not necessarily mean he would use forever.

Other components of CBT of substance use in adolescents include problem-solving, assertiveness training, improving communication skills and anger management. The decision to use particular interventions with an individual client depends on the formulation of their problems and the goals negotiated. CBT can be a useful treatment approach in adolescents with dual diagnoses (substance use disorder with mental health problems) as there is evidence for its effectiveness in various psychological disorders.

26.6 Practical considerations for cognitive behavioural interventions in adolescent substance use disorders

26.6.1 Developmental factors unique to adolescence

The cognitive behavioural interventions used in adolescents are often similar to those used in adults. However, they may not always be appropriate to the developmental needs of adolescents.

Developmental factors pertinent to adolescence are important in influencing substance use in this group (Botvin and Botvin, 1992). Increasing influence of the peer group, and the adolescent's need to belong to a group, resulting in increased conformity behaviour and dependency on peers, can make them vulnerable to peer-influenced substance use. Therefore, these factors should be considered in the formulation of their problems followed by appropriate interventions to target them.

Factors related to cognitive development can influence substance use behaviour (Wagner and Kassel, 1995). As adolescents acquire formal operations, they become aware of grey areas and contradictions in the actions of adults, actions that they had not previously questioned. These changes can make them question some of the knowledge, such as the negative effects of substance use, they may have acquired from adults. This may affect their motivation to reduce or stop substance use. Hence, the therapist should be aware of this and the techniques of MET could be used to enhance motivation.

The ability of abstract thinking, subtle language and speech problems, short-term memory and other developmental aspects are crucial to consider when using CBT in this group. Young people may not have sophisticated language development, are inclined to exaggerate and may over-report drug and alcohol use. Hence, it is essential that the therapist use language that can be under-stood by the adolescent and be specific and concrete. Developing a common vocabulary helps both to understand what the adolescent means and strengthen collaboration.

It is important that effort is made during therapy to clarify what the adolescents mean when they say something and not just to assume meaning. For example, if the adolescent says he drank large amounts of alcohol the previous day, it should be clarified exactly how much, what, where and how he consumed it.

26.6.2 Developing a collaborative relationship in therapy

Collaboration is central to CBT and requires the therapist and the patient to work together to deal with a problem. This is important in all age groups but particularly so when treating young people.

Adolescents who are referred for treatment of substance abuse are quite often brought to therapy by concerned parents or carers, sometimes against their wishes. Also, adolescents tend to view themselves as lower in hierarchical status than the therapist. They expect to be told by the therapist what is right for them and what they should do just as other adults in their life have done. This can make collaboration difficult. Those with comorbidity, such as attention deficit hyperactivity disorder and conduct disorder, may find it difficult to collaborate.

It is essential that the therapist makes an effort to create an atmosphere of cooperation and conveys that he/she is willing to work with the adolescent to understand and find ways to tackle the substance abuse. The therapist should be careful not to adopt a patronizing attitude. It is quite easy to be patronizing and adopt a preaching attitude when treating young people with substance abuse. It is important that the therapist consciously and actively avoids this attitude.

Listening empathetically, summarizing and reflecting on what the patient has said, eliciting feedback from the patient regarding content of therapy regularly, allowing the patient to make choices, etc. can facilitate a collaborative atmo-sphere. The techniques used in MET can be used to help the therapist engage the young person. It is also crucial that the therapist is attuned to working with young people, understands the developmental context and uses appropriate techniques to engage the client.

26.6.3 Homework assignments

Acquisition of skills required for change entails active participation by the client and compliance with treatment-related assignments. In CBT, compliance with treatment in and out of sessions (homework) is assumed to be central to therapeutic change.

Adolescents tend to equate homework with schoolwork and tend not to like doing it. There are several reasons for not complying with homework: they may not have enough time, they are attending multiple other appointments, circumstances such as chaotic lifestyle are not conducive to completing assignments, there is a lack of understanding of the rationale for the tasks, too much is given to do or they simply find the assignments boring. They may have learning difficulties with literacy skills problems, little support at home and have been disaffected from the education system for some years.

It is essential when setting homework tasks with adolescents that a number of steps are taken to foster compliance. It should be relevant to the adolescent's problems and fit into their lifestyle. It should be developed collaboratively with the adolescent and the rationale explained clearly. Wherever possible, the task should be practised within sessions first so that the adolescent is clear about what to do. Exploration of difficulties that can affect compliance and ways to overcome these might facilitate compliance.

The adolescent can be offered various choices or alternative ways of completing a homework assignment. For example, record keeping of environmental events, thoughts and feelings associated with substance use can be done in the usual adult way (daily thought record). Alternatively, some adolescents prefer to record this in a narrative fashion from which the therapist can identify the different components. Some adolescents do not like to write or have difficulties with literacy skills and so may prefer to dictate it onto a tape recorder. Some adolescents like to create their own format using a computer. Using the adolescent's creativity to design the assignments can facilitate compliance. Prizes for completion of assignments may be given to aid compliance.

The authors' clinical experience suggests that adolescents appreciate more visual aids and materials, and are more likely to engage if these aids are more personalized. Flip charts or white boards can be used in sessions to illustrate concepts.

26.6.4 Identification of different emotional states, cognitions and establishing the link between them

Identification of different emotional states experienced by a client is an important component of CBT. In order to learn to manage and change emotions, adolescents must be able to distinguish between them. Adolescents can experience difficulties in this and some may not be able to give a name to what they feel. For example, they may say they feel 'good' or 'bad' and not specify exactly what they feel.

The therapist may need to provide education about different moods or emotions by listing different moods a person can experience. The adolescent can then be asked to identify various moods he/she experiences in a day. Vignettes can be used to help the adolescent identify different emotional states. Education about common physical sensations or bodily changes associated with some emotions can help in the identification of emotions – e.g. breathlessness and palpitations associated with anxiety and panic, heaviness and tiredness with depression.

Recognition of emotions is also important in facilitating the access of key cognitions. Adolescents may have difficulties in accessing cognitions and monitoring them. They may believe that situations lead to feelings/emotions. They may need to be given vignettes to illustrate that it is the interpretation of a situation (i.e. thoughts) that influences their emotions and not the situation itself.

Once they are able to recognize that thoughts can influence feelings, they can then use feelings as a window to their cognitions. Practising the identification and monitoring of thoughts in therapy sessions using their own experiences will help adolescents monitor their thought processes outside sessions.

The above techniques are similar to those used in adults. However, for adolescents, the vignettes used must interest them and be appropriate for their age. Using examples from popular films or television programmes to illustrate concepts can be useful.

26.7 Conclusions and recommendations

There is an increasing interest in and evidence base for the application of CBT in addictions in general and now in adolescents with substance use disorders. CBT in substance use disorders has largely drawn from Marlatt's model, which is essentially a relapse prevention model. The interventions used in adolescent substance use disorder are adapted from those used in adults and comprise diverse behavioural and cognitive techniques rather than formulation-driven treatment.

The emphasis of most interventions is behavioural and the cognitive component is limited. This reflects the dearth of specific empirically validated CBT models for substance use disorders. There is a need to develop theoretical models that can be empirically tested on the basis of which possibly more effective interventions can be applied to substance abuse in this age group.

Further research is also needed to evaluate the efficacy of existing cognitive behavioural interventions to establish the evidence for them more firmly. These can then be applied to clinical practice. Manual-driven therapies can aid delivery and dissemination of effective interventions that can be evaluated. Individualizing manual-based approaches by selecting interventions that are personally relevant to the client and adapting them may be a practical and effective solution in clinical practice.

However, one must be aware of the complexities and comorbidity that often presents in these adolescents, and thus CBT is but one part of an overall care plan. The issue for treatment units is the need for comprehensiveness, treating not just the drug abuse/dependence but also ensuring that developmental needs are met. This requires a multi-component approach to the multiple issues.

26.8   REFERENCES

Abrams, D. B. and Niaura, R. S. (1987). Social learning theory. In H. T. Blane and K. E. Leonard (eds.), *Psychological Theories of Drinking and Alcoholism*. New York: Guilford Press, pp. 131–78.

American Psychiatric Association (1994). *Diagnostic and Statistical Manual of Mental Disorders*, 4th edn. Washington DC: American Psychiatric Association.

American Psychiatric Association Work Group on Substance Use Disorders (1995). Practice guidelines for the treatment of patients with substance use disorders: alcohol, cocaine, opioids. *American Journal of Psychiatry*, **152** (suppl), 2–59.

Azrin, N. H., McMahon, P. T., Donohue, B. *et al.* (1994). Behaviour therapy for drug abuse: a controlled treatment outcome study. *Behaviour Research and Therapy*, **32**, 857–66.

Bandura, A. (1977). Self-efficacy: towards a unifying theory of behaviour change. *Psychological Review*, **84**, 191–215.

Beck, A. T., Rush, A. J., Shaw, B. F and Emery, G. (1979). *Cognitive Therapy of Depression*. New York: Guilford Press.

Beck, A. T., Wright, F. D., Newman, C. F. and Liese, B. S (1993). *Cognitive Therapy of Substance Abuse*. New York: Guilford Press.

Botvin, G. J. and Botvin, E. M. (1992). Adolescent tobacco, alcohol and drug use: prevention strategies, empirical findings and assessment issues. *Developmental and Behavioural Paediatrics*, **13**, 290–301.

Brown, S. A., Christiansen, B. A. and Goldman, M. S. (1987). The alcohol expectancy questionnaire. An instrument for the assessment of adolescent and adult alcohol expectancies. *Journal of Studies on Alcohol*, **48**, 483–91.

Bukstein, O and the Work Group on Quality Issues (1997). Practice parameters for the assessment and treatment of children and adolescents with substance use disorders. *Journal of the American Academy of Child and Adolescent Psychiatry*, **36** (suppl), 140s–56s.

Dennis, M. L., Babor, T. F., Diamond, G. *et al.* (2000). *The Cannabis Youth Treatment (CYT) Experiment: Preliminary Findings*. Rockville, MD: Substance Abuse and Mental Health Services and Administration, Centre for Substance Abuse Treatment.

Gilvarry, E. (2000). Substance abuse in young people. *Journal of Child Psychology and Psychiatry*, **41**, 55–80.

Gilvarry, E., Christian, J., Crome, I., Johnson, P., McArdle and McCarthy, S. (2001). *The Substance of Young Needs: Review*. Home Office, London: Health Advisory Service. Available at http://www.dpas.gov.uk.

Hser, Y. I., Grella, C. E., Hubbard, R. L. *et al.* (2001). An evaluation of drug treatments for adolescents in four US cities. *Archives of General Psychiatry*, **58**, 689–95.

Kaminer, Y. and Burkstein, O. G. (1992). Inpatient behavioural and cognitive therapy for substance abuse in adolescents. In V. B. Van Hasselt and D. J. Kolko (eds.), *Inpatient Behaviour Therapy for Children and Adolescents*. New York: Plenum Press.

Kaminer, Y. and Burleson, J. (1999). Psychotherapies for adolescent substance abusers: 15 month follow-up of a pilot study. *American Journal of Addiction*, **8**, 114–19.

Kaminer, Y., Burleson, J., Blitz, C., Sussman, J. and Rounsaville, B. J. (1998). Psychotherapies for adolescent substance abusers: a pilot study. *Journal of Nervous and Mental Disease*, **186**, 684–90.

Kandel, D. B., Kessler, R. C. and Margulies, R. Z. (1978). Antecedents of adolescent initiation into stages of drug use. A developmental analysis. In D. B. Kandel (ed.), *Longitudinal Research on Drug Use: Empirical Findings and Methodological Issues*. Washington, DC: Hemisphere- Wiley.

Lewinsohn, P. M. and Clarke, G. N. (1999). Psychosocial treatments for adolescent depression. *Clinical Psychology Review*, **19**, 329–42.

March, J. S. (1995). Cognitive behavioural psychotherapy for children and adolescents with OCD: a review and recommendations for treatment. *Journal of the American Academy of Child and Adolescent Psychiatry*, **34**, 7–17.

March, J. S., Amaya-Jackson, L., Murray, M. C. and Schulte, A. (1998). Cognitive behavioural psychotherapy for children and adolescents with posttraumatic stress disorder after a single incident stressor. *Journal of the American Academy of Child and Adolescent Psychiatry*, **37**, 585–93.

Marlatt, G. A. and Gordon, J. R. (1980). Determinants of relapse: implications for the maintenance of behaviour change. In P. O. Davidson and S. M. Davidson (eds.), *Behavioural Medicine: Changing Health Life Styles*. New York: Pergamon, pp. 410–52.

(1985). *Relapse Prevention: Maintenance Strategies in the Treatment of Addictive Behaviours*. New York: Guilford Press.

Martin, C. S., Pollock, N. K., Bukstein, O. G. and Lynch, K. (2000). Interrater reliability of the SCID alcohol and substance use disorders sections among adolescents. *Drug and Alcohol Dependence*, **59**, 173–6.

Miller, W. R. and Rollnick, S. (1992). *Motivational Interviewing: Preparing People to Change Addictive Behaviour*. New York: Guilford Press.

National Institute on Drug Abuse (1998). *A Cognitive-Behavioural Approach: Treating Cocaine Addiction*. Rockville, MD: National Institutes of Health.

Nowinski, J. (1990). *Substance Abuse in Adolescents and Young Adults: A Guide to Treatment*. New York: W. W. Norton.

Prochaska, J. and DiClemente, C. (1984). *The Transtheoretical Approach: Crossing Traditional Boundaries of Therapy*. Homewood, IL: Dow Jones/Irwin.

Project Match Research Group. (1997). Matching alcoholism treatment to client heterogeneity: Project Match post treatment drinking outcomes. *Journal of Studies on Alcohol*, **58**, 7–29.

Rounsaville, B. J. and Carroll, K. M. (1992). Individual psychotherapy for drug users. In J. H. Lowinsohn, P. Ruiz and R. B. Millman (eds.), *Comprehensive Textbook of Substance Abuse*, 2nd edn. New York: Williams and Wilkins, pp. 496–508.

Sampl, S. and Kadden, R. (2001). *Motivational Enhancement Therapy and Cognitive Behavioural Therapy for Adolescent Cannabis Users: Five sessions. CYT Cannabis Youth Treatment Series, Volume 1*. Rockville MD: Centre for Substance Abuse Treatment, Substance Abuse and Mental Health Services Adminstration.

Silverman, W. K., Kurtines, W. M., Ginsburg, G. S., Weems, C. F., Lumpkin, P. W. and Carmichael, D. H. (1999). Treating anxiety disorders in children with group cognitive behavioural therapy: a randomised clinical trial. *Journal of Consulting and Clinical Psychology*, **67**, 995–1003.

Wagner, E. F. and Kassel, J. D. (1995). Substance use and abuse. In R. T. Ammerman and M. Hersen (eds.), *Handbook of Child Behaviour Therapy in the Psychiatric Setting*. New York: John Wiley and Sons, pp. 367–88.

Waldron, H. B., Slesnick, N., Brody, J. L., Turner, C. W. and Peterson, T. R. (2001). Treatment outcomes for adolescent substance abuse at 4- and 7-month assessments. *Journal of Consulting and Clinical Psychology*, **69**, 802–13.

Part VI

CBT applications in preventive interventions

27

The prevention of conduct problems

Robert J. McMahon and Dana M. Rhule

University of Washington, Seattle, Washington, USA

Conduct problems in children constitute a broad spectrum of 'acting-out' behaviours, ranging from relatively minor oppositional behaviours such as yelling and temper tantrums to more serious forms of antisocial behaviour such as aggression, physical destructiveness and stealing. These behaviours typically co-occur as a complex or syndrome, and there is strong evidence to suggest that oppositional behaviours (e.g. non-compliance) are developmental precursors to more serious antisocial behaviour. In this chapter, the term 'conduct problems' (CP) is used to refer to this constellation of behaviours. The authors' conceptualization of CP is consistent with, but not isomorphic with, the *Diagnostic and Statistical Manual of Mental Disorders-IV* (American Psychiatric Association, 2000) diagnostic categories of oppositional defiant disorder and conduct disorder.

27.1 The early starter developmental pathway for serious CP

The prevention of CP has received increasing interest and attention over the past 10 years. This has been partly due to advances made in the delineation of developmental pathways of CP and the risk and protective factors associated with progression on this pathway. Identification of such pathways and associated risk and protective factors can provide guidance for interventions with developmental precursors (e.g. oppositional behaviour) that may be more amenable to change.

The pathway with the most negative long-term prognosis, and which is the most salient for prevention, has been referred to as the 'early starter' (Patterson *et al.*, 1991) or 'life-course persistent' (Moffitt, 1993) pathway. As described in previous chapters (Chapters 13 and 25), the early starter pathway is characterized by the onset of CP in the preschool and early school-age years, by increasing severity and diversity of CP behaviours and by a high degree of continuity

Cognitive Behaviour Therapy for Children and Families, ed. Philip J. Graham.
Published by Cambridge University Press. © Cambridge University Press 2004.

throughout childhood and into adolescence and adulthood. Furthermore, there is an expansion of the settings in which the CP behaviours occur over time, from the home to other settings such as the school and the broader community. The risk for continuing on this pathway may be as high as 50% or greater (e.g. Campbell, 2002) for children between the ages of 5 and 8 years who are displaying CP behaviours. Therefore, many of the children who are at risk can be identified early in the developmental progression.

What are the implications of this developmental model for intervention (Conduct Problems Prevention Research Group (CPPRG), 1992)? First, interventions should address multiple skill domains of the child (e.g. emotional/behavioural regulation, adaptive interpersonal relationships and academic achievement). Secondly, this necessitates a focus on multiple socialization support systems such as the family, peer group and the school. Thirdly, given the chronic nature of serious CP, interventions may need to be sustained and the intervention components should be well integrated. Finally, the intervention should be developmentally and culturally informed. By this, it is meant that the focus, content and structure of the intervention should be developmentally sensitive, and that, ideally, the intervention should permit options for individualized tailoring of content and intensity.

27.2   Treatment versus prevention of CP

Increased interest in prevention has also evolved from the successes and limitations of the treatment-focused interventions described in earlier sections of this volume (see Chapters 13 and 25). With a few exceptions (such as parent training with young children with CP), the effects of single-component treatments have demonstrated limited generalizability, especially over time. Nonetheless, it has been argued that well-designed treatment research with single-intervention components lays the foundation for the selection of components in multi-component preventive interventions (Dodge, 1993).

Proponents of a preventive approach argue that there will never be adequate numbers of mental health professionals to treat the large number of individuals with a disorder, that effective prevention is cost-effective compared with treatment and that preventing the human suffering and loss of productivity caused by mental disorder is an important goal in its own right (Coie *et al.*, 2000). The field of prevention science has developed in response to the need to develop evidence-based preventive interventions, and has spawned a heuristic model to guide research in this area. The preventive intervention research cycle (Mrazek and Haggerty, 1994) describes a: '. . . recursive process in which new learning emerges from clinical trials, field trials, and community implementations, and this new learning in turn influences the direction of the more 'basic' science steps in the model' (Coie *et al.*, 2000, p. 96) – steps which focus on the identification of risk and protective factors central to the development and maintenance of the disorder.

There are three categories of preventive interventions: universal, selected and indicated (Mrazek and Haggerty, 1994). A universal intervention is administered to an entire population (e.g. a school or neighbourhood), whereas selected and indicated interventions are targeted to individuals who are at risk, either because of environmental risk factors (e.g. poverty) or individual risk factors (e.g. low levels of CP), respectively. Some preventive interventions include both universal and targeted components.

To a certain extent, the distinction between treatment and prevention of CP is often difficult to make, since preventive interventions have usually (although not always) targeted younger children who are already engaging in some type of CP behaviour (i.e. an indicated intervention) (Coie and Dodge, 1998). One distinction is that treatment involves referral for assistance, whereas participation in prevention is usually done by screening. This is a somewhat tenuous distinction. For example, a number of family-based interventions that were developed as treatments for CP have been identified as model family programmes for delinquency prevention (Alvarado *et al.*, 2000).

In this chapter, the authors have organized the presentation of preventive interventions by the developmental period at which the programme is implemented: infancy/preschool, early elementary school age and late elementary/early middle-school age. Space considerations preclude a detailed description of the many programmes that have been developed or that are in progress for the prevention of CP. (For reviews, see Yoshikawa, 1994; LeMarquand *et al.*, 2001; Webster-Stratton and Taylor, 2001.) The focus is primarily on programmes that include cognitive and behavioural components, and which have been empirically validated. Those programmes (usually school based) designed to prevent the onset of substance use in youth are not discussed.

27.3   Identification and screening

One of the first steps in prevention research involves identifying and selecting intended participants. The nature of this process depends on whether the intervention will be universally implemented or, instead, targeted at specific populations. In general, less expensive interventions with a lower potential of unintended negative side effects have a greater potential to be implemented universally. However, as the costs and risks increase, targeted interventions are often employed to direct services towards those most at risk. In universal prevention, the primary decision to be made concerns the particular geographical location, neighbourhood or school(s) that will receive the intervention. Demographic and school information (average income, percentage with reduced lunches, test scores, etc.) and crime statistics are often employed to select schools and/or neighbourhoods with higher levels of risk and fewer resources that may benefit more from services.

Targeted interventions offer several advantages, including a greater coverage of at-risk children, in comparison with clinical interventions, and a more efficient allocation of resources, in comparison with universal interventions. However, the success of targeted interventions depends on the ability to identify high-risk children accurately (Bennett et al., 1998). The first step in implementation involves establishing marker variables and developing a screening method that will identify high-risk children. The presence of early externalizing behaviours has been widely used for screening purposes and is considered by many to be the single best predictor of risk for future CP (Loeber, 1990; Yoshikawa, 1994). It has been suggested that high-risk children can be identified as early as elementary school (e.g. CPPRG, 1992). Thus, kindergarten and/or first grade may be optimal times for early screening, given that school entry marks a stressful period in development and provides the first opportunity for high-risk children to be evaluated in comparison with most of their same-age peers (Lochman and CPPRG, 1995; L. G. Hill et al., unpublished data).

Until more recently, most selection methods have utilized a sole criterion of externalizing symptoms exceeding an arbitrary cut-off point to identify high-risk groups. However, Bennett and colleagues (1998, 1999) demonstrated that risk classification based on a single assessment of externalizing problems alone does not offer sufficient accuracy, as the sensitivity and positive predictive value are below preset criteria of >50%, particularly under the low prevalence conditions of normal populations. The 'multiple-gating' method, an alternative approach to screening using multiple, step-wise assessment measures, may offer greater classification accuracy and prove to be cost-effective (Feil et al., 1995). In this approach, a less costly assessment procedure is utilized with a specified population, generating a pool of possible high-risk children (first gate). A second assessment is then conducted with this subgroup, often using a more expensive or extensive screening measure (second gate). Children who meet criteria at each screening gate would then become part of the high-risk group. Ideally, different reporters would provide ratings at each gate in order to diminish bias and error in the ratings and to select children demonstrating behaviour problems across settings who are more likely to show later negative outcomes (Loeber, 1990).

One possible two-gate approach employs teacher ratings as a broad, initial screening instrument and parent ratings of child behaviour as a second gate. Implemented and tested with 382 kindergarten boys, this screening method proved to be an effective means of predicting behaviour problems at first grade across home and school settings (Lochman and CPPRG, 1995). Furthermore, the addition of the second gate (parent ratings) increased the predictive accuracy of the teacher ratings, and long-term analyses have revealed the validity of the screening procedure in identifying children at risk for problem outcomes (Jones et al., 2002).

Unfortunately, multiple-gating approaches still demonstrate the inherent limitations in predictive accuracy of early, behavioural screening methods (Offord, 1997). Screening for future disorder involves trade-offs between the sensitivity and the positive predictive value (PPV) of the screening measure. Thus, attempts to increase the proportion of children identified who will eventually show antisocial behaviour (PPV) can decrease the proportion of children with antisocial behaviour who are identified by the screen (sensitivity), and vice versa. Such inaccuracies have significant implications: the presence of false positives is associated with possible stigmatization, adverse effects and wasted resources, whereas the presence of false negatives represents a failure to deliver the intervention to children who may desperately need, and could benefit from, services. Girls appear to be at a particular disadvantage in that they are more likely to be under-identified but, due to the lower prevalence of CP in girls (Bennett et al., 1999; L. G. Hill et al., unpublished data), thus are also at a greater risk of being incorrectly identified. These limitations signal the need for more accurate screening methods and stress the importance of considering the nature of the intervention programme, including potency, potential risk, costs and available resources, when setting goals for selection accuracy (Offord, 1997).

27.4 Illustrative preventive interventions

In this section, a number of programmes that have been designed either explicitly to prevent the development or exacerbation of CP or which have noted such effects as part of their evaluations will be described. The programmes described here are meant to be representative, rather than exhaustive, examples of well-designed, empirically evaluated preventive interventions, with an emphasis on those that have cognitive/behavioural components. Two broad classes of interventions are applicable to the prevention of CP: early intervention programmes with infants and preschool-age children that are not focused on CP *per se* and interventions that specifically target the prevention of CP (McMahon and Wells, 1998). The latter types of interventions have focused on children ranging from preschool to adolescence.

27.4.1   Interventions during the infancy/preschool period
27.4.1.1   Broad-based early interventions

There is a growing body of evidence that early intervention programmes can have long-term effects on the reduction of CP in adolescence and into adulthood (see Yoshikawa, 1994). This is of particular import, because these programmes have not explicitly targeted the prevention of CP. Yoshikawa (1994) noted four elements common to the early intervention programmes described in his review that have demonstrated long-term preventive effects with respect to CP: (1) each intervention included both family support and child education components; (2) the intervention was implemented during the child's first 5 years; (3) the intervention lasted for at least 2 years; and (4) the intervention had short- to medium-term effects on risk factors shown to be associated with CP. A brief description of another successful broad-based programme will be provided below.

27.4.1.1.1   Elmira Home Visitation Project
The Infancy and Early Childhood Visitation Programme developed by Olds and colleagues (Olds *et al.*, 1997) offered extensive home visits from nurses to low-income, first-time mothers and their babies. In order to reduce risk factors for infant prematurity, low birthweight and neurodevelopmental impairment, visits during pregnancy addressed women's health behaviours such as smoking, drug and alcohol use and nutrition. Visitation continued until the children were 2 years old and focused on improving caregiving and reducing child maltreatment, preventing future unplanned pregnancies and promoting the mothers' completion of school and participation in the work force.

Several controlled studies have demonstrated the programme's effectiveness in meeting these objectives. In comparison with mothers in the control groups, mothers who received visitation had heavier and fewer preterm babies and showed a greater reduction in smoking. Fifteen years later, visited mothers had fewer subsequent births, fewer reports of child maltreatment and child injuries, a greater increase in labour force participation and decrease in welfare dependence and fewer arrests. Of particular interest, the visitation programme (although not specifically targeting child CP) successfully reduced the children's early antisocial behaviour and juvenile delinquency, including arrests, running away, adolescent sexual behaviour, smoking and alcohol use and substance-related behavioural problems (see Olds *et al.*, 1999). However, the programme appeared to have the greatest impact on the most at-risk families (low-income, unmarried women) and offered relatively little benefit for the broader population.

27.4.1.2 Family-based intervention with young children

A second preventive approach with preschool-aged children has been to employ family-based interventions designed to address early manifestations of child CP and the associated risk and protective factors. Given the primacy of the family in the early development of CP, so-called parent-training interventions may have significant preventive effects, especially if they are applied during the preschool period (Reid, 1993; Sanders, 1996) or if they are a component of broader preventive interventions for school-age children at risk for CP (e.g. CPPRG, 1992; Tremblay *et al.*, 1992). Descriptions of two cognitive behavioural parent-training programmes are presented below as examples of family-based interventions for preschool- and early school-aged children with CP. Descriptions of the clinical procedures utilized in these programmes are widely available in therapist manuals, and each of the programmes has been extensively evaluated.

27.4.1.2.1 *Helping the non-compliant child (HNC)*

The HNC parent-training programme (Forehand and McMahon, 1981; McMahon and Forehand, 2003) is specifically designed to treat non-compliance in younger children (3–8 years of age). Non-compliance (i.e. excessive disobedience to adults) is considered to be a keystone behaviour in the early starter pathway of CP, given its early appearance in the progression of CP, duration and association with referral for treatment. The programme presents a number of discrete parenting skills that are taught to the parent by didactic instruction, modelling and role playing. The parent practises the skills in the clinic with the child while receiving prompting and feedback from the therapist, and then employs these newly acquired skills in the home in structured practice settings.

The treatment programme consists of two phases. During the differential–attention phase of treatment (phase I), the parent learns to break out of the coercive cycle of interaction and establish a positive, mutually reinforcing relationship with the child. To do so, the parent is taught to increase the frequency and range of social attention (attending and praise), reduce the frequency of competing verbal behaviour and ignore minor inappropriate behaviours. Phase II of the treatment programme consists of teaching the parent to use appropriate commands, positive attention for compliance and a time-out procedure to decrease non-compliant behaviour exhibited by the child.

The HNC parent-training programme has been extensively evaluated in terms of its effectiveness, generalization and social validity (see McMahon and Forehand, 2003 for a detailed summary). It has documented short-term effectiveness and setting generalization from the clinic to the home for parent and child behaviour and for parents' perception of the child's adjustment. Furthermore, these improvements occur regardless of families' socioeconomic status or age of the children (within the 3–8-year old range). Maintenance of effects for the HNC programme has been demonstrated for up to 14 years after treatment (e.g. Long *et al.*, 1994). The HNC programme has demonstrated sibling generalization at the end of treatment, as well as behavioural generalization from the treatment of child non-compliance to other deviant behaviours (e.g. aggression and temper tantrums). Finally, HNC has been shown to be more effective than systems family therapy (Wells and Egan, 1988).

27.4.1.2.2   *Triple-P Positive Parenting Program*

Triple-P (Sanders, 1999) is a five-level system of parenting and family support that offers a tiered continuum of services, with an increase in intensity according to need. Guided by behavioural family intervention principles, the programme aims to promote caring and supportive parent–child relationships and to provide parents with effective management skills for dealing with childhood behavioural and developmental issues. Level 1 of the Triple-P model is a universal intervention offering parenting information to interested parents through a media and promotional campaign. The next level, Selected Triple-P, includes the provision of advice on how to deal with common behavioural difficulties and developmental transitions. The third level, Primary Care Triple-P, is a moderate-intensity intervention consisting of a brief programme of parenting skills training, advice and feedback to promote the effective management of discrete child behaviour problems. The highest two levels of Triple-P (Standard Triple P and Enhanced Triple-P) are intended for parents of children with more severe CP and thus provide intensive parent training focusing on positive parenting skills and generalization strategies. In addition, level 5 addresses familial dysfunction by offering individually tailored behavioural family intervention and home visits to promote stress-coping and partner support skills.

Triple-P has been, and/or is currently being, evaluated in several efficacy and effectiveness trials in community, university and hospital settings in Australia, Singapore, the USA, New Zealand, the UK, Switzerland and Germany. Overall, research findings have demonstrated positive benefits of many of the various levels of Triple-P intervention (see Sanders, 1999 for a comprehensive review), including a reduction in observed and parent-reported child behaviour problems maintained up to 1 year later (e.g. Sanders *et al.*, 2000).

27.4.2 Early elementary school-age interventions

Several different types of preventive interventions have been implemented during the elementary school period. School-based universal interventions for the prevention of CP are typically administered by teachers to all students in the classroom. Below is described one such programme: PATHS (Kusche and Greenberg, 1994). In contrast, a number of multi-component interventions that target either at-risk or universal populations have been implemented during early elementary school. 'First generation' interventions implemented in the 1980s have now reported on long-term outcomes, while 'second generation' interventions implemented in the 1990s have reported short- to medium-term outcomes to date. Examples of both generations of interventions are presented below. In addition, a widely disseminated programme designed to reduce bullying in schools is described.

27.4.2.1 School-based single-component universal interventions

27.4.2.1.1 PATHS

One of the most widely known universal prevention programmes is the Promoting Alternative THinking Strategies (PATHS) classroom curriculum (Kusche and Greenberg, 1994), which can be implemented in kindergarten through to grade 6. Originally formulated for deaf children, the programme has been widely implemented and tested. The classroom-based programme consists of systematic developmentally based lessons promoting greater development of emotional understanding, self-control, positive self-esteem, prosocial relationships and interpersonal problem-solving skills. Teachers are trained by programme staff in the implementation of the curriculum, which they provide to their students approximately three times a week. The lessons utilize didactic presentation, discussion, modelling and role playing of skills. The programme also incorporates techniques to promote the use of self-control, emotion regulation and problem-solving skills during real-life conflicts, as well as parent updates and home activities to engage parents and facilitate generalization. Finally, teachers are taught strategies to manage classroom disruptive behaviour effectively (see Bierman *et al.*, 1996 for more detail).

Multiple evaluations of the programme have demonstrated positive effects, including improvements in adaptive functioning (teacher- and self-report), emotional and cognitive skills, self-control, conflict resolution, CP and problem-solving, which have been maintained at 1–2 year follow-ups (see Greenberg *et al.*, 1998). The PATHS curriculum has also been tested as a component of the comprehensive Fast Track intervention (CPPRG, 1992, 2000) (see below). Initial analyses after first grade revealed a significant effect of the curriculum on observed classroom atmosphere and peer nominations of aggression and hyperactive–disruptive behaviour, but not on teacher ratings (CPPRG, 1999b).

27.4.2.2   Multi-component interventions

The Montreal and Seattle prevention trials were conducted in the 1980s and are representative of the first generation of preventive interventions.

27.4.2.2.1   *Montreal Longitudinal Experimental Study*

The Montreal Longitudinal Experimental Study (Tremblay *et al.*, 1992) evaluated the effects of a two-component intervention in preventing antisocial behaviour in boys identified as disruptive at kindergarten. The programme offered parent training, based on the Oregon Social Learning Model developed by Patterson and colleagues (Patterson *et al.*, 1975), and classroom-based child social skills training, focusing on prosocial skills and self-control. Services were provided for 2 years, beginning when boys were 7 years old.

Results of a randomized study indicated that intervention boys were less disruptive, showed better elementary school adjustment and reported fewer delinquent behaviours (including theft, gang membership and substance use) 3 and 5 years later than boys in the control condition (Tremblay *et al.*, 1992; Tremblay *et al.*, 1995). However, the intervention did not significantly affect delinquency, as measured by juvenile court records (Tremblay *et al.*, 1995).

27.4.2.2.2   *Seattle Social Development Project (SSDP)*

The Seattle Social Development Project (Hawkins *et al.*, 1992, 2002) was a universal intervention implemented in regular classrooms in the Seattle public school system. The intervention offered a combination of teacher training, parent training and social–cognitive skills training for children in grades 1–6. Teachers were instructed in the use of proactive classroom management, interactive teaching and cooperative learning and in the implementation of a social–cognitive skills training programme, based on the Interpersonal Cognitive Problem-Solving Curriculum (Shure and Spivack, 1980). Tailored to the children's developmental level, the parent component provided skills training in effective monitoring, reinforcement and consequences, having clear expectations and the encouragement of greater parental involvement and support of the children's academic success.

At the end of grade 6, girls in the intervention programme reported significantly more classroom participation, bonding and commitment to school, and showed a trend towards less initiation of alcohol and marijuana use. Boys showed better social and academic skills, reported more commitment and bonding to school and less initiation of delinquency and were rated as having fewer antisocial friends (O'Donnell *et al.*, 1995). Six years after the programme ended, intervention students reported less school misbehaviour, violent delinquent behaviour, alcohol use and sexual activity, as well as greater academic achievement and commitment to school (Hawkins *et al.*, 1999). Additionally, the intervention demonstrated a dose-dependent effect, in that the group who received the comprehensive 6-year intervention showed better outcomes than those who received the intervention in grades 5 and 6 only.

Two interventions that are representative of the more recent second generation of prevention trials will now be described. A third example, the Incredible Years Training Series (Webster-Stratton, 2000), is not described here as there is a description of a very similar programme in Chapter 13.

27.4.2.2.3   First Step to success

Walker and colleagues (Walker *et al.*, 1998) have developed and tested a preventive intervention for at-risk kindergarteners that includes three main components: universal screening, a classroom intervention and parent training. The school-based component utilizes a behavioural management strategy (adapted from Hops and Walker's 1988 Contingencies for Learning Academic and Social Skills (CLASS) Programme) that is initially implemented by a First Step consultant and then continued by the classroom teacher. The home-based parent training is conducted by the same consultant who facilitates communication and cooperation between the home and school in order to promote cross-setting skills acquisition by the child. This component focuses on building child competencies necessary for school success.

Post-test and 2-year follow-up analyses of a controlled trial in Oregon have demonstrated positive effects of the programme in increasing adaptive behaviour and academically engaged time and reducing aggressive and maladaptive behaviour (Walker *et al.*, 1998a). Additionally, the intervention appeared to be most effective for children with the most serious behavioural problems. Subsequent studies, including a large-scale effectiveness trial, have replicated these findings (Golly *et al.*, 1998; Walker *et al.*, in press).

27.4.2.2.4   Linking the interests of families and teachers (LIFT)

The LIFT Project (Reid *et al.*, 1999; Reid and Eddy, 2002) is a school-based, universal prevention programme focusing on the transitions into elementary and middle schools. At these key developmental periods, the programme provides an interpersonal skills training programme and a playground behavioural programme for first and fifth graders and a parent-training programme for their parents. The parent-training programme emphasizes appropriate discipline and supervision strategies and promotes greater communication between teachers and parents. The school-based programme included classroom lessons emphasizing social and problem-solving skills and playground use of the Good Behavior Game (Kellam *et al.*, 1994), which is a team-based behaviour management strategy.

A randomized intervention trial in 12 elementary schools demonstrated immediate positive effects across reporters (teacher, parent and observer), including a decrease in physical aggression on the playground and aversive behaviour at home, as well as an improvement in classroom behaviour (Reid *et al.*, 1999). Additionally, these effects appeared strongest for children at higher risk at the beginning of the intervention (Stoolmiller *et al.*, 2000). Follow-up analyses have indicated that, compared with the control group, intervention children were less likely to show an increase in the severity of attention deficit symptoms, to affiliate with deviant peers, to show patterned alcohol use and to be arrested 30 months later (Eddy *et al.*, 2000).

27.4.2.3   Core Programme Against Bullying and Antisocial Behaviour

Over the past two decades, Olweus (1993) has developed and tested an intervention designed to reduce bullying in schools. Targeting school, classroom and individual levels, this programme aims to 'restructure the social environment' in order to provide fewer opportunities and rewards for aggression and bullying. Specifically, the intervention emphasizes positive teacher and parent involvement, enhanced communication, awareness and supervision, firm limits to unacceptable behaviour and consistent, non-physical sanctions for rule breaking. Components at the school level include dissemination of an anonymous student questionnaire that assesses the extent of bullying in each school, formalized discussion of the problem, formation of a committee to plan and deliver the programme and a system of supervision of students between classes and during recess. At the classroom level, teachers provide clear, 'no tolerance' rules for bullying and hold regular classroom meetings for students, as well as parents. Finally, individual interventions are provided for bullies, victims and parents to ensure that the bullying stops and that victims are supported and protected.

Implemented and evaluated in Bergen, Norway between 1983 and 1985, the original project included 2500 youths in grades 4 through to 7 across 42 schools. The programme has since been replicated in other countries, including the USA. Across grades, the intervention has demonstrated positive effects on bully / victim problems, including reductions of more than 50% in the frequency of bullying in the 2 years following the programme. Additionally, student satisfaction with school and classroom social climate (order and discipline, social relationships and attitude to school and schoolwork) improved, while the rate of general antisocial behaviour (theft, vandalism, fighting and truancy) dropped during the 2-year period (Olweus, 1991, 1993). Furthermore, marked reductions in aggressive behaviour have been demonstrated in a subsequent intervention trial, with effects maintained 2 years later (see Olweus, 2001 for an overview).

27.4.3   Late elementary/early middle-school interventions

In addition to LIFT, there are a number of other preventive interventions that have been successfully implemented with at-risk children during the late elementary school period: the Anger Coping/Coping Power Program (Lochman *et al.*, 1987), and its more recent adaptation, the Coping Power program (Lochman and Wells, 1996), and, during middle school, the Adolescent Transitions Program (Dishion and Kavanagh, 2000). These interventions may be appropriate for youths who display either early starting or adolescent-limited patterns of CP (i.e. 'late starters') (Moffitt, 1993), although, to the authors' knowledge, this has not been addressed empirically. Both of these interventions are described in Chapter 25.

27.4.4   A multi-component, long-term preventive intervention: fast track

The final example of a preventive intervention is the Fast Track programme (CPPRG, 1992, 2000). The Fast Track project design involves a randomized, controlled trial of a multifaceted, long-term prevention programme embedded within a longitudinal study of normative and high-risk youths at four sites in the USA (CPPRG, 1992, 2000).

The Fast Track project is unique in the size, scope and duration of the intervention. The prevention programme involved a 10-year span of prevention activities covering the important developmental transitions of entry into elementary, middle and high school. It included both universal and targeted interventions. The latter were directed to one-half of the children in the high-risk sample (identified in kindergarten as the most disruptive children in school and at home). The intervention began in first grade and continued through tenth grade. However, there were two periods of most intensive intervention: school entry (first and second grade) and the transition into middle school (fifth and sixth grades). The intervention at school entry targeted proximal changes in six domains: (1) disruptive behaviours in the home; (2) disruptive and off-task behaviours in the school; (3) social–cognitive skills pertaining to affect regulation and social problem-solving skills; (4) peer relations; (5) academic skills; and (6) the family–school relationship. Integrated intervention components included parent training, home visiting, social skills training, academic tutoring and a universal teacher-administered intervention designed to increase social and emotional competence in the classroom (PATHS; see above). The intervention at the entry into middle school in grades 5 and 6 (and through grade 10) included interventions with increasing emphasis on parent/adult monitoring and positive involvement, peer affiliation and peer influence, academic achievement and orientation to school and social cognition and identity development.

Early results of the Fast Track intervention have indicated significant positive effects for high-risk children and their families, as well as classroom effects from the universal intervention (PATHS) described above (CPPRG, 1999a,b, 2002a,b). At the end of first grade, compared with children in the control condition, there were consistent, moderate effects for children in the intervention condition in the following areas: social, emotional and academic skills, peer interactions and social status, CP and special education resource use. Parents in the intervention condition reported less use of physical discipline and greater parenting satisfaction/ease of parenting, and they demonstrated more appropriate/consistent discipline and warmth/positive involvement when interacting with their children. Teachers reported that the parents had more positive involvement with their children's school. Intervention effects for parenting and child behaviour were generally maintained at the end of third and fourth grade.

27.5   Issues

In this section, five important issues facing practitioners and researchers alike concerning interventions for the prevention of CP in children and adolescents will be briefly discussed: (1) the need to assess and account for the mechanisms of effectiveness (i.e. mediation and moderation); (2) the possibility of iatrogenic effects as a function of screening, the intervention or both; (3) the need for greater cultural sensitivity in the development, implementation and evaluation of preventive interventions; (4) the need for appropriately designed economic analyses of preventive interventions; and (5) the need to attend to issues concerning the effective dissemination of these empirically supported interventions.

27.5.1   Mechanisms of effectiveness

As the efficacy of many interventions for the prevention of CP has become established, increased attention is now being paid to questions concerning the extent to which the intervention effects may be limited to particular groups of individuals (i.e. moderation and e.g. boys versus girls and European-American children versus children of colour) and the processes that may account for the intervention outcomes (i.e. mediation). Space considerations preclude a thorough review of moderation and mediation in the prevention of CP. However, a few examples will be provided to illustrate the diversity of findings to date. With respect to moderation, a recent meta-analysis of school-based programmes for the prevention of aggressive behaviour found that, while child gender and ethnicity did not moderate the intervention effects, these programmes tended to demonstrate larger effect sizes for high-risk than low-risk children, for preschool-aged children and adolescents than elementary school-aged children and for programmes with high levels of implementation quality as opposed to low implementation quality (Wilson *et al.*, 2003). With respect to mediation, proximal goals of the Fast Track intervention at grade 3 (e.g. hostile attributional bias, problem-solving skill, harsh parental discipline and aggressive and prosocial behaviour at home and school) were found to partially mediate outcomes 1 year later (CPPRG, 2002b). Of particular importance was that the findings were largely consistent with the early starter model of CP; furthermore, the patterns of mediation were domain specific (e.g. parenting behaviour mediated the intervention effect on the child's behaviour at home but not at school) rather than sequential.

27.5.2   Iatrogenic effects

Iatrogenic effects (i.e. negative effects caused by the intervention) may potentially manifest themselves in two aspects of the prevention enterprise: in screening and during the intervention itself. With respect to screening, a major criticism of targeted approaches to prevention that identify at-risk groups of children or families is that such identification may lead to stigmatization (Kerns and Prinz, 2002). This may be especially salient when the intervention occurs in the school setting, and a particular child's participation in the intervention is clear to the child's classmates and teachers. To the authors' knowledge, this concern has not been empirically verified. Furthermore, the authors' experiences in working with at-risk children and families in the Fast Track project (CPPRG, 1992, 2000) has been that, if the intervention is presented as a skill- and competency-enhancing intervention, then such stigmatization is less likely to occur.

In contrast, there is clear empirical evidence to support at least one type of iatrogenic effect that is a function of a particular type of intervention at a particular developmental period. Dishion and colleagues (Dishion *et al.*, 1999) have reviewed evidence suggesting that the placement of high-risk adolescents in at least some peer-group interventions may result in increases in both CP behaviour and negative life outcomes compared with control youths. For example, Poulin *et al.* (2001) demonstrated that increases in both teacher-reported delinquency and self-report of smoking were associated with participation in prevention-orientated groups of high-risk youths 3 years earlier. The putative mechanism of influence is so-called 'deviancy training', in which youths receive group attention for engaging in various problem behaviours. These findings have led to the development and promotion of interventions that minimize the influence of groups of high-risk adolescent peers and involve the youngsters in conventional peer activities (e.g. sports teams and school clubs) with low-risk peers. At this point, it is not known whether such iatrogenic effects occur with groups of younger children at risk for CP, or the extent to which this phenomenon is occurring in other interventions with at-risk adolescents. Nevertheless, these findings send a clear message to interventionists of the need to consider alternatives to group-based interventions when working with adolescents at risk for CP.

27.5.3   Cultural sensitivity

It is well established that most interventions for the prevention of CP have been based primarily on research with European–American, middle-class families (Kerns and Prinz, 2002; Kumpfer *et al.*, 2002). Important questions that need to be addressed are the extent to which these generic programmes work with other cultural groups, whether there is a need to adapt these interventions or whether culturally specific interventions need to be developed. Unfortunately, there is a paucity of data that address these questions, and the field is divided on this issue (Kumpfer *et al.*, 2002). It is the case that many of the interventions described in this chapter have included other ethnic groups in their programme evaluations, and some have noted the generalization of effects across groups (i.e. a lack of moderation; e.g. CPPRG, 1999a). However, that is not to say that culturally adapted versions of these interventions would not be even more effective.

27.5.4   Economic analyses

According to an analysis conducted by Cohen (1998), an individual career criminal in the USA costs society approximately $1.3 million (1997 dollars, discounted at 2%). In the UK, the average cost was £15 382 in a single year for a sample of 4–10-year-old children with CP (Knapp *et al.*, 1999). Given these astounding figures, it is apparent that effective prevention programmes may not only be beneficial from a human services context but from an economic one as well, if they are successful in diverting young people from the early starter pathway of CP. To date, there have been relatively few economic analyses done with evidence-based preventive interventions, although that is changing (e.g. Greenwood *et al.*, 1996; Chatterji *et al.*, 2001). These types of analyses are likely to be especially influential in gaining social and political support for interventions that may, at first glance, seem quite expensive.

27.5.5   Intervention delivery

It is clear from the review in this chapter that there are a variety of interventions that have shown great promise in the prevention of CP. However, a major challenge to the field is the dissemination and diffusion of these evidence-based interventions to communities. A few programmes, such as Triple-P (Sanders, 1999), have designed dissemination and diffusion strategies into their model. A very promising strategy for addressing this challenge is the Communities That Care operating system for the selection and delivery of a range of effective prevention programmes (Hawkins *et al.*, 2002). Communities collect local data on risk and protective factors, which are then used to select the most appropriate preventive interventions for reducing these risk factors and increasing protective factors. There is a strong emphasis on community mobilization and education, which is posited to lead to commitment and ownership among a broad spectrum of the community. Such a 'bottom up' approach to prevention has also been employed in the Better Beginnings, Better Futures Project (Peters *et al.*, 2003), which is a community-based, universal project designed to promote positive development and prevent emotional and behavioural maladjustment in young children. Emphasizing community involvement in its development and implementation, the project focuses on strengthening families and neighbourhoods and establishing coordinated partnerships with new and existing services. The individualized nature of this project is unique and offers community members a fundamental role in determining the type and structure of services and/or programmes that would best meet local needs and, therefore, receive funding.

27.6   Conclusions

In this chapter, a number of interventions that have been developed and evaluated with respect to the prevention of CP in children and adolescents have been presented and described. Those intervention programmes have varied with respect to the age of children for whom they are intended, the level of prevention (i.e. universal, selected or indicated) and the type of intervention(s) employed. A variety of issues that are important in the prevention of CP have also been described, including the identification and screening of children, mechanisms of effectiveness, the possibility of iatrogenic effects, cultural sensitivity, economic analyses and intervention delivery. It is hoped that the information presented in this chapter will be of use to clinicians and other interventionists as they consider the prevention of CP in children and adolescents.

27.7 Acknowledgements

Preparation of this manuscript was supported in part by grant R18 MH50951 from the National Institute of Mental Health.

27.8 REFERENCES

Alvarado, R., Kendall, K., Beesley, S. and Lee-Cavaness, C. (2000). *Strengthening America's Families: Model Family Programs for Substance Abuse and Delinquency Prevention*. Salt Lake City, UT: University of Utah.

American Psychiatric Association (2000). *Diagnostic and Statistical Manual of Mental Disorders*, 4th edn. Washington, DC: American Psychiatric Association.

Bennett, K. J., Lipman, E. L., Brown, S., Racine, Y., Boyle, M. H. and Offord, D. R. (1999). Predicting conduct problems: can high-risk children be identified in kindergarten and grade 1? *Journal of Consulting and Clinical Psychology*, **67**, 470–80.

Bennett, K. J., Lipman, E. L., Racine, Y. and Offord, D. R. (1998). Annotation: do measures of externalizing behaviour in normal populations predict later outcome? Implications for targeted interventions to prevent conduct disorder. *Journal of Child Psychology and Psychiatry*, **39**, 1059–70.

Bierman, K. L., Greenberg, M. T. and the Conduct Problems Prevention Research Group (1996). Social skills training in the Fast Track program. In R. DeV. Peters and R. J. McMahon (eds.), *Preventing Childhood Disorders, Substance Abuse, and Delinquency*. Thousand Oaks, CA: Sage, pp. 65–89.

Campbell, S. B. (2002). *Behavior Problems in Preschool Children: Clinical and Developmental Issues*, 2nd edn. New York: Guilford Press.

Chatterji, P., Caffray, C. M., Jones, A. S., Lillie-Blanton, M. and Werthamer, L. (2001). Applying cost analysis methods to school-based prevention programs. *Prevention Science*, **2**, 45–55.

Cohen, M. A. (1998). The monetary value of saving a high-risk youth. *Journal of Quantitative Criminology*, **14**, 5–33.

Coie, J. D. and Dodge, K. A. (1998). Aggression and antisocial behavior. In W. Damon and N. Eisenberg (eds.), *Handbook of Child Psychology, Volume 3. Social, Emotional, and Personality Development*, 5th edn. New York: Wiley, pp. 779–862.

Coie, J. D., Miller-Johnson, S. and Bagwell, C. (2000). Prevention science. In A. J. Sameroff, M. Lewis, and S. M. Miller (eds.), *Handbook of Developmental Psychopathology*, 2nd edn. New York: Kluwer Academic/Plenum Publishers, pp. 93–112.

Conduct Problems Prevention Research Group (1992). A developmental and clinical model for the prevention of conduct disorder: the FAST Track program. *Development and Psychopathology*, **4**, 509–27.

  (1999a). Initial impact of the Fast Track prevention trial of conduct problems: II. The high-risk sample. *Journal of Consulting and Clinical Psychology*, **67**, 631–47.

(1999b). Initial impact of the Fast Track prevention trial of conduct problems: II. Classroom effects. *Journal of Consulting and Clinical Psychology*, **67**, 648–57.

(2000). Merging universal and indicated prevention programs: the Fast Track model. *Addictive Behaviors*, **25**, 913–27.

(2002a). Evaluation of the first three years of the Fast Track prevention trial with children at high risk for adolescent conduct problems. *Journal of Abnormal Child Psychology*, **30**, 19–35.

(2002b). Using the Fast Track randomized prevention trial to test the early-starter model of the development of serious conduct problems. *Development and Psychopathology*, **14**, 925–43.

Dishion, T. J. and Kavanagh, K. (2000). A multilevel approach to family-centered prevention in schools: process and outcome. *Addictive Behaviors*, **25**, 899–911.

Dishion, T. J., McCord, J. and Poulin, F. (1999). When interventions harm: peer groups and problem behavior. *American Psychologist*, **54**, 755–64.

Dodge, K. A. (1993). The future of research on the treatment of conduct disorder. *Development and Psychopathology*, **5**, 311–19.

Eddy, J. M., Reid, J. B. and Fetrow, R. A. (2000). An elementary school-based prevention program targeting modifiable antecedents of youth delinquency and violence: linking the Interests of Families and Teachers (LIFT). *Journal of Emotional and Behavioral Disorders*, **8**, 165–76.

Feil, E. G., Walker, H. M. and Severson, H. H. (1995). The Early Screening Project for young children with behavior problems. *Journal of Emotional and Behavioral Disorders*, **3**, 194–202.

Forehand, R. and McMahon, R. J. (1981). *Helping the Noncompliant Child: A Clinician's Guide to Parent Training*. New York: Guilford Press.

Golly, A., Stiller, B. and Walker, H. M. (1998). First Step to Success: replication and social validation of an early intervention program for achieving secondary prevention goals. *Journal of Emotional and Behavioral Disorders*, **6**, 243–50.

Greenberg, M. T., Kusche, C. A. and Mihalic, S. F. (1998). *Blueprints for Violence Prevention, Book Ten: Promoting Alternative Thinking Strategies (PATHS)*. Boulder, CO: Center for the Study and Prevention of Violence.

Greenwood, P. W., Model, K. E., Rydell, C. P. and Chiesa, J. (1996). *Diverting Children from a Life of Crime: Measuring Costs and Benefits*. Santa Monica, CA: The RAND Corporation.

Hawkins, J. D., Catalano, R. F. and Arthur, M. W. (2002). Promoting science-based prevention in communities. *Addictive Behaviors*, **27**, 951–76.

Hawkins, J. D., Catalano, R. F., Kosterman, R., Abbott, R. and Hill, K. G. (1999). Preventing health-risk behaviors by strengthening protection during childhood. *Archives of Pediatrics and Adolescent Medicine*, **153**, 226–234.

Hawkins, J. D., Catalano, R. F., Morrison, D. M. *et al.* (1992). The Seattle Social Development Project: effects of the first four years on protective factors and problem behaviors. In J. McCord and R. E. Tremblay (eds.), *Preventing Antisocial Behavior: Interventions from Birth through Adolescence*. New York: Guilford Press, pp. 139–61.

Hawkins, J. D., Smith, B. H., Hill, K. G., Kosterman, R., Catalano, R. F. and Abbott, R. D. (2002). Understanding and preventing crime and violence. In T. P. Thornberry and M. D. Krohn (eds.), *Taking Stock of Delinquency: An Overview of Findings from Contemporary Longitudinal Studies*. New York: Kluwer Academic/Plenum Publishers, pp. 255–312.

Hops, H. and Walker, H. M. (1988). *CLASS: Contingencies for Learning Academic and Social Skills.* Seattle, WA: Educational Achievement Systems.

Jones, D., Dodge, K. A., Foster, E. M., Nix, R. and the Conduct Problems Prevention Research Group. (2002). Early identification of children at risk for costly mental health service use. *Prevention Science*, **3**, 247–56.

Kellam, S. G., Rebok, G. W., Ialongo, N. and Mayer, L. S. (1994). The course and malleability of aggressive behavior from early first grade into middle school: results of a developmental epidemiologically-based preventive trial. *Journal of Child Psychology and Psychiatry*, **35**, 259–81.

Kerns, S. E. and Prinz, R. J. (2002). Critical issues in the prevention of violence-related behavior in youth. *Clinical Child and Family Psychology Review*, **5**, 133–60.

Knapp, M., Scott, S. and Davies, J. (1999). The cost of antisocial behaviour in younger children. *Clinical Child Psychology and Psychiatry*, **4**, 457–73.

Kumpfer, K. L., Alvarado, R., Smith, P. and Bellamy, N. (2002). Cultural sensitivity and adaptation in family-based prevention interventions. *Prevention Science*, **3**, 241–6.

Kusche, C. and Greenberg, M. (1994). *The PATHS Curriculum: Promoting Alternative THinking Strategies.* Seattle, WA: Developmental Research and Programs.

LeMarquand, D., Tremblay, R. E. and Vitaro, F. (2001). The prevention of conduct disorder: a review of successful and unsuccessful experiments. In J. Hill and B. Maughan (eds.), *Conduct Disorders in Childhood and Adolescence.* New York: Cambridge University Press, pp. 449–77.

Lochman, J. E. and the Conduct Problems Prevention Research Group. (1995). Screening of child behavior problems for prevention programs at school entry. *Journal of Consulting and Clinical Psychology*, **63**, 549–59.

Lochman, J. E. and Wells, K. C. (1996). A social-cognitive intervention with aggressive children: prevention effects and contextual implementation issues. In R. D. Peters and R. J. McMahon (eds.), *Preventing Childhood Disorders, Substance Abuse, and Delinquency.* Thousand Oaks, CA: Sage, pp. 111–43.

Lochman, J. E., Lampron, L. B., Gemmer, T. C. and Harris, S. R. (1987). Anger coping intervention with aggressive children: a guide to implementation in school settings. In P. A. Keller and S. R. Heyman (eds.), *Innovations in Clinical Practice: A Source Book*, Volume 6. Sarasota, FL: Professional Resource Exchange, pp. 339–56.

Loeber, R. (1990). Development and risk factors of juvenile antisocial behavior and delinquency. *Clinical Psychology Review*, **10**, 1–41.

Long, P., Forehand, R., Wierson, M. and Morgan, A. (1994). Does parent training with young noncompliant children have long-term effects? *Behaviour Research and Therapy*, **32**, 101–7.

McMahon, R. J. and Forehand, R. L. (2003). *Helping the Noncompliant Child: Family-Based Treatment for Oppositional Behavior*, 2nd edn. New York: Guilford Press.

McMahon, R. J. and Wells, K. C. (1998). Conduct problems. In E. J. Mash and R. A. Barkley (eds.), *Treatment of Childhood Disorder*, 2nd edn. New York: Guilford Press, pp. 111–207.

Moffitt, T. E. (1993). 'Adolescence-limited' and 'life-course-persistent' antisocial behavior: a developmental taxonomy. *Psychological Review*, **100**, 674–701.

Mrazek, P. J. and Haggerty, R. J. (1994). *Reducing Risks for Mental Disorders: Frontiers for Prevention Intervention Research*. Washington, DC: National Academy Press.

O'Donnell, J., Hawkins, J. D., Catalano, R. F., Abbott, R. D. and Day, L. E. (1995). Preventing school failure, drug use, and delinquency among low-income children: long-term intervention in elementary schools. *American Journal of Orthopsychiatry*, **65**, 87–100.

Offord, D. R. (1997). Bridging development, prevention, and policy. In D. M. Stoff, J. Breiling, and J. D. Maser (eds.), *Handbook of Antisocial Behavior*. New York: Wiley, pp. 357–64.

Olds, D. L., Henderson, C. R., Kitzman, H. J., Eckenrode, J. J., Cole, R. E. and Tatelbaum, R. C. (1999). Prenatal and infancy home visitation by nurses: recent findings. *The Future of Children*, **9**, 44–65.

Olds, D., Kitzman, H., Cole, R. and Robinson, J. (1997). Theoretical foundations of a program of home visitation for pregnant women and parents of young children. *Journal of Community Psychology*, **25**, 9–25.

Olweus, D. (1991). Bully/victim problems among schoolchildren: basic facts and effects of a school based intervention program. In D. J. Pepler and K. H. Rubin (eds.), *The Development and Treatment of Childhood Aggression*. Hillsdale, NJ: Erlbaum, pp. 411–88.

   (1993). *Bullying at School: What We Know and What We Can Do*. Maiden, MA: Blackwell Publishers.

   (2001). Peer harassment: a critical analysis and some important issues. In J. Juvonen and S. Graham (eds.), *Peer Harassment in School: The Plight of the Vulnerable and Victimized*. New York: Guilford Press, pp. 1–20.

Patterson, G. R., Capaldi, D. and Bank, L. (1991). An early starter model for predicting delinquency. In D. J. Pepler and K. H. Rubin (eds.), *The Development and Treatment of Childhood Aggression*. Hillsdale, NJ: Erlbaum, pp. 139–68.

Patterson, G. R., Reid, J. B., Jones, R. R. and Conger, R. R. (1975). *A Social Learning Approach to Family Intervention: Families with Aggressive Children*, Volume 1. Eugene, OR: Castalia.

Peters, R. DeV., Petrunka, K. and Arnold, R. (2003). The Better Beginnings, Better Futures Project: a universal, comprehensive, community-based prevention approach for primary school children and their families. *Journal of Clinical Child and Adolescent Psychology*, **32**, 215–27.

Poulin, F., Dishion, T. J. and Burraston, B. (2001). Three-year iatrogenic effects associated with aggregating high-risk adolescents in cognitive-behavioral preventive interventions. *Applied Developmental Science*, **5**, 214–24.

Reid, J. B. (1993). Prevention of conduct disorder before and after school entry: relating interventions to developmental findings. *Development and Psychopathology*, **5**, 243–62.

Reid, J. B. and Eddy, J. M. (2002). Preventive efforts during the elementary school years: the Linking the Interests of Families and Teachers (LIFT) Project. In J. R. Reid, G. R. Patterson and J. Snyder (eds.), *Antisocial Behavior in Children and Adolescents: A Developmental Analysis and Model for Intervention*. Washington, DC: American Psychological Association, pp. 219–33.

Reid, J. B., Eddy, J. M., Fetrow, R. A. and Stoolmiller, M. (1999). Description and immediate impacts of a preventive intervention for conduct problems. *American Journal of Community Psychology*, **27**, 483–517.

Sanders, M. R. (1996). New directions in behavioral family intervention with children. In T. H. Ollendick and R. J. Prinz (eds.), *Advances in Clinical Child Psychology*, Volume 18. New York: Plenum Press, pp. 283–331.

(1999). The Triple P–Positive Parenting Program: towards an empirically validated multilevel parenting and family support strategy for the prevention of behavior and emotional problems in children. *Clinical Child and Family Psychology Review*, **2**, 71–90.

Sanders, M. R., Markie-Dadds, C., Tully, L. and Bor, B. (2000). The Triple P-Positive Parenting Program: a comparison of enhanced, standard, and self-directed behavioral family intervention for parents of children with early onset conduct problems. *Journal of Consulting and Clinical Psychology*, **68**, 624–40.

Shure, M. B. and Spivack, G. (1980). Interpersonal problem solving as a mediator of behavioral adjustment in preschool and kindergarten children. *Journal of Applied Developmental Psychology*, **1**, 29–44.

Stoolmiller, M., Eddy, J. M. and Reid, J. B. (2000). Detecting and describing preventive intervention effects in an universal school-based randomized trial targeting violent and delinquent behaviour. *Journal of Consulting and Clinical Psychology*, **68**, 296–306.

Tremblay, R. E., Pagani-Kurtz, L., Masse, L. C., Vitaro, F. and Pihl, R. O. (1995). A bimodal preventive intervention for disruptive kindergarten boys: its impact through mid-adolescence. *Journal of Consulting and Clinical Psychology*, **63**, 560–8.

Tremblay, R. E., Vitaro, F., Bertrand, L. *et al.* (1992). Parent and child training to prevent early onset of delinquency: the Montreal longitudinal-experimental study. In J. McCord and R. E. Tremblay (eds.), *Preventing Antisocial Behavior: Interventions from Birth through Adolescence*. New York: Guilford Press, pp. 117–38.

Walker, H. M., Kavanagh, K., Stiller, B., Golly, A., Severson, H. H. and Feil, E. G. (1998a). First Step to Success: an early intervention approach for preventing school antisocial behavior. *Journal of Emotional and Behavioral Disorders*, **6**, 66–80.

Walker, H. M., Sprague, J. R., Perkins-Rowe, K. A. *et al.* (in press). The First Step to Success Program: achieving secondary prevention outcomes for behaviorally at-risk children through early intervention. In M. Epstein, K. Kutash and A. Duchnowski (eds.), *Outcomes for Children and Youth with Behavioral and Emotional Disorders*, 2nd edn. Austin, TX: PRO-ED.

Walker, H. M., Stiller, B., Severson, H. H., Feil, E. G. and Golly, A. (1998b). First Step to Success: intervening at the point of school entry to prevent antisocial behavior patterns. *Psychology in the Schools*, **35**, 259–69.

Webster-Stratton, C. (2000). *The Incredible Years Training Series Bulletin*. Washington, DC: US Department of Justice, Office of Justice Programs, Office of Juvenile Justice and Delinquency Prevention.

Webster-Stratton, C. and Taylor, T. (2001). Nipping early risk factors in the bud: preventing substance abuse, delinquency, and violence in adolescence through interventions targeted at young children (0–8 years). *Prevention Science*, **2**, 165–92.

Wells, K. C. and Egan, J. (1988). Social learning and systems family therapy for childhood oppositional disorder: comparative treatment outcome. *Comprehensive Psychiatry*, **29**, 138–46.

Wilson, S. J., Lipsey, M. W. and Derzon, J. H. (2003). The effects of school-based intervention
programs on aggressive behavior: a meta-analysis. *Journal of Consulting and Clinical Psychology*,
71, 136–49.

Yoshikawa, H. (1994). Prevention as a cumulative protection: effects of early family support and
education on chronic delinquency and its risks. *Psychological Bulletin*, **115**, 28–54.

Index